Ovarian Cancer - Updates in Tumour Biology and Therapeutics

Edited by Gwo-Yaw Ho and Kate Webber

Published in London, United Kingdom

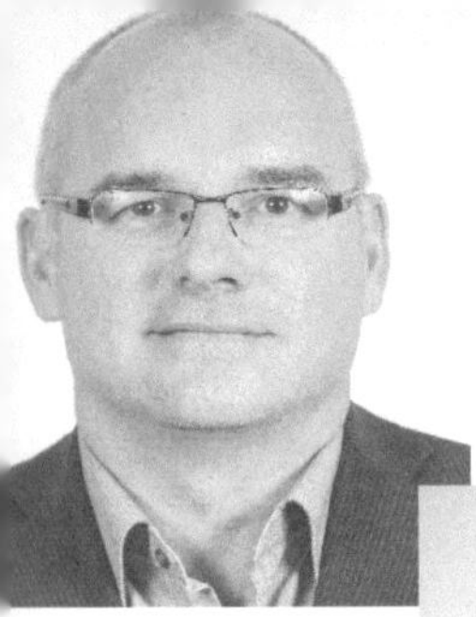
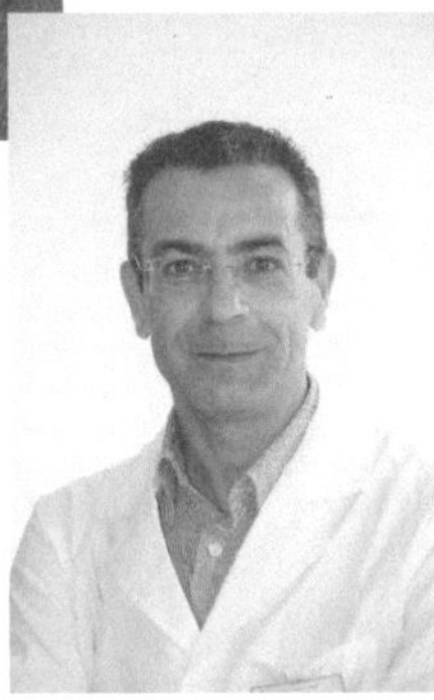
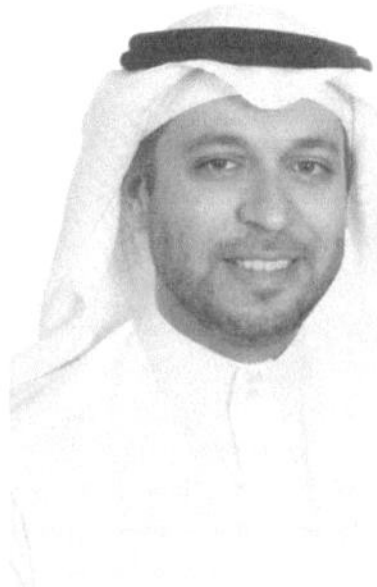
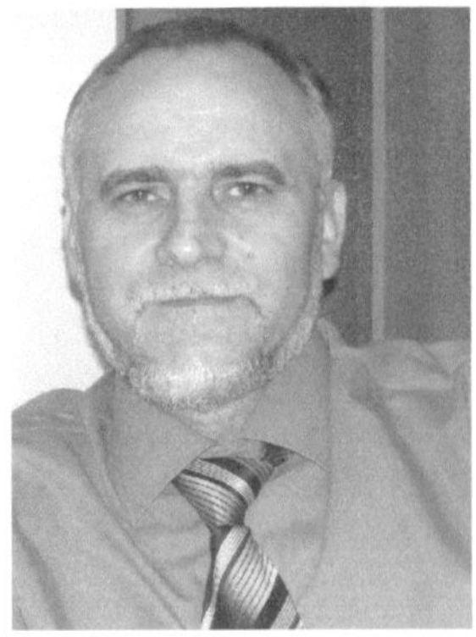
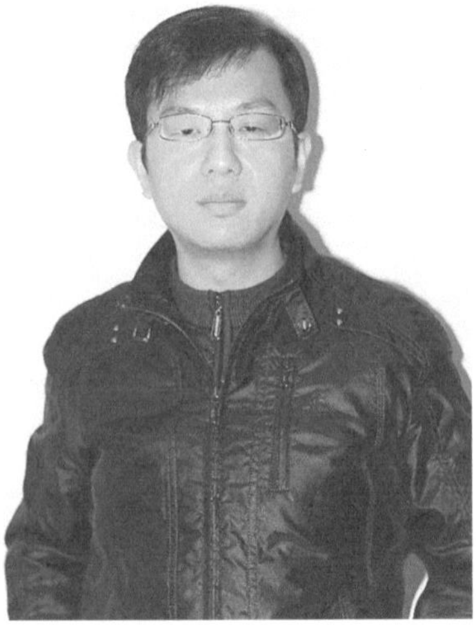
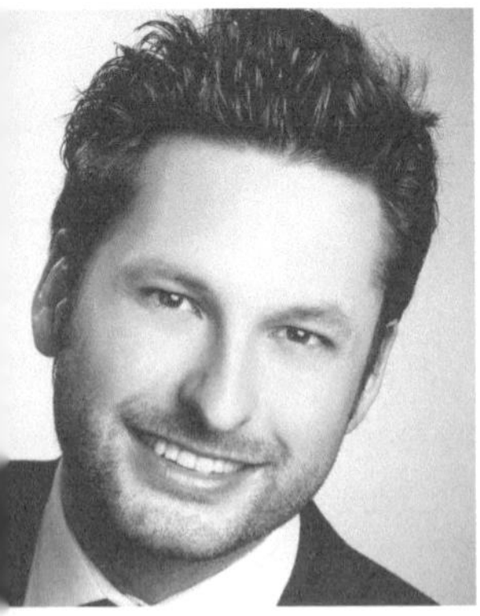
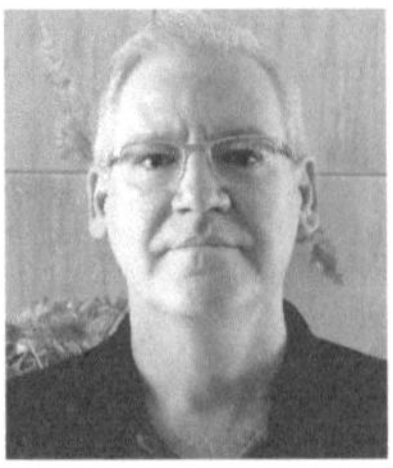

IntechOpen

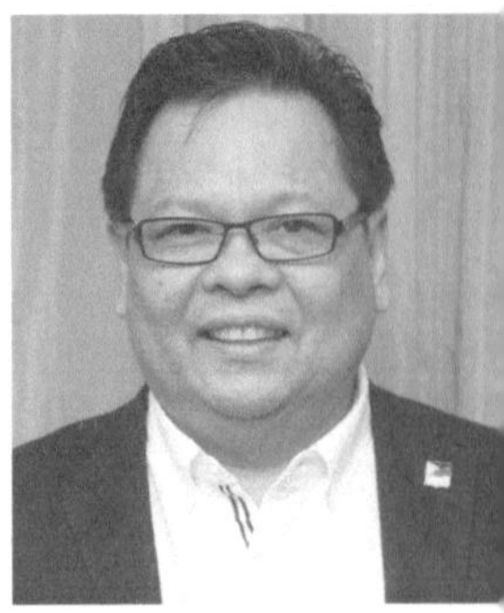
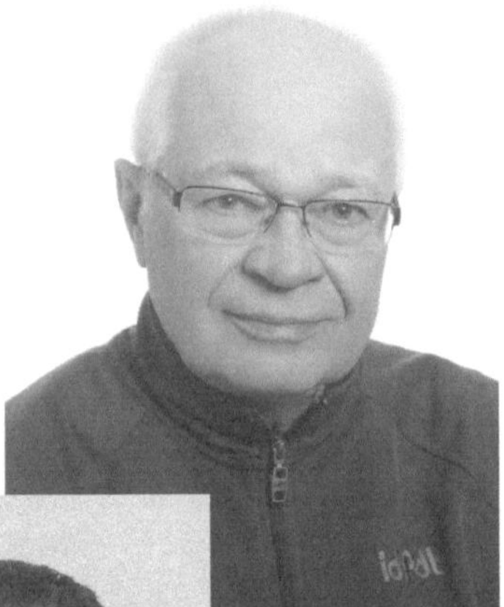
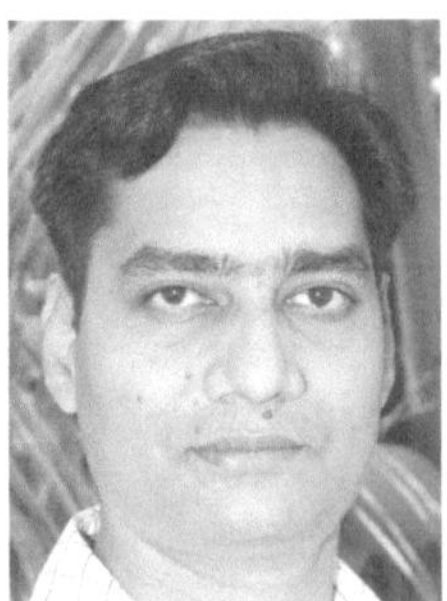
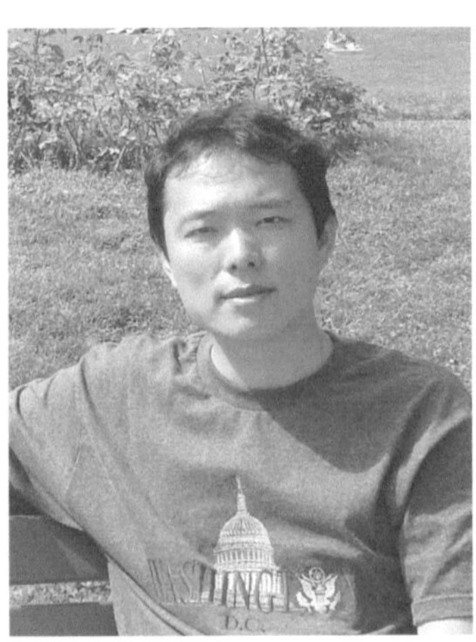
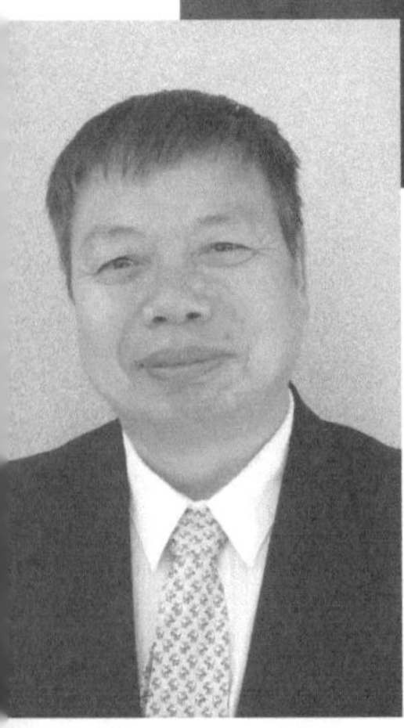
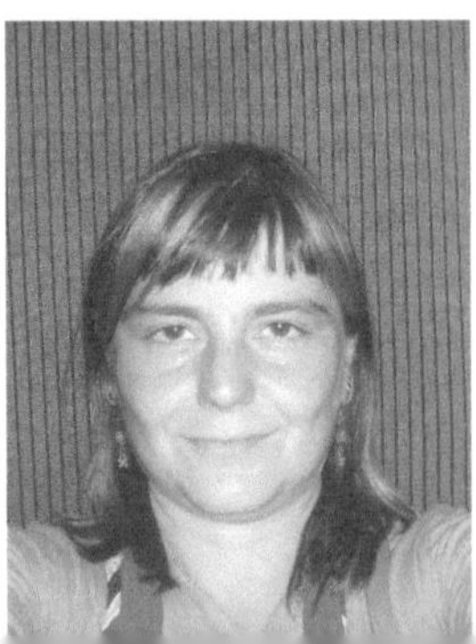

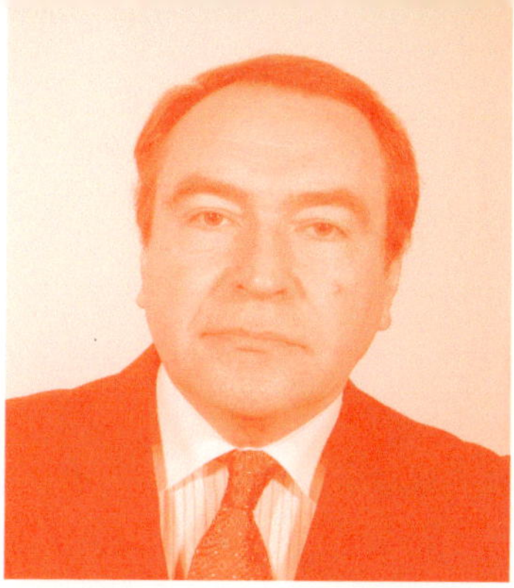
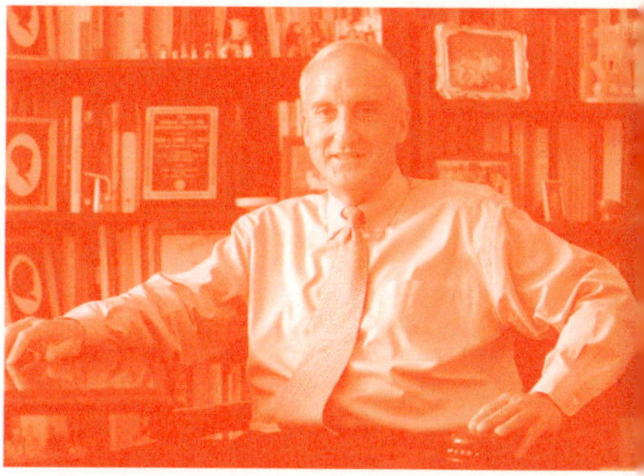
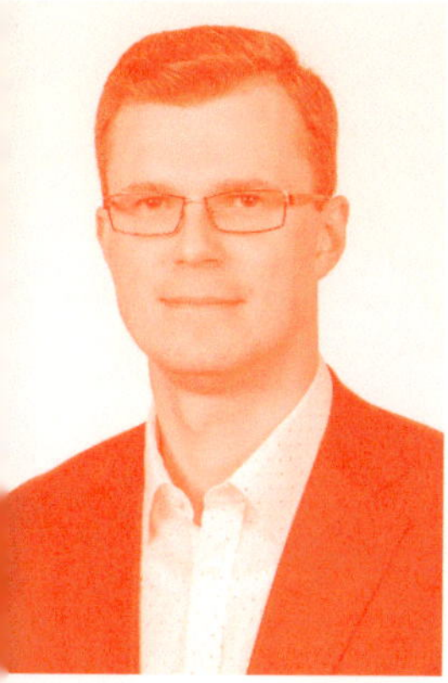
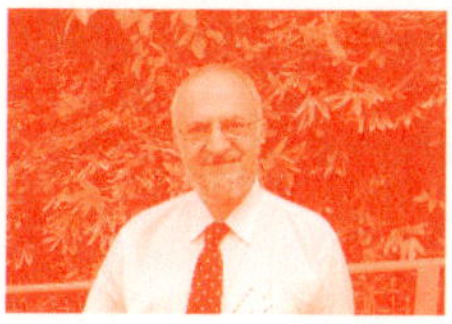
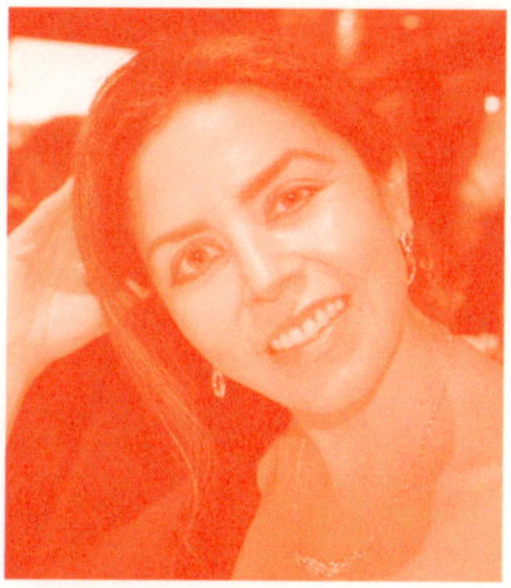

Supporting open minds since 2005

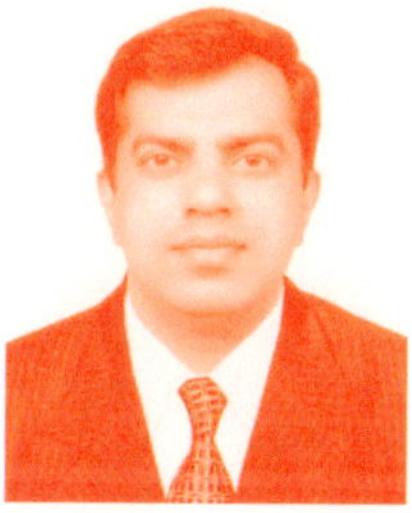
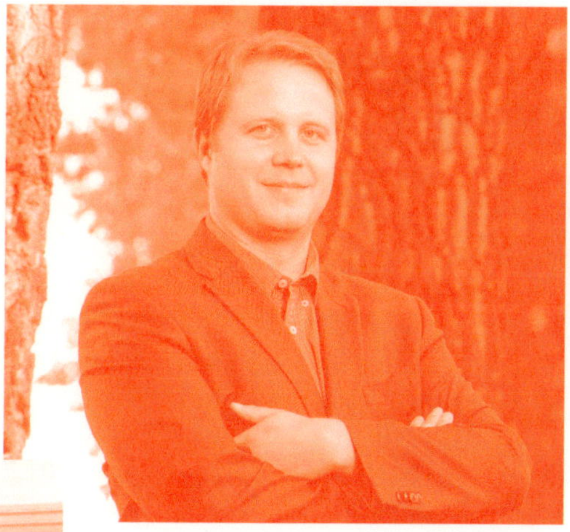
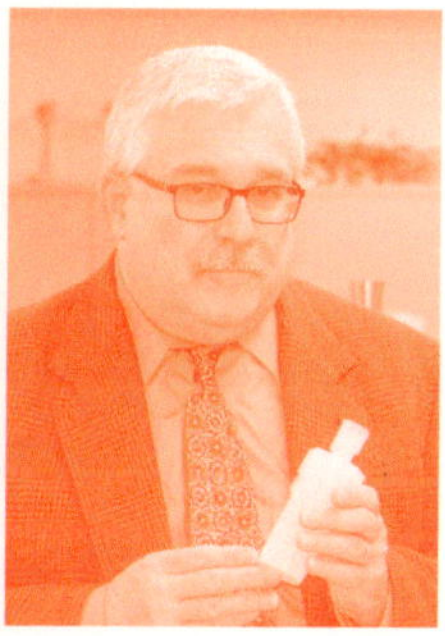
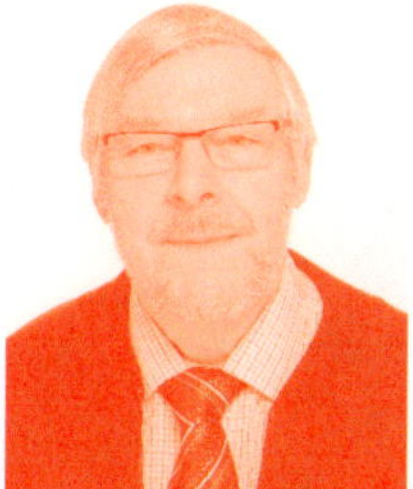
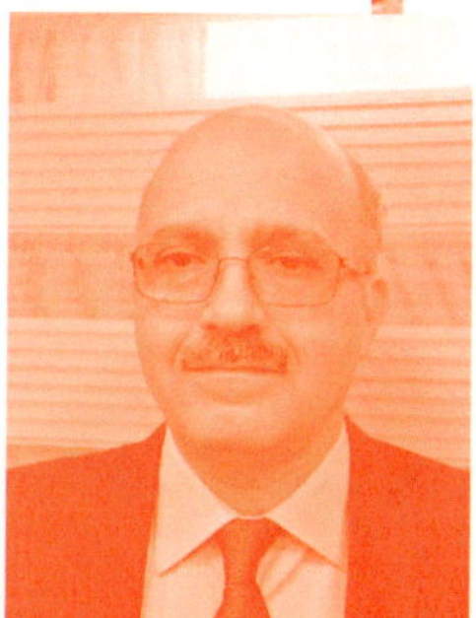
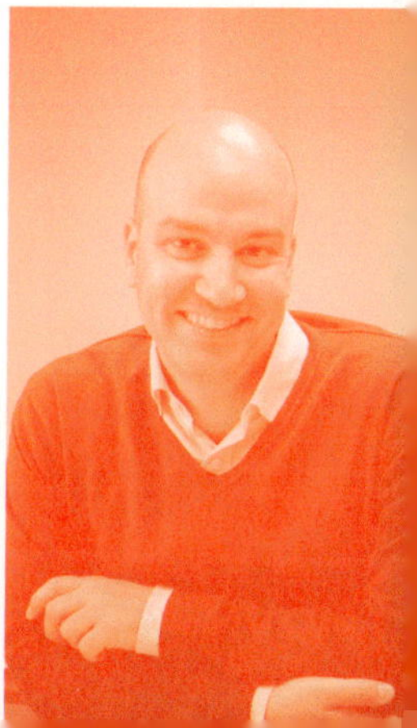
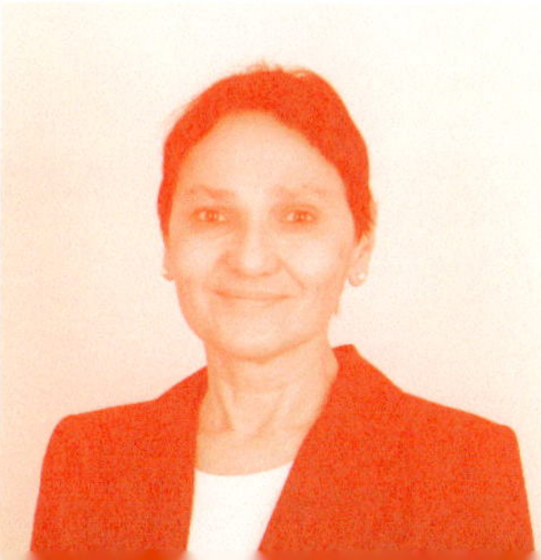

Ovarian Cancer - Updates in Tumour Biology and Therapeutics
http://dx.doi.org/10.5772/intechopen.91528
Edited by Gwo-Yaw Ho and Kate Webber

Assistant to the Editors: Elizabeth Kyran

Contributors
Felicia Elena Buruiana, Lamiese Ismail, Hooman Soleymani Majd, Federico Ferrari, Takol Chareonsirisuthigul, Yanisa Rattanapan, Xianquan Zhan, Na Li, Michael Friedrich, Dominique Friedrich, Stefan Krämer, Clayton Kraft, Walther Kuhn, Silviu-Tiberiu Makkai-Popa, Bogdan Moldovan, Costel Rad, Radu Pisica, Vlad Untaru, Doly Stoica, Bibha Choudhary, Febina Ravindran, shyamika Mirisse Acharige, Cheng Yeoh, Ján Varga, Mohammed E. Mansur, Olga Ostrovsky, Courtney Griffiths, Michelle Bilbao, Lauren Krill, Simon Chu, Peter J. Fuller, Trang Nguyen, Maria Alexiadis, Trang Minh Tran, Yee Shen Choo, Milad Rasouli, Nadia Fallah, Kostya (Ken) Ostrikov, Gwo-Yaw Ho, Maree Bilandzic, Nazanin Karimnia, Andrew N. Stephens

First published in London, United Kingdom, 2021 by IntechOpen
IntechOpen is the global imprint of INTECHOPEN LIMITED, registered in England and Wales, registration number: 11086078, 5 Princes Gate Court, London, SW7 2QJ, United Kingdom
Printed in Croatia

British Library Cataloguing-in-Publication Data
A catalogue record for this book is available from the British Library

Additional hard and PDF copies can be obtained from orders@intechopen.com

Ovarian Cancer - Updates in Tumour Biology and Therapeutics
Edited by Gwo-Yaw Ho and Kate Webber
p. cm.
Print ISBN 978-1-83968-743-3
Online ISBN 978-1-83968-744-0
eBook (PDF) ISBN 978-1-83968-745-7

Meet the editors

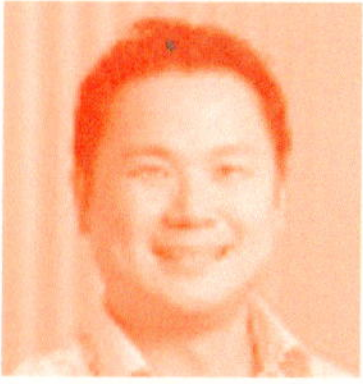

Gwo-Yaw Ho is a senior medical oncologist at Monash Health and specialises in treating women with breast and gynaecologic cancer. He has an academic appointment with Monash University, Australia, as a research fellow and was awarded the Monash University, School of Clinical Science Clinician-scientist Fellowship in 2020. He completed his Ph.D. study in 2019 at the Walter and Eliza Hall (WEHI) Institute of Medical Research whilst practicing as a medical oncologist at the Peter MacCallum Cancer Centre and Royal Women's Hospital, Melbourne. The focus of his research is a subset of high-grade ovarian cancer, including carcinosarcoma, with the poorest outcome which is associated with increased activity of the oncogenic MYCN pathway and the development of pre-clinical cancer models.

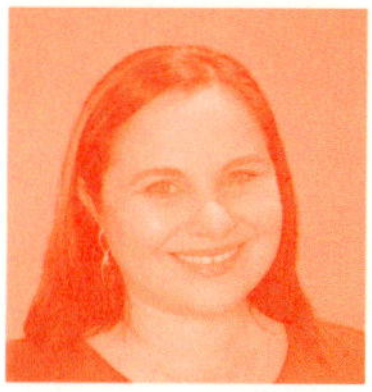

Kate Webber is a senior medical oncologist at Monash Health and an adjunct senior lecturer at Monash University, Australia. She has a keen interest in breast and gynaecological oncology, cancer survivorship and clinical trials. She graduated from the University of New South Wales in 2002 with first-class honours and completed her specialty training in medical oncology at St. George and Prince of Wales Hospitals in Sydney. She completed a Ph.D. in 2016 at the University of New South Wales examining long-term health and psychosocial issues affecting cancer survivors whilst looking at novel models of care for these patients. Dr. Webber is the current co-chair of the Cancer Institute NSW eviQ Medical Oncology Reference Committee.

Contents

Preface

Ovarian cancer (OC) is a heterogeneous disease composed of multiple distinct molecular and clinical subtypes. Women with OC, in particular high-grade serous ovarian cancer (HGSOC), face a formidable challenge as fatal resistance to therapies commonly occurs within a few years of diagnosis, with the exception of rare subtypes such as ovarian germ cell tumour. Improvement in our ability to target the underlying drivers and vulnerabilities of OC, together with advances in surgical techniques, are essential to developing effective treatments for women battling this disease.

HGSOC accounts for much of the lethality of epithelial OC and is the OC subtype of focus in this book. However, the book also covers the genetics and mutational landscape of a rare and lesser-known ovarian cancer, granulosa cell tumour. In general, the molecular characterisation of HGSOC has revealed several subtypes associated with distinct phenotypes and clinical outcomes. The first section of this book explores the utility of OC molecular subtyping for directing therapeutic decisions, the implications of ovarian cancer genetic profiling for the patient, the current understanding of OC tumorigenesis and the role of epigenetic events in this disease.

Most OC is diagnosed at an advanced stage and, in particular for HGSOC, often regarded as a systemic disease. Despite this, the role of surgical cytoreduction remains paramount in the management of OC diagnosed at any stage. Although there has been a significant shift in the management paradigm for women with more advanced OC from primary cytoreductive surgery (PCS) to neoadjuvant chemotherapy (NACT) followed by interval surgery, maximum cytoreduction of tumour to microscopic residual disease, also known as R0 resection or complete resection (CR), is one of the most important positive prognostic factors for women with OC. R0 resection is the current gold standard for optimal debulking surgery. The second section of the book focuses on the role of ultra-radical surgery and hyperthermic intraperitoneal chemotherapy (HIPEC) in the management of women with more advanced OC.

Unfortunately, it is inevitable that most OC will recur. More than 70% of women with HGSOC will relapse within three years, and almost all patients with the recurrent disease will eventually succumb to their cancer. The focus of any treatment is therefore mainly palliative. Chemotherapy with platinum-based or non-platinum-based agents has remained the mainstay of treatment for affected women, despite minimal gains in OC overall survival for the last three decades. It is only recently, with the introduction of poly adenosine diphosphate(ADP)-ribose polymerase inhibitors (PARPi) for treatment of patients with homologous recombination deficient (HRD) tumours, that improvements in OC overall survival is observed. To develop more effective treatments for HGSOC, an in-depth understanding of the early genetic events in HGSOC tumorigenesis is crucial. The last section of the book highlights several potential novel OC therapeutic approaches including targeting the leader cell population to increase chemotherapy sensitivity, use of nanoparticle and gas plasma technologies, and exploration of anti-parasitic drug and epigenetic therapies.

In summary, this book brings together many leading specialists' discoveries and opinions in exploring novel concepts in OC tumour biology and management. It also highlights the rapidly evolving landscape in the understanding and treatment of this devastating disease.

Gwo-Yaw Ho
School of Clinical Sciences,
Monash University,
Department of Medical Oncology,
Monash Health,
Melbourne, Australia

Kate Webber
Monash University,
Australia

Section 1

Ovarian Cancer Genomics

Chapter 1

Ovarian Cancer: Molecular Classification and Targeted Therapy

Febina Ravindran and Bibha Choudhary

Abstract

Ovarian cancer is the deadliest gynecological cancer among women with an overall 5-year survival rate below 50% due to its asymptomatic nature, diagnosis at advanced stages, and a high recurrence rate after standard therapy in 70% of cases. Ovarian cancers are heterogenous cancers where each subtype possesses a varied morphology and biologic behavior. Accumulating evidence has identified each of these subtypes characterized with specific pathways activated in each along with specific gene alterations. For example, high-grade serous ovarian cancer is characterized by universal *TP53* mutation, mucinous ovarian cancer with *KRAS* mutation and clear cell or endometrioid ovarian cancers with *ARID1A* mutations. With the current focus of molecular-targeted therapies for cancer, such druggable markers serve as excellent targets for precision therapy and combination therapy. This chapter, provides an overview of the critical molecular pathways activated in the ovarian cancer subtypes with its druggable targets studied in ovarian cancer. We also highlight the implications of miRNAs in chemoresistance and sensitivity in the regulation of ovarian cancer.

Keywords: ovarian cancer subtypes, targeted therapy, miRNAs in ovarian cancers

1. Introduction

Ovaries are the prime female reproductive organ that produces the oocyte or the egg cell for fertilization. It is also an endocrine gland that produces the female sex hormones estrogen and progesterone responsible for ovulation and pregnancy maintenance. Some of the diseases that affect the ovaries are ovarian cysts, primary ovarian insufficiency, ovarian torsion and more recently ovarian cancer (OC). OC was first detected in the 1950s and is now one of the deadliest gynecological cancers among women [1, 2]. According to the latest Global Cancer Observatory: CANCER TODAY (GLOBOCAN 2018), the incidence and mortality rates of OC vary globally and ranks at the 8th and 7th position respectively [3]. The highest mortality rates are reported in Oceania and Europe and the lowest are from Latin America, the Caribbean and Asia [3]. OCs are also prevalent in countries with a high human development index (HDI) but with lower mortality rates due to increased diagnostic and therapeutic support [4].

Most OCs manifest post menopause and the increased incidence is reported in women older than 65 years [5]. Considering the ethnicity, non-Hispanic white women are reported to have the highest incidence and mortality rates [6]. OCs are heterogeneous cancer, hence the risk factors for each histological subtype vary. In general, some of the major risk factors for OC include Hereditary Breast and Ovarian Cancer (HBOC) syndrome [7], Lynch syndrome [8], menopausal hormonal therapy [9, 10], endometriosis [11], IVF treatment [12], use of fertility drugs [13], late menopause [14] and null parity [15]. Interestingly, high parity [16], hysterectomy [17] and usage of hormonal contraceptive pills for prolonged periods [18] are reported to have a protective effect since these conditions confer in the suppression of ovulatory cycles [19]. The sterilization treatment, tubal ligation is also reported to reduce the risk of OCs [17, 20]. Recently reported other emerging risk factors for OCs are the use of talc powders [21], asbestos exposure [22] and pelvic inflammatory disease [23].

OCs are difficult to detect;therefore almost 60% of OC cases are diagnosed at advanced stages [24]. It is often called the "whispering cancer" or "silent cancer" due to its asymptomatic nature and late presentation [25, 26]. Late-stage OC symptoms are very nonspecific and diffuse but may include abdominal bloating or swelling, pelvic pain, increased urinary urgency, weight loss, or fatigue [27, 28]. Although a biopsy is the only reliable diagnosis for OC, screening for serum cancer antigen 125 (CA-125) levels combined with ultrasound imaging are used for women with increased risk [29]. The emerging technique of liquid biopsy is being explored for identifying serum biomarkers for early detection of OCs. It holds great promise being non-invasive and is utilized to diagnose, prognose and predict surgical outcomes. One such serum biomarker identified is the Human Epididymis Protein 4 (HE4) which is reported to have high specificity for OCs [30, 31]. 2011 FDA approved, ROMA index (risk of ovarian malignancy algorithm) deduced from HE4, CA-125 and the menopausal status is used for diagnosis and prognosis of OCs with a specificity of 90% [32–34]. Another recent 2016 FDA approved serum-based screening test, Overa also uses HE4 levels along with other serum proteins is reported to show a sensitivity of 94% along with pathological diagnosis [35]. The mutational status of multiple cancer-causing genes are also being developed as screening tests for various cancers like PapSEEK and CancerSEEK and are reported to detect OC with a specificity of 63% and 98%, respectively [36, 37].

According to the World cancer report 2020, OC five-year survival rate is below 30% [38]. This is mainly because this cancer gets diagnosed at stage III or IV with metastasis and the recurrence rate high despite standard therapy. Cytoreductive surgery followed by chemotherapy based on cancer's surgical stage remains the gold standard treatment for OCs. The most commonly administered chemotherapy drugs are platinum derivatives e.g. cisplatin and carboplatin and are often combined with taxane-based drugs like paclitaxel or docetaxel. These drugs induce apoptosis in the tumor cells by creating double-stranded breaks in the DNA [39]. Despite chemotherapy being effective for advanced cancers in the initial phases, cancer relapses in 70% of cases due to drug resistance [40]. In the case of recurrent OCs, the second line of the chemotherapy treatment regimen is based on the platinum-free interval and the tumor's molecular profile [41]. Furthermore, the treatment options include combinations of carboplatin with gemcitabine, topotecan, vinorelbine, trabectedin, belotecan or pegylated liposomal doxorubicin [42].

Despite intensive combination chemotherapy, the survival rate decreases with chemoresistance and subsequent OC metastasis. The lack of anatomical barrier around the ovaries facilitates the dissemination of OC cells into the peritoneal cavity, metastasizing onto abdominal organs resulting in bowel obstruction, which is the major cause of OC morbidity and mortality [43, 44]. Currently, there are no preventive measures for OCs, and options for the high-risk category are prophylactic surgeries like hysterectomy (removal of the uterus) combined with bilateral salpingo-oophorectomy (removal of both ovaries and fallopian tube) or bilateral salpingectomy (removal of both fallopian tubes) [45]. Women with average risk can opt for oral contraceptive treatment [46].

Presently, there is no effective cure for advanced OC. Though these cancers vary histologically, clinical treatment therapies neglect these differences and are treated as a single disease. Each OC subtype is characterized by specific genetic mutations that deregulate specific signaling pathways that should be utilized for personalized or tailored therapeutics. Precision therapy is the need of the hour for OC treatment in improving the current survival rate. In the following sections of the chapter, we describe the various OC subtypes, their histological classification and the key molecular pathways activated in each subtype along with its druggable targets.

2. Ovarian cancer subtypes

OC neoplasms arise from distinct regions of the ovary. They are termed heterogeneous as each OC subtype is unique with varied morphology, biologic behavior and even prognosis. High throughput sequencing technologies have identified each OC subtype as distinct even on a molecular level with unique genomic characteristics. OCs are broadly classified into epithelial and non-epithelial cancers. Non-epithelial cancer comprises germ cell cancer, stromal cell cancer, and the rare small cell carcinoma. The origin of the various subtypes of OCs and the sub-classifications are depicted in **Figure 1**.

2.1 Epithelial ovarian cancer (EOC)

Epithelial ovarian cancers (EOCs) comprise 90% of all OCs and are among the most well-characterized forms of OC. EOCs are thought to arise from the epithelium, the outer lining of the ovary. EOC is an age-related disease and is considered mainly a postmenopausal disease. Based on tumor cell morphology, they are further subdivided into high grade serous ovarian carcinoma (HGSOC), low grade serous ovarian carcinoma (LGSOC), mucinous ovarian carcinoma (MOC), endometrioid carcinoma (EC), and clear-cell carcinoma (CCC). The histological image, epidemiology, molecular alterations and pathways affecting each EOC variant are outlined in **Figure 2**.

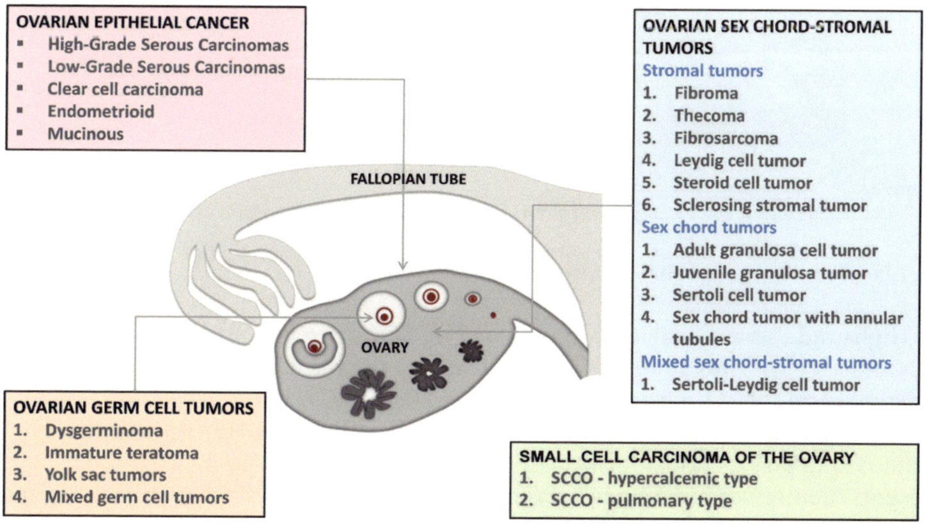

Figure 1.
Origin of the various ovarian cancer subtypes and their sub-classifications.

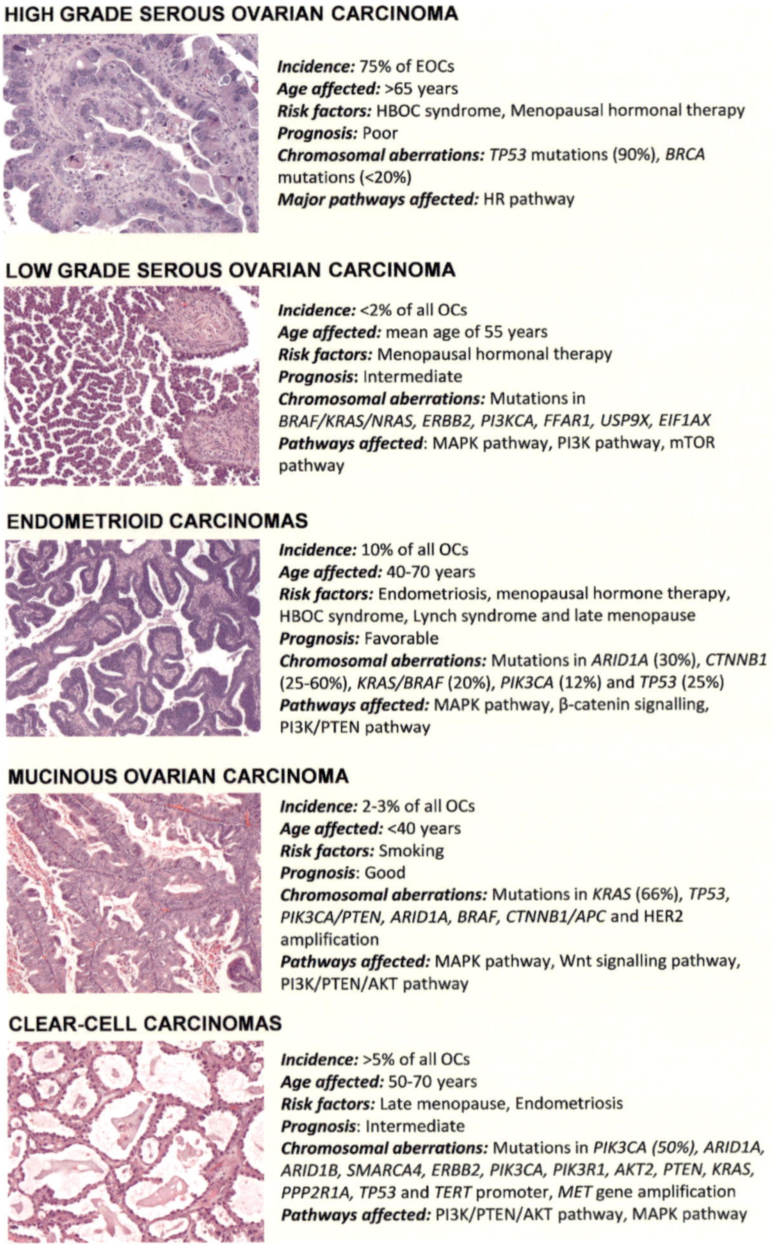

Figure 2.
EOC subtypes: histology, epidemiology, and molecular alterations. Histology images courtesy [47].

2.1.1 High grade serous ovarian carcinoma (HGSOC)

High grade serous ovarian carcinomas (HGSOCs) are the most lethal forms of OCs and account 75% of all EOCs [48]. They are the most aggressive and chemo-resistant forms of EOCs responsible for 70–80% of OC related deaths. HGSOCs are thought to be derived from the fallopian tube [49]. These cancers are mainly diagnosed in postmenopausal women and due to its asymptomatic character presents themselves in advanced stages. Familial HBOC syndrome, and menopausal hormonal therapy predispose women towards this cancer [25, 50].

HGSOCs are characterized by a high frequency (90%) of somatic *TP53* mutations. These mutations are present in the DNA binding domain of TP53 which render its tumor-suppressive function inactive, leading to enhanced cell proliferation and metastasis. The drug APR-246 targeting TP53 resulting in its wild type stabilization is under clinical trial and has shown favorable results [51]. Another drug, nutlin-3a targeting MDM2, a negative regulator of TP53, has also entered clinical trials with positive outcomes [52]. Moreover, combination therapy using nutlin-3 and RG7388 (another MDM2-TP53 antagonist) have reported cytotoxic effects in various OC cell lines [53].

15–20% of HGSOC patients harbor germline mutations in *BRCA1* or *BRCA2* [48]. The *BRCA* genes are involved in the repair of double-strand DNA breaks through homologous recombination (HR). Besides, most HGSOCs with the germline *BRCA* mutation are also reported to harbor somatic mutations in other HR-related genes conferring an HR deficient (HRD) phenotype [54]. The Cancer Genome Atlas Research Network (TCGA) has reported almost 50% HGSOCs cases as HR deficient [55]. HRD conferring genes besides *BRCA1/2* include Fanconi anemia genes (*PALB2, FANCA, FANCI, FANCL, FANCC*), RAD family genes (*RAD50, RAD51, RAD51C, RAD54L*), MRN complex genes (*Mre11-Rad50-Nbs1*), and also DNA damage response genes (*ATM, ATR, CHEK1, CHEK2*) [54, 56]. This manifestation of inactivating *BRCA* gene mutations and other HRD genes confer a DNA repair-deficient phenotype leading to genomic instability [57].

One of the most remarkable developments for OC therapy has been the PARP (poly (ADP-ribose) polymerase) inhibitors. PARP is an excision repair enzyme involved in the repair of single DNA strand breaks. PARP inhibitor treatment in BRCA-deficient cancer induces synthetic lethality and cell death [58]. The PARP inhibitor olaparib has been reported to show increased progression-free survival (PFS) and is currently approved as first-line maintenance therapy for *BRCA*-mutant individuals [59, 60]. Another PARP inhibitor, niraparib, improved PFS regardless of *BRCA* or HRD status is also approved for first-line maintenance of advanced OCs [61]. CDK4/6 inhibitors (palbociclib, ribociclib and abemaciclib) are also under clinical trials as maintenance and combination therapy for HGSOCs [62]. Cyclin-dependent kinase 4 and 6 (CDK4/6) are key kinases that regulate the cell cycle. CDK4/6 inhibitors hinder G1-S transition inducing cell cycle arrest at the G1 phase. PI3K/AKT and NOTCH pathways are reported to be deregulated in HGSOCs which could also be targeted via combination therapies using PI3K inhibitors or the AKT inhibitor, afuresertib [63].

One of the first targeted therapy used to treat advanced OCs is Bevacizumab, an anti-angiogenic agent that targets vascular endothelial growth factor (VEGF) [64]. Angiogenesis plays a pivotal role in tumor progression and metastasis in many malignant cancers. This drug acts by neutralizing VEGF-A, thereby inhibiting tumor growth and invasion. Bevacizumab is currently approved as a combination therapy along with platinum/taxane drugs for advanced HGSOCs and has been reported to show a significant improvement in progression-free survival [57].

2.1.2 Low grade serous ovarian carcinoma (LGSOC)

As the name suggests, LGSOCs are indolent and less aggressive tumors with relatively better prognosis than HGSOC. They are prevalent in younger women with a median age of 55 years and constitute less than 5% of all OCs [65]. Though LGSOCs are chemoresistant they are treated the same way as HGSOCs with platinum/taxane drugs. The increased survival rate in LGSOCs is attributed to its longer disease trajectory and complete resection of the tumor post-primary cytoreductive surgery [66].

LGSOCs are characterized by activation of the mitogen-activated protein kinase (MAPK) pathway in 80% cases. *KRAS* (54%), *BRAF* (33%), *NRAS* (26%), and

ERBB2, the upstream regulators of MAPK pathways are reported to be mutated, with mutations in *BRAF/KRAS* considered as good prognostic markers [67]. Due to the high prevalence of activated MAPK pathway in LGSOCs, MEK inhibitors (Trametinib, Selumetinib, Pimasertib, Binimetinib) are among the druggable targets for these cancers and some are under evaluation [65]. Recurrent mutations in *PIK3CA*, *FFAR1*, *USP9X* (11%) and *EIF1AX* (15%) are reported as driver mutations [68]. *USP9X* and *EIF1AX* are regulators of the mTOR pathway which are downstream effectors of the MAPK pathway. The use of Metformin, an inhibitor of the mTOR pathway, along with MEK inhibitor (Trametinib) has been reported to show an inhibitory effect in various LGSOCs cell lines [69]. Taken together, MEK inhibitors and Metformin are potential candidates for targeted therapies. CDK4/6 inhibitors, (ribociclib and abemaciclib) are under clinical trials for LGSOCs [65]. Endocrine therapy using letrozole, anastrozole or tamoxifen used as maintenance therapy has been reported to be beneficial in LGSOCs due to estrogen and progesterone receptors expressions [70].

2.1.3 Endometrioid carcinomas

Endometrioid carcinomas (ECs) are the second most common EOCs representing 10% of all OCs [71]. They are diagnosed in women in the age range of 40–70 years and are associated with a good prognosis. As its name suggests they are associated with endometriosis and are thought to be derived from the endometrium [72]. Endometriosis, menopausal hormone therapy, HBOC syndrome, Lynch syndrome and late menopause are some of the risk factors associated with ECs [14, 73].

One of the most mutated genes reported in ECs is *ARID1A* at a frequency of 30%. *ARID1A* is a component of the SWI/SNF chromatin remodeling complex. Targeting *ARID1A* with HDAC inhibitors have been reported to be effective in mice models harboring *ARID1A* tumor mutation [74]. *CTNNB1*, of the β-catenin signaling is also reported to be mutated at a rate of 25–60%. β-catenin signaling is a conserved pathway involved in development implicated in other epithelial cancers but its oncogenic role is less understood [75]. Other less frequent mutations are *KRAS/BRAF* (20%), which are regulators of MAPK pathways, *PIK3CA* (12%), and *TP53* (25%) [76]. *PTEN* mutations with frequent loss of heterozygosity (45–75%) is also reported [52]. *PTEN* is a tumor-suppressor gene that is a negative regulator of the PI3K pathway and is also the most mutated in the related endometrial cancers [77]. The multiple mutational spectra of ECs warrants the investigation of combination therapy using MEK inhibitors (trametinib, MEK162), TP53 activators (APR-246), and PI3K inhibitors (idelalisib, voxtalisib). Only 14% of EC cases are reported to be *BRCA* mutation carriers [78], and HBOC syndrome being one of the risk factors for ECs, PARP inhibitors are a viable option for targeted therapies.

2.1.4 Mucinous ovarian carcinomas

Mucinous carcinomas (MOCs) are a rare subset of EOCs accounting for 2–3% of all OCs. They are histologically characterized by high levels of intracellular mucin. MOCs are more prevalent in women below 40 years and unlike other EOC types, the only risk factor identified is smoking [14, 79]. Early-stage MOCs have an excellent prognosis and beyond stage II, they are addressed by standard chemotherapeutic agents with poor outcomes, as these tumors are chemoresistant.

Though rare, MOCs have been well characterized. The predominant mutation present in MOCs is *KRAS* mutations reported in 66% of cases [79, 80]. A recent large cohort study identified many other mutations in MOCs besides *KRAS* in varying degrees which are *TP53* mutation, HER2 amplification (a member of the epidermal growth factor receptor family), *PIK3CA/PTEN* (regulator of PI3K-PTEN-AKT pathway), *BRAF* mutation, *CTNNB1/APC* mutations (regulator of Wnt-signaling pathway), and *ARID1A* mutation (a member of the SWI/SNF family) [79, 80]. One of the potential drugs for the treatment of MOCs is 5-fluorouracil. MOCs and mucinous colorectal cancer (CRC) share a similar mutational profile with unfavorable outcome [81]. 5-fluorouracil, which is currently utilized for CRC treatment has been effective in various MOC cell lines in combination with oxaliplatin [82]. Moreover, the multiple mutational spectra reported in MOCs are a great avenue for identifying the most potent target for tailored therapies. Some targeted drugs like BRAF inhibitors, PI3K inhibitors are already being investigated in various other cancer types. Combinatorial therapy using dual inhibitors is warranted for MOC treatment due to its varied mutational landscape.

2.1.5 Clear-cell carcinomas

Clear cell carcinomas (CCCs) of the ovary constitute >5% of all OCs and 10% of all EOCs [83]. The incidence rates of CCCs vary by ethnicity; the majority of the cases are reported in East Asian countries (mainly Japan) for unknown reasons [84]. They are mostly diagnosed in younger women with an option of fertility-sparing surgery before standard chemotherapy. These are chemoresistant tumors with a poor prognosis if diagnosed at an advanced stage, but most of these cases are diagnosed early with a good prognosis [83]. They are a distinct class of EOCs thought to arise from endometriosis or clear cell adenofibroma, hence they are associated with endometriosis which is thought to be the precursor for CCC manifestation and this association is considered a good prognosis [85]. Late menopause and endometriosis are considered to be the highest risk factors for developing CCCs.

The most common genomic alterations identified in CCCs are activating mutations in *PIK3CA*, a regulator of the PI3K-PTEN-AKT pathway (50%), and loss of function in *ARID1A*, component of SWI/SNF chromatin remodeling complex (50%) [86]. Other mutations reported in varying degrees are *MET* gene amplification, mutations in *ARID1B, SMARCA4*, *ERBB2, PIK3CA, PIK3R1, AKT2, PTEN, KRAS, PPP2R1A, TP53, TERT* promoter, and ZNF217 overexpression [85, 87]. Antioxidant genes like *Glutathione peroxidase 3 (GPX3)*, *glutaredoxin (GLRX),* and *superoxide dismutase 2 (SOD2)* are reported to be highly expressed in CCCs rendering them resistant to chemotherapy [88]. A recent report on the pharmacological inhibition of EZH2 for loss of function of *ARID1A* has shown considerable promise in treating CCCs [89]. The overexpression of the transcription factor ZNF217 is a poor prognostic marker. In-vitro studies in ZNF217-overexpressing cells treated with triciribine, a DNA synthesis inhibitor, have shown inhibitory effects suggesting ZNF217 be a druggable target [90]. Targeting PI3K/AKT/mTOR pathways using PI3K inhibitor (idelalisib, Voxtalisib) or mTOR pathway inhibitor (Metformin) are other viable options.

2.2 Sex cord-stromal tumors (SCSTs)

The rare ovarian sex cord-stromal tumors (SCSTs) constitute 8% of all OCs and are diagnosed in broad age groups with mixed prognosis [91]. These neoplasms originate from the stromal cells and/or the sex chord cells of the ovary, which are involved in the endocrine function of producing the female sex hormones, therefore unlike EOCs, they present with hormone-related disorders. Certain hereditary cancer syndromes predispose patients towards SCST. Based on the WHO classification of OCs, the various subtypes of SCSTs with their incidence, risk factors, prognosis, and molecular alterations are outlined in **Table 1** [92].

SCST subtypes	Incidence rates	Incident age groups	Risk factors	Prognosis	Chromatic alteration
Stromal tumors					
Fibroma	4% of all OCs	~ 40 years	Meigs' syndrome	Good	
Thecoma	0.5–1% of all OCs	26–86 years		Poor	*FOXL2* (~21%)
Fibrosarcoma		20–73 years		Poor	
Leydig cell tumor	0.1% of all SCST	Post-menopausal women		Good	
Steroid cell tumor	0.1% of all SCST	~ 43 years	Cushing syndrome	Good	
Sclerosing stromal tumor	>0.1% of all SCST	<30 years		Good	
Sex-chord tumors					
Adult granulosa cell tumor	5% of all OCs, 70% of all SCSTs	24–84 years	Peutz Jeghers syndrome, Potters syndrome	Poor	*FOXL2* mutation (> 95%), *TERT* mutations (~40%), AKT1 amplification (~60%)
Juvenile granulosa tumor	5% of all GCTs	8–45 years	Ollier disease, Maffucci disease	Good	AKT1 amplification (~60%), *GNAS* mutations (~30%)
Sertoli cell tumor		2–76 years	Peutz Jeghers syndrome	Good	
Sex chord tumor with annular tubules	1.4% of all SCST	5–39 years	Peutz Jeghers syndrome	Favorable	
Mixed sex chord-stromal tumors					
Sertoli-Leydig cell tumor	0.5% of all OCs	>30 years	Dicer syndrome	Good	Germline and somatic *DICER1* mutations (60%)

Table 1.
Sex cord-stromal tumors subtypes: epidemiology, and molecular alterations.

Due to the rarity of these tumor types, the molecular characteristics of only a few of these subtypes are reported. The cancers arising in the ovary's granulosa cells are the most common in this group comprising 2–5% of all OCs [93]. Granulosa cells are somatic cells involved in folliculogenesis and ovulation, the variant adult granulosa cell tumors (AGCTs), which are estradiol producing are the most common in this group constituting 70% of all SCSTs [94]. Inhibin, a gonadal hormone secreted by granulosa cells, is reported to be elevated in GCT patients [95]. Inhibin level and CA-125 are utilized as a diagnostic biomarker to assess disease progression in GCTs [96]. 97% of AGCTs are characterized by the ubiquitous presence of *FOXL2* mutations, a component of the TGFβ pathway [95]. The pleiotropic TGFβ pathway is reported to be deregulated in many cancers conferring chemoresistance and metastasis [97]. Moreover, *TERT* promoter mutations are reported in 40% of recurrent AGCT cases with poor prognosis [98]. Few small cohort studies of AGCTs, and juvenile granulosa cell tumors (JGCTs), have reported amplification in

AKT leading to possible dysregulations in PI3K/AKT pathways [99, 100]. Activating GNAS mutations involved in tumor invasion are reported in 30% of JGCTs with aggressive nature [101]. The notch signaling pathway is also reported to be altered in GCTs [102]. Estrogen producing thecomas, composed of pure stromal cells are also reported to harbor *FOXL2* mutation at a rate of 21% [103]. Sertoli-Leydig cell tumors (SLCTs), which belong to mixed-sex chord and stromal cells are androgen-secreting tumors that induce varying degrees of virilization (male physical characteristics) [104]. Mutation in *DICER1*, an endoribonuclease involved in microRNA biogenesis, is reported with a high frequency of 88% in undifferentiated SLCTs [105].

Targeting Activin A of the TGFβ pathway and aromatase, a downstream target of FOXL2 has been reported promising for targeted therapies [106, 107]. *TERT* promoter mutations are present in various cancer types and are reported to activate the oncogenic MAPK pathway; targeting this pathway using MEK inhibitors (trametinib, MEK162) are potential treatment options [108]. Besides, other druggable pathways for GCTs include PI3K and NOTCH pathways. Identifying drugs targeting DICER1 is warranted which could provide novel modalities for tailored therapies for SLCTs.

2.3 Ovarian germ cell tumors (OGCTs)

Ovarian germ cell tumors (OGCTs) of the ovary are rare ovarian neoplasms comprising 2–3% of all OCs [109]. These histologically variant heterogeneous neoplasms arise in the egg or ovum, the ovary's primordial germ cell. They primarily manifest in young and adolescent women with excellent prognosis if diagnosed in earlier stages [110]. These tumors are chemosensitive allowing fertility-sparing surgery in most cases [111]. A recent small cohort study reported a low mutational burden in OGCTs explaining their chemosensitive disposition [112]. OGCTs are classified into dysgerminomas, immature teratomas, yolk sac tumors, and mixed germ cell tumors in order of their frequency. Embryonal carcinomas, choriocarcinomas, and malignant struma ovarii tumors are other very rare forms of OGCTs [113]. The understudied, very rare mixed germ cell tumors are the only aggressive OGCT subtype with poor prognosis [114]. There are no risk factors identified for OGCTs but certain genetic diseases like Turner's syndrome, Triple X syndrome, and Swyer syndrome are reported to be high-risk factors for dysgerminomas [115]. The incidence rate, prognosis, risk factors, and their molecular characteristics are outlined in **Table 2**.

OGCT subtypes	Incidence rates	Incident age groups	Prognosis	Chromatic alteration
Dysgerminoma	40% of OGCTs	19–23 years	Good	*KIT* mutation (30–50%), 12p amplifications harboring *KRAS* (80%)
Immature teratoma	~35% of OGCTs	18–36 years	Good	
Yolk sac tumors	15% of OGCTs	15–40 years	Good	*PIK3CA* or *AKT1* mutation (72%), 12p amplifications harboring *KRAS* (60%)
Mixed germ cell tumors	5% of OGCTs	<20 years	Poor	12p amplifications harboring *KRAS* (~40%)

Table 2.
Ovarian germ cell tumors subtypes: epidemiology and molecular alterations.

SCCO subtypes	Incidence rates	Incident age groups	Prognosis	Chromatic alteration
SCCO-hypercalcemic type	<1% of all OCs	<40 years	Poor	*SMARCA* mutation (90%)
SCCO- pulmonary type	<1% of all OCs	<59 years	Poor	None reported

Table 3.
Small cell carcinoma of the ovary subtypes: Epidemiology, and molecular alterations.

The most frequent mutations reported in OGCTs are *KIT* mutations and 12p amplification, which harbor KRAS [112]. The OGCT subtype, dysgerminomas harbor 12p amplification and *KIT* mutation at a frequency of 80% and 30–50%, respectively [116]. *KIT* is a proto-oncogene involved in PI3K/AKT/mTOR, JAK/STAT and MAPK pathways [117], whereas the oncogene *KRAS* is involved in the tumor development pathway of Ras/Raf/MEK/ERK pathway [118]. The aneuploid, yolk sac tumors are reported to harbor PI3K and AKT1 mutations, besides *KRAS* altering PI3K/AKT/mTOR pathway. The TGFβ/BMP and Wnt/β-catenin signaling pathways are also reported to be activated in yolk sac tumors [116]. Few druggable targets of these pathways like AKT inhibitor (afuresertib) and MEK inhibitor (trametinib) are already under clinical trials for various OCs [119].

2.4 Small cell carcinoma of the ovary (SCCO)

Small cell carcinoma of the ovary (SCCO) is a group of extremely rare OCs accounting for <1% of all OCs [120]. Their biology is poorly understood as their cellular lineage is unknown. Based on histologic characterization, SCCO is classified into hypercalcemic type (SCCO-HT), which is chemoresistant and pulmonary type (SCCO-PT) which is chemo-sensitive. These are highly malignant cancers with an average survival of 5.7 years. The incidence rate, prognosis, risk factors and molecular characteristics are outlined in **Table 3**.

One of the significant mutations identified in 90% of cases of SCCOHT is germline or somatic mutations of *SMARCA4* [121]. *SMARCA4* mutation is considered one of the hallmarks of SCCOHT, it is a key component of the switching/sucrose non-fermenting (SWI/SNF) chromatin remodeling complex [122, 123]. The loss of function of *SMARCA4* leads to the upregulation of EZH2, the catalytic subunit of the PRC2 complex which is utilized as a druggable target for SCCOHT [124]. Targeting EZH2 using tazemetostat has reported antiproliferative and antitumor effects in SCCOHT cell lines [125]. Moreover, a recent study has reported oncolytic viruses' effect on SCCOHT derived cell line BIN-1 in reducing its proliferation >75%, which holds promise in developing targeted therapies [126]. Some of the broad categories of drugs being investigated for SCCOHT and some of which are already in clinical trials, include tyrosine kinase inhibitors, immune checkpoint inhibitors and HDAC inhibitors [127]. There are no studies reported on the molecular characterization and pathogenesis of SCCO-PT due to its rarity.

3. Potential drugs for targeted therapies in OCs

Presently, targeted therapy is employed only to improve the efficacy of standard therapy in OC treatment with drugs such as bevacizumab, an anti-angiogenic agent which is licensed for use as front-line therapy for advanced OCs [57] and olaparib, a PARP inhibitor which is now approved for first-line maintenance therapy for patients with relapsed *BRCA*-mutated OCs [128]. Very recently, the combination of bevacizumab and olaparib is FDA approved for first-line maintenance treatment in advanced OCs with HRD positive status [129].

Generic drugs being investigated for a variety of OC types are receptor tyrosine kinase (RTK) inhibitors. RTK inhibitors have been reported to be efficacious in treating a variety of malignant cancers by inhibiting tumor cell proliferation via blocking the signal transduction cascade. For e.g., Ponatinib is a multi-tyrosine kinase inhibitor that targets pathways like EGFR, FGFR, PDGFR, and VEGFR all of which are aberrantly activated in various cancer types [130]. Other RTK inhibitors being investigated for OCs are Palbociclib, Abemaciclib and Ribociclib [131, 132]. Likewise, immunotherapy using immune checkpoint inhibitors like Pembrolizumab and Nivolumab has been revolutionary in oncology research. These are monoclonal antibodies that trigger the immune T-cell activation to attack the cancer cells and Pembrolizumab is already under clinical trial for various cancer types [133, 134]. Epigenetic abnormalities being the hallmarks of cancers, epigenetic modulators like HDAC inhibitors have shown great promise as anti-cancer drugs. HDAC inhibitors like Vorinostat, Panobinostat, Quisinostat, and Trichostatin are under investigation for targeted therapies for OCs [126, 135].

4. Role of miRNAs in ovarian cancer

miRNAs are single-stranded RNA nucleotides that regulate gene expression. In the human body, they are reported to be involved in regulating around 60% of genes affecting various cellular and biological processes. Each miRNA has multiple gene targets or multiple miRNAs can act on one target gene. They can function either as an oncogene or a tumor suppressor and their expressions in cancer cells are deregulated [136]. The miRNA expression profile for each OC subtype is reported to be distinct, with a subset of miRNAs downregulated or upregulated [137]. The miRNA signatures identified in various cancer types are being investigated for their utility as cancer biomarkers in tumor diagnosis, prognosis and therapeutic outcome.

Ovarian cancer subtype	Upregulated	Downregulated	References
Serous Ovarian cancer	miR-429, miR-141, miR-200c, miR-93, miR-16, miR-20a, miR-21, miR-27a, miR-200a, miR-200b, miR-200c, miR-203, miR-205, miR-375, miR-145	miR-320c, miR-383, let-7b, miR-99a, miR-125b, miR-145, miR-100, miR-31, miR-137, miR-132, miR-26a	[138, 139]
Clear-cell carcinomas	miR-93, miR-126, miR-338, miR-200a, miR-200b, miR-30a, miR-141, miR-182, miR-200a, miR-510, miR-509,	miR-383, miR-424, miR-127, miR-155, miR-99b	[138, 139]
Mucinous ovarian carcinoma	miR-192, miR-194	—	[137]
Endometrioid carcinomas	miR-7, miR-429, miR-21, miR-29a, miR-92, miR-30c1, miR-126, miR-126, miR-29a	miR-342, miR-181a, miR-450b, miR-155, miR-25, miR-93, miR-127, miR-99b	[136–138]
Ovarian Germ cell tumors	miR-373-3p, miR-372-3p and miR-302c-3p, mir-302–367 cluster, mir-371–373 cluster, miR-146b, miR-155, miR-182	miR-199a-5p, miR-214-5p and miR-202-3p, Let-7	[139, 140]

Table 4.
Deregulated miRNAs in ovarian cancer subtypes.

The sensitivity of a cancer drug profoundly affects treatment efficacy and prognosis. miRNAs are involved in conferring chemo-sensitive or chemoresistant phenotype by regulating the drug-resistance related genes [138]. Therefore, manipulating the expression levels of specific miRNAs can aid in drug sensitivity. As previously mentioned, the sensitivity for platinum drugs varies among each OC subtype, and this profoundly affects the treatment efficacy and prognosis. Though still in its infancy, targeting miRNA holds great promise for a more customized therapeutic approach. Here, we highlight the key miRNAs reported in recent literature, which are deregulated in the various OC subtypes (**Table 4**).

5. Conclusion

The global incidence rate for OC is expected to increase by 47% by 2040 [141]. Except for the emergence of PARP inhibitors in women with HRD HGSOC tumors, the conventional treatment protocol for other OC subtypes has remained the same since the 1980s, with no significant impact on survival rates. Screening for high-grade OCs remains a challenge. With the advances in the high throughput screening technologies, the focus is warranted to shift towards translational research to treat each OC subtype for their underlying genomic aberrations.

Author details

Febina Ravindran* and Bibha Choudhary
Institute of Bioinformatics and Applied Biotechnology, Bangalore, India

*Address all correspondence to: vibha@ibab.ac.in

References

[1] Swerdlow M. Mesothelioma of the pelvic peritoneum resembling papillary cystadenocarcinoma of the ovary; case report. Am J Obstet Gynecol 1959; 77: 197-200.

[2] Jacobs IJ, Menon U. Progress and challenges in screening for early detection of ovarian cancer. Mol Cell Proteomics 2004; 3: 355-366.

[3] Ferlay J, Colombet M, Soerjomataram I, et al. Estimating the global cancer incidence and mortality in 2018: GLOBOCAN sources and methods. Int J Cancer 2019; 144: 1941-1953.

[4] Shabir S, Gill PK. Global scenario on ovarian cancer – Its dynamics, relative survival, treatment, and epidemiology. AUJMSR 2020; 2: 17-25.

[5] Mohammadian M, Ghafari M, Khosravi B, et al. Variations in the Incidence and Mortality of Ovarian Cancer and Their Relationship with the Human Development Index in European Countries in 2012. Biomedical Research and Therapy 2017; 4: 1541.

[6] Torre LA, Trabert B, DeSantis CE, et al. Ovarian cancer statistics, 2018. CA Cancer J Clin 2018; 68: 284-296.

[7] Nielsen FC, van Overeem Hansen T, Sørensen CS. Hereditary breast and ovarian cancer: new genes in confined pathways. Nat Rev Cancer 2016; 16: 599-612.

[8] Nakamura K, Banno K, Yanokura M, et al. Features of ovarian cancer in Lynch syndrome (Review). Mol Clin Oncol 2014; 2: 909-916.

[9] Collaborative Group On Epidemiological Studies Of Ovarian Cancer, Beral V, Gaitskell K, et al. Menopausal hormone use and ovarian cancer risk: individual participant meta-analysis of 52 epidemiological studies. Lancet 2015; 385: 1835-1842.

[10] Trabert B, Wentzensen N, Yang HP, et al. Ovarian cancer and menopausal hormone therapy in the NIH-AARP diet and health study. Br J Cancer 2012; 107: 1181-1187.

[11] Pearce CL, Templeman C, Rossing MA, et al. Association between endometriosis and risk of histological subtypes of ovarian cancer: a pooled analysis of case-control studies. Lancet Oncol 2012; 13: 385-394.

[12] D Farhud D, Zokaei S, Keykhaei M, et al. Strong Evidences of the Ovarian Carcinoma Risk in Women after IVF Treatment: A Review Article. Iran J Public Health 2019; 48: 2124-2132.

[13] Practice Committee of the American Society for Reproductive Medicine. Electronic address: ASRM@asrm.org, Practice Committee of the American Society for Reproductive Medicine. Fertility drugs and cancer: a guideline. Fertil Steril 2016; 106: 1617-1626.

[14] Wentzensen N, Poole EM, Trabert B, et al. Ovarian Cancer Risk Factors by Histologic Subtype: An Analysis From the Ovarian Cancer Cohort Consortium. J Clin Oncol 2016; 34: 2888-2898.

[15] Lundberg FE, Iliadou AN, Rodriguez-Wallberg K, et al. The risk of breast and gynecological cancer in women with a diagnosis of infertility: A nationwide population-based study. Eur J Epidemiol 2019; 34: 499-507.

[16] McGuire V, Hartge P, Liao LM, et al. Parity and Oral Contraceptive Use in Relation to Ovarian Cancer Risk in Older Women. Cancer Epidemiol Biomarkers Prev 2016; 25: 1059-1063.

[17] Rice MS, Murphy MA, Tworoger SS. Tubal ligation, hysterectomy and ovarian cancer: A meta-analysis. J Ovarian Res 2012; 5: 1-16.

[18] Michels KA, Brinton LA, Pfeiffer RM, et al. Oral Contraceptive Use and Risks of Cancer in the NIH-AARP Diet and Health Study. Am J Epidemiol 2018; 187: 1630-1641.

[19] Fathalla MF. Incessant ovulation and ovarian cancer - a hypothesis re-visited. Facts Views Vis Obgyn 2013; 5: 292-297.

[20] Madsen C, Baandrup L, Dehlendorff C, et al. Tubal ligation and salpingectomy and the risk of epithelial ovarian cancer and borderline ovarian tumors: a nationwide case-control study. Acta Obstet Gynecol Scand 2015; 94: 86-94.

[21] Kadry Taher M, Farhat N, Karyakina NA, et al. Critical review of the association between perineal use of talc powder and risk of ovarian cancer. Reprod Toxicol 2019; 90: 88-101.

[22] Steffen JE, Tran T, Yimam M, et al. Serous Ovarian Cancer Caused by Exposure to Asbestos and Fibrous Talc in Cosmetic Talc Powders-A Case Series. J Occup Environ Med 2020; 62: e65–e77.

[23] Zhou Z, Zeng F, Yuan J, et al. Pelvic inflammatory disease and the risk of ovarian cancer: a meta-analysis. Cancer Causes Control 2017; 28: 415-428.

[24] Siegel RL, Miller KD, Jemal A. Cancer Statistics, 2017. CA Cancer J Clin 2017; 67: 7-30.

[25] Momenimovahed Z, Tiznobaik A, Taheri S, et al. Ovarian cancer in the world: epidemiology and risk factors. Int J Womens Health 2019; 11: 287-299.

[26] Jasen P. From the 'silent killer' to the 'whispering disease': ovarian cancer and the uses of metaphor. Med Hist 2009; 53: 489-512.

[27] Gajjar K, Ogden G, Mujahid MI, et al. Symptoms and risk factors of ovarian cancer: a survey in primary care. ISRN Obstet Gynecol 2012; 2012: 754197.

[28] Ebell MH, Culp MB, Radke TJ. A Systematic Review of Symptoms for the Diagnosis of Ovarian Cancer. Am J Prev Med 2016; 50: 384-394.

[29] Menon U, Karpinskyj C, Gentry-Maharaj A. Ovarian Cancer Prevention and Screening. Obstet Gynecol 2018; 131: 909-927.

[30] Dochez V, Caillon H, Vaucel E, et al. Biomarkers and algorithms for diagnosis of ovarian cancer: CA125, HE4, RMI and ROMA, a review. J Ovarian Res 2019; 12: 28.

[31] Shen Y, Zhao L, Lu S. Diagnostic performance of HE4 and ROMA among Chinese women. Clin Chim Acta 2020; 500: 42-46.

[32] Kadija S, Stefanovic A, Jeremic K, et al. The utility of human epididymal protein 4, cancer antigen 125, and risk for malignancy algorithm in ovarian cancer and endometriosis. Int J Gynecol Cancer 2012; 22: 238-244.

[33] Zhang L, Chen Y, Wang K. Comparison of CA125, HE4, and ROMA index for ovarian cancer diagnosis. Curr Probl Cancer 2019; 43: 135-144.

[34] Cui R, Wang Y, Li Y, et al. Clinical value of ROMA index in diagnosis of ovarian cancer: meta-analysis. Cancer Manag Res 2019; 11: 2545-2551.

[35] Shulman LP, Francis M, Bullock R, et al. Clinical Performance Comparison of Two In-Vitro Diagnostic Multivariate Index Assays (IVDMIAs) for Presurgical Assessment for Ovarian Cancer Risk. Adv Ther 2019; 36: 2402-2413.

[36] Wang Y, Li L, Douville C, et al. Evaluation of liquid from the Papanicolaou test and other

liquid biopsies for the detection of endometrial and ovarian cancers. Sci Transl Med; 10. Epub ahead of print 21 March 2018. DOI: 10.1126/scitranslmed.aap8793.

[37] Cohen JD, Li L, Wang Y, et al. Detection and localization of surgically resectable cancers with a multi-analyte blood test. Science 2018; 359: 926-930.

[38] Wild CP, Weiderpass E, Stewart BW, editors (2020). World Cancer Report: Cancer Research for Cancer Prevention. Lyon, France: International Agency for Research on Cancer. Available from: http://publications.iarc.fr/586. Licence: CC BY-NC-ND 3.0 IGO.

[39] Chen X, Wu Y, Dong H, et al. Platinum-based agents for individualized cancer treatment. Curr Mol Med 2013; 13: 1603-1612.

[40] Targeted therapy of ovarian cancer including immune check point inhibitor. Korean J Intern Med. DOI: 10.3904/kjim.2017.008.

[41] Corrado G, Salutari V, Palluzzi E, et al. Optimizing treatment in recurrent epithelial ovarian cancer. Expert Rev Anticancer Ther 2017; 17: 1147-1158.

[42] Monk BJ, Coleman RL. Changing the paradigm in the treatment of platinum-sensitive recurrent ovarian cancer: from platinum doublets to nonplatinum doublets and adding antiangiogenesis compounds. Int J Gynecol Cancer 2009; 19 Suppl 2: S63–S67.

[43] Motohara T, Masuda K, Morotti M, et al. An evolving story of the metastatic voyage of ovarian cancer cells: cellular and molecular orchestration of the adipose-rich metastatic microenvironment. Oncogene 2018; 38: 2885-2898.

[44] Mitra AK. Ovarian Cancer Metastasis: A Unique Mechanism of Dissemination. Tumor Metastasis. Epub ahead of print 2016. DOI: 10.5772/64700.

[45] Temkin SM, Bergstrom J, Samimi G, et al. Ovarian Cancer Prevention in High-risk Women. Clin Obstet Gynecol 2017; 60: 738-757.

[46] Grimbizis GF, Tarlatzis BC. The use of hormonal contraception and its protective role against endometrial and ovarian cancer. Best Pract Res Clin Obstet Gynaecol 2010; 24: 29-38.

[47] WebPathology, https://www.webpathology.com/contact.asp (accessed 6 December 2020).

[48] Lheureux S, Gourley C, Vergote I, et al. Epithelial ovarian cancer. Lancet 2019; 393: 1240-1253.

[49] Karst AM, Levanon K, Drapkin R. Modeling high-grade serous ovarian carcinogenesis from the fallopian tube. Proc Natl Acad Sci U S A 2011; 108: 7547-7552.

[50] George SHL, Garcia R, Slomovitz BM. Ovarian Cancer: The Fallopian Tube as the Site of Origin and Opportunities for Prevention. Front Oncol 2016; 6: 108.

[51] Zhang Q, Bykov VJN, Wiman KG, et al. APR-246 reactivates mutant p53 by targeting cysteines 124 and 277. Cell Death Dis 2018; 9: 439.

[52] Moufarrij S, Dandapani M, Arthofer E, et al. Epigenetic therapy for ovarian cancer: promise and progress. Clin Epigenetics 2019; 11: 7.

[53] Zanjirband M, Gentles L, Curtin NJ, et al. 55P Evaluation of MDM2-p53 antagonists, nutlin-3 and RG7388, combined with the PARPi rucaparib in primary cultures of ovarian cancer. Annals of Oncology 2020; 31: S1234.

[54] Frey MK, Pothuri B. Homologous recombination deficiency (HRD) testing

in ovarian cancer clinical practice: a review of the literature. Gynecol Oncol Res Pract 2017; 4: 4.

[55] Network TCGAR, The Cancer Genome Atlas Research Network. Integrated genomic analyses of ovarian carcinoma. Nature 2011; 474: 609-615.

[56] Konstantinopoulos PA, Ceccaldi R, Shapiro GI, et al. Homologous Recombination Deficiency: Exploiting the Fundamental Vulnerability of Ovarian Cancer. Cancer Discov 2015; 5: 1137-1154.

[57] Gadducci A, Guarneri V, Peccatori FA, et al. Current strategies for the targeted treatment of high-grade serous epithelial ovarian cancer and relevance of BRCA mutational status. J Ovarian Res 2019; 12: 1-8.

[58] Dziadkowiec KN, Gąsiorowska E, Nowak-Markwitz E, et al. PARP inhibitors: review of mechanisms of action and BRCA1/2 mutation targeting. Prz Menopauzalny 2016; 15: 215-219.

[59] Kaufman B, Shapira-Frommer R, Schmutzler RK, et al. Olaparib monotherapy in patients with advanced cancer and a germline BRCA1/2 mutation. J Clin Oncol 2015; 33: 244-250.

[60] Banerjee SN, Lord CJ. First-line PARP inhibition in ovarian cancer — standard of care for all? Nature Reviews Clinical Oncology 2020; 17: 136-137.

[61] Ethier J-L, Lheureux S, Oza AM. The role of niraparib for the treatment of ovarian cancer. Future Oncology 2018; 14: 2565-2577.

[62] Iyengar M, O'Hayer P, Cole A, et al. CDK4/6 inhibition as maintenance and combination therapy for high grade serous ovarian cancer. Oncotarget 2018; 9: 15658-15672.

[63] Lisio M-A, Fu L, Goyeneche A, et al. High-Grade Serous Ovarian Cancer: Basic Sciences, Clinical and Therapeutic Standpoints. Int J Mol Sci; 20. Epub ahead of print 22 February 2019. DOI: 10.3390/ijms20040952.

[64] Pfisterer J, Shannon CM, Baumann K, et al. Bevacizumab and platinum-based combinations for recurrent ovarian cancer: a randomised, open-label, phase 3 trial. Lancet Oncol 2020; 21: 699-709.

[65] Gadducci A, Cosio S. Therapeutic Approach to Low-Grade Serous Ovarian Carcinoma: State of Art and Perspectives of Clinical Research. Cancers; 12. Epub ahead of print 23 May 2020. DOI: 10.3390/cancers12051336.

[66] Grisham RN, Iyer G. Low-Grade Serous Ovarian Cancer: Current Treatment Paradigms and Future Directions. Curr Treat Options Oncol 2018; 19: 496.

[67] Kaldawy A, Segev Y, Lavie O, et al. Low-grade serous ovarian cancer: A review. Gynecol Oncol 2016; 143: 433-438.

[68] Hunter SM, Anglesio MS, Ryland GL, et al. Molecular profiling of low grade serous ovarian tumours identifies novel candidate driver genes. Oncotarget 2015; 6: 37663-37677.

[69] Mert I, Chhina J, Allo G, et al. Synergistic effect of MEK inhibitor and metformin combination in low grade serous ovarian cancer. Gynecologic Oncology 2017; 146: 319-326.

[70] Gershenson DM, Bodurka DC, Coleman RL, et al. Hormonal Maintenance Therapy for Women With Low-Grade Serous Cancer of the Ovary or Peritoneum. Journal of Clinical Oncology 2017; 35: 1103-1111.

[71] Nasioudis D, Latif NA, Simpkins F, et al. Adjuvant chemotherapy for early

stage endometrioid ovarian carcinoma: An analysis of the National Cancer Data Base. Gynecol Oncol 2020; 156: 315-319.

[72] Terada T. Endometrioid adenocarcinoma of the ovary arising in atypical endometriosis. Int J Clin Exp Pathol 2012; 5: 924-927.

[73] Helder-Woolderink JM, Blok EA, Vasen HFA, et al. Ovarian cancer in Lynch syndrome; a systematic review. Eur J Cancer 2016; 55: 65-73.

[74] Fukumoto T, Park PH, Wu S, et al. Repurposing Pan-HDAC Inhibitors for ARID1A-Mutated Ovarian Cancer. Cell Rep 2018; 22: 3393-3400.

[75] Kim S, Jeong S. Mutation Hotspots in the β-Catenin Gene: Lessons from the Human Cancer Genome Databases. Mol Cells 2019; 42: 8-16.

[76] Elsherif S, Javadi S, Viswanathan C, et al. Low-grade epithelial ovarian cancer: what a radiologist should know. Br J Radiol 2019; 92: 20180571.

[77] Papa, Papa, Pandolfi. The PTEN–PI3K Axis in Cancer. Biomolecules 2019; 9: 153.

[78] Lynch HT, Casey MJ, Snyder CL, et al. Hereditary ovarian carcinoma: heterogeneity, molecular genetics, pathology, and management. Mol Oncol 2009; 3: 97-137.

[79] Babaier A, Ghatage P. Mucinous Cancer of the Ovary: Overview and Current Status. Diagnostics 2020; 10: 52.

[80] Gorringe KL, Cheasley D, Wakefield MJ, et al. Therapeutic options for mucinous ovarian carcinoma. Gynecol Oncol 2020; 156: 552-560.

[81] Kelemen LE, Köbel M. Mucinous carcinomas of the ovary and colorectum: different organ, same dilemma. The Lancet Oncology 2011; 12: 1071-1080.

[82] Sato S, Itamochi H, Kigawa J, et al. Combination chemotherapy of oxaliplatin and 5-fluorouracil may be an effective regimen for mucinous adenocarcinoma of the ovary: a potential treatment strategy. Cancer Sci 2009; 100: 546-551.

[83] Liu H, Xu Y, Ji J, et al. Prognosis of ovarian clear cell cancer compared with other epithelial cancer types: A population-based analysis. Oncology Letters. Epub ahead of print 2020. DOI: 10.3892/ol.2020.11252.

[84] Fujiwara K, Shintani D, Nishikawa T. Clear-cell carcinoma of the ovary. Ann Oncol 2016; 27 Suppl 1: i50–i52.

[85] Iida Y, Okamoto A, Hollis RL, et al. Clear cell carcinoma of the ovary: a clinical and molecular perspective. Int J Gynecol Cancer. Epub ahead of print 18 September 2020. DOI: 10.1136/ijgc-2020-001656.

[86] Huang H-N, Lin M-C, Huang W-C, et al. Loss of ARID1A expression and its relationship with PI3K-Akt pathway alterations and ZNF217 amplification in ovarian clear cell carcinoma. Mod Pathol 2014; 27: 983-990.

[87] Matsuzaki S, Yoshino K, Ueda Y, et al. Potential targets for ovarian clear cell carcinoma: a review of updates and future perspectives. Cancer Cell Int 2015; 15: 117.

[88] Takano M, Tsuda H, Sugiyama T. Clear cell carcinoma of the ovary: Is there a role of histology-specific treatment? Journal of Experimental & Clinical Cancer Research; 31. Epub ahead of print 2012. DOI: 10.1186/1756-9966-31-53.

[89] Bitler BG, Aird KM, Garipov A, et al. Synthetic lethality by targeting EZH2 methyltransferase activity in

ARID1A-mutated cancers. Nat Med 2015; 21: 231-238.

[90] Littlepage LE, Adler AS, Kouros-Mehr H, et al. The transcription factor ZNF217 is a prognostic biomarker and therapeutic target during breast cancer progression. Cancer Discov 2012; 2: 638-651.

[91] Fuller PJ, Leung D, Chu S. Genetics and genomics of ovarian sex cord-stromal tumors. Clin Genet 2017; 91: 285-291.

[92] Horta M, Cunha TM. Sex cord-stromal tumors of the ovary: a comprehensive review and update for radiologists. Diagn Interv Radiol 2015; 21: 277-286.

[93] Khosla D, Dimri K, Pandey AK, et al. Ovarian granulosa cell tumor: clinical features, treatment, outcome, and prognostic factors. N Am J Med Sci 2014; 6: 133-138.

[94] Hodeib M, Tsui I, Sinno A, et al. Adult Granulosa Cell Tumor of the Ovary: Initial Evaluation and Current Treatment Paradigm. Journal of Cancer Science and Clinical Therapeutics 2018; 01: 6-18.

[95] Kottarathil VD, Antony MA, Nair IR, et al. Recent advances in granulosa cell tumor ovary: a review. Indian J Surg Oncol 2013; 4: 37-47.

[96] Robertson DM, Pruysers E, Jobling T. Inhibin as a diagnostic marker for ovarian cancer. Cancer Letters 2007; 249: 14-17.

[97] Colak S, ten Dijke P. Targeting TGF-β Signaling in Cancer. Trends in Cancer 2017; 3: 56-71.

[98] Alexiadis M, Rowley SM, Chu S, et al. Mutational Landscape of Ovarian Adult Granulosa Cell Tumors from Whole Exome and Targeted TERT Promoter Sequencing. Molecular Cancer Research 2019; 17: 177-185.

[99] Caburet S, Anttonen M, Todeschini A-L, et al. Combined comparative genomic hybridization and transcriptomic analyses of ovarian granulosa cell tumors point to novel candidate driver genes. BMC Cancer 2015; 15: 1-11.

[100] Auguste A, Bessière L, Todeschini A-L, et al. Molecular analyses of juvenile granulosa cell tumors bearing AKT1 mutations provide insights into tumor biology and therapeutic leads. Hum Mol Genet 2015; 24: 6687-6698.

[101] Kalfa N, Ecochard A, Patte C, et al. Activating mutations of the stimulatory g protein in juvenile ovarian granulosa cell tumors: a new prognostic factor? J Clin Endocrinol Metab 2006; 91: 1842-1847.

[102] Li J, Bao R, Peng S, et al. The molecular mechanism of ovarian granulosa cell tumors. J Ovarian Res 2018; 11: 1-8.

[103] Shah SP, Köbel M, Senz J, et al. Mutation of FOXL2 in granulosa-cell tumors of the ovary. N Engl J Med 2009; 360: 2719-2729.

[104] Abu-Zaid A, Azzam A, Alghuneim LA, et al. Poorly Differentiated Ovarian Sertoli-Leydig Cell Tumor in a 16-Year-Old Single Woman: A Case Report and Literature Review. Case Reports in Obstetrics and Gynecology 2013; 2013: 1-6.

[105] de Kock L, Terzic T, McCluggage WG, et al. DICER1 Mutations Are Consistently Present in Moderately and Poorly Differentiated Sertoli-Leydig Cell Tumors. Am J Surg Pathol 2017; 41: 1178-1187.

[106] Bonilla L, Oza AM. Targeting TGFβ Pathway in Adult Granulosa Cell

Tumor: Opening Pandora's Box? Clinical Cancer Research 2019; 25: 5432-5434.

[107] Yang AD, Curtin J, Muggia F. Ovarian adult-type granulosa cell tumor: focusing on endocrine-based therapies. International Journal of Endocrine Oncology 2018; 5: IJE08.

[108] Bell RJA, Rube HT, Xavier-Magalhaes A, et al. Understanding TERT Promoter Mutations: A Common Path to Immortality. Molecular Cancer Research 2016; 14: 315-323.

[109] Brown J, Friedlander M, Backes FJ, et al. Gynecologic Cancer Intergroup (GCIG) consensus review for ovarian germ cell tumors. Int J Gynecol Cancer 2014; 24: S48–S54.

[110] Smith HO, Berwick M, Verschraegen CF, et al. Incidence and survival rates for female malignant germ cell tumors. Obstet Gynecol 2006; 107: 1075-1085.

[111] Iavazzo C, Vorgias G, Iavazzo PE, et al. Is fertility sparing surgery a treatment option for premenopausal patients with dysgerminoma? Bratisl Lek Listy 2016; 117: 738-740.

[112] Van Nieuwenhuysen E, Busschaert P, Neven P, et al. The genetic landscape of 87 ovarian germ cell tumors. Gynecol Oncol 2018; 151: 61-68.

[113] Shaaban AM, Rezvani M, Elsayes KM, et al. Ovarian malignant germ cell tumors: cellular classification and clinical and imaging features. Radiographics 2014; 34: 777-801.

[114] Lee Y-L, Lai C-R, Yen M-S. Recurrent ovarian mixed germ cell tumor with unusual malignant transformation: a case report. J Ovarian Res 2019; 12: 1-6.

[115] Kota S, Pani J, Meher L, et al. Dysgerminoma in a female with turner syndrome and Y chromosome material: A case-based review of literature. Indian Journal of Endocrinology and Metabolism 2012; 16: 436.

[116] Maoz A, Matsuo K, Ciccone MA, et al. Molecular Pathways and Targeted Therapies for Malignant Ovarian Germ Cell Tumors and Sex Cord–Stromal Tumors: A Contemporary Review. Cancers 2020; 12: 1398.

[117] Cardoso HJ, Figueira MI, Socorro S. The stem cell factor (SCF)/c-KIT signalling in testis and prostate cancer. J Cell Commun Signal 2017; 11: 297-307.

[118] Guo Y, Pan W, Liu S, et al. ERK/MAPK signalling pathway and tumorigenesis (Review). Experimental and Therapeutic Medicine. Epub ahead of print 2020. DOI: 10.3892/etm.2020.8454.

[119] Maoz A, Ciccone MA, Matsuzaki S, et al. Emerging serine-threonine kinase inhibitors for treating ovarian cancer. Expert Opin Emerg Drugs 2019; 24: 239-253.

[120] Oneda E, Zorzi F, Gorio A, et al. Differential Diagnosis of Small Cell Carcinoma of the Ovary or Ovarian Metastases of Small Cell Carcinoma of the Lung: A Case Report and Review of the Literature. Case Rep Oncol 2020; 13: 822-828.

[121] Auguste A, Blanc-Durand F, Deloger M, et al. Small Cell Carcinoma of the Ovary, Hypercalcemic Type (SCCOHT) beyond Mutations: A Comprehensive Genomic Analysis. Cells; 9. Epub ahead of print 19 June 2020. DOI: 10.3390/cells9061496.

[122] Bailey S, Murray MJ, Witkowski L, et al. Biallelic somatic SMARCA4 mutations in small cell carcinoma of the ovary, hypercalcemic type (SCCOHT). Pediatr Blood Cancer 2015; 62: 728-730.

[123] Lu B, Shi H. An In-Depth Look at Small Cell Carcinoma of the Ovary, Hypercalcemic Type (SCCOHT): Clinical Implications from Recent Molecular Findings. J Cancer 2019; 10: 223-237.

[124] Wang Y, Chen SY, Karnezis AN, et al. The histone methyltransferase EZH2 is a therapeutic target in small cell carcinoma of the ovary, hypercalcaemic type. J Pathol 2017; 242: 371-383.

[125] Chan-Penebre E, Armstrong K, Drew A, et al. Selective Killing of SMARCA2- and SMARCA4-deficient Small Cell Carcinoma of the Ovary, Hypercalcemic Type Cells by Inhibition of EZH2: and Preclinical Models. Mol Cancer Ther 2017; 16: 850-860.

[126] Gamwell LF, Gambaro K, Merziotis M, et al. Small cell ovarian carcinoma: genomic stability and responsiveness to therapeutics. Orphanet J Rare Dis 2013; 8: 33.

[127] Tischkowitz M, Huang S, Banerjee S, et al. Small-Cell Carcinoma of the Ovary, Hypercalcemic Type–Genetics, New Treatment Targets, and Current Management Guidelines. Clinical Cancer Research 2020; 26: 3908-3917.

[128] Banerjee S, Gonzalez-Martin A, Harter P, et al. First-line PARP inhibitors in ovarian cancer: summary of an ESMO Open - Cancer Horizons round-table discussion. ESMO Open 2020; 5: e001110.

[129] Ray-Coquard I, Pautier P, Pignata S, et al. Olaparib plus Bevacizumab as First-Line Maintenance in Ovarian Cancer. N Engl J Med 2019; 381: 2416-2428.

[130] Tan FH, Putoczki TL, Stylli SS, et al. Ponatinib: a novel multi-tyrosine kinase inhibitor against human malignancies. Onco Targets Ther 2019; 12: 635-645.

[131] Lang JD, Hendricks WPD, Orlando KA, et al. Ponatinib Shows Potent Antitumor Activity in Small Cell Carcinoma of the Ovary Hypercalcemic Type (SCCOHT) through Multikinase Inhibition. Clin Cancer Res 2018; 24: 1932-1943.

[132] Xue Y, Meehan B, Macdonald E, et al. CDK4/6 inhibitors target SMARCA4-determined cyclin D1 deficiency in hypercalcemic small cell carcinoma of the ovary. Nat Commun 2019; 10: 558.

[133] Lee EK, Esselen KM, Kolin DL, et al. Combined CDK4/6 and PD-1 Inhibition in Refractory SMARCA4-Deficient Small-Cell Carcinoma of the Ovary, Hypercalcemic Type. JCO Precis Oncol 2020; 4: 736-742.

[134] Jelinic P, Ricca J, Van Oudenhove E, et al. Immune-Active Microenvironment in Small Cell Carcinoma of the Ovary, Hypercalcemic Type: Rationale for Immune Checkpoint Blockade. J Natl Cancer Inst 2018; 110: 787-790.

[135] Mottamal M, Zheng S, Huang TL, et al. Histone deacetylase inhibitors in clinical studies as templates for new anticancer agents. Molecules 2015; 20: 3898-3941.

[136] Gandellini P, Giovannetti E, Nicassio F. MicroRNAs in Cancer Management: Big Challenges for Small Molecules. BioMed Research International 2015; 2015: 1-2.

[137] Alshamrani AA. Roles of microRNAs in Ovarian Cancer Tumorigenesis: Two Decades Later, What Have We Learned? Front Oncol 2020; 10: 1084.

[138] Chen S-N, Chang R, Lin L-T, et al. MicroRNA in Ovarian Cancer: Biology, Pathogenesis, and Therapeutic Opportunities. Int J Environ Res Public Health; 16. Epub ahead of print 29 April 2019. DOI: 10.3390/ijerph16091510.

[139] Kraggerud SM, Hoei-Hansen CE, Alagaratnam S, et al. Molecular characteristics of malignant ovarian germ cell tumors and comparison with testicular counterparts: implications for pathogenesis. Endocr Rev 2013; 34: 339-376.

[140] Chang RK, Li X, Mu N, et al. MicroRNA expression profiles in non-epithelial ovarian tumors. Int J Oncol 2018; 52: 55-66.

[141] Ferlay J, Ervik M, Lam F, Colombet M, Mery L, Piñeros M, Znaor A, Soerjomataram I, Bray F (2018). Global Cancer Observatory: Cancer Tomorrow. Lyon, France: International Agency for Research on Cancer. Available from: https://gco.iarc.fr/tomorrow, accessed [01 Dec 2020].

Chapter 2

Ovarian Cancer Genetics and the Implications

Shyamika Mirisse Acharige and Chit Cheng Yeoh

Abstract

Ovarian cancers mostly arise sporadically, however about 20–25% of the cases arise as a part of hereditary syndromes. There are numerous mutations involved in the ovarian cancer development and more to be discovered. Knowing the pathogenic variants of the mutations present in the ovarian cancers are important in developing and practising of risk reduction strategies in asymptomatic carriers, genetic counselling, prognostication and decision on treatment. This chapter will focus on the various types of mutations found in ovarian cancers and their implications- when considering testing, treatment options and insight for the next level of Improvement in cancer care.

Keywords: ovarian cancer, somatic BRCA mutation, germline BRCA mutations, PARP inhibitors, homologous recombination

1. Introduction

BRCA1/2 somatic and germline, *PTEN* deletion, *CCNE* amplification and *RB1/NF1* loss, *RAD51C, RAD51D, BRIP 1* are some of the known mutations causing the ovarian cancers [1]; the *BRCA1/2* gene mutations are the most common and deleterious to find in this spectrum. From women who inherit a pathogenic *BRCA1* variant and *BRCA2* variant at risk of developing ovarian cancer 39–44% and 11–17% respectively by the age of 70–80 years [2, 3].

The current recommended guidelines for all high grade serous ovarian cancer patients at the diagnosis, apart from mucinous adenocarcinoma of Ovaries, are screen upfront for pathogenic *BRCA1/2* genes, regardless whether they have family history or not. The uptake of this screen is 1:10 patient, and if we extend the screening to tumour somatic testing, the uptake becomes 17% of all ovarian cancer diagnosis with germline and somatic BRCA mutations. Difference between the somatic and the germline BRCA mutations are discussed later in this chapter.

The following is a schematic representation of the various known mutation prevalence in the ovarian Cancers particularly in High grade serous ovarian carcinoma. As obvious *BRCA1* and *BRCA2* are the most common type of mutations found in the OC and signifies the importance, hence this chapter mainly focus on the BRCA mutations (**Figure 1**).

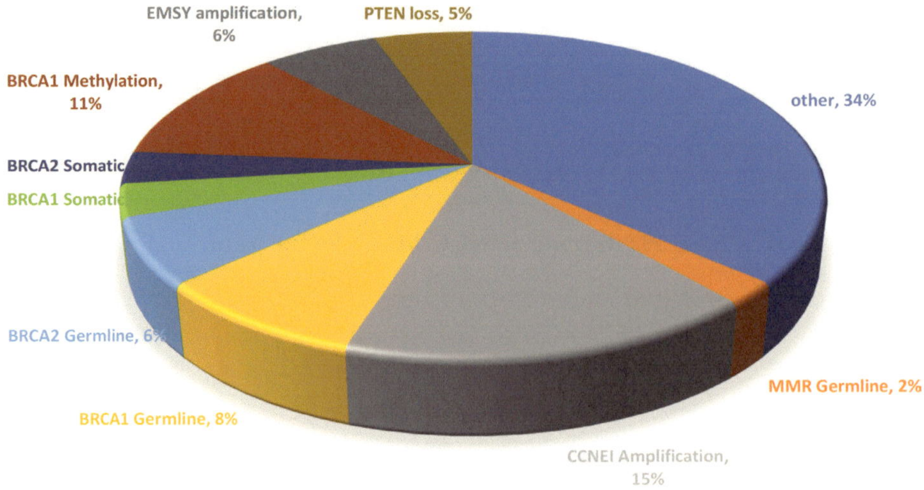

Figure 1.
Common Pathogenic mutations in high grade serous ovarian cancer.

2. Genetics of sporadic ovarian cancers

There's a multitude of genetics involved in the sporadic ovarian cancers, involving multiple cellular pathways. There are 2 types of sporadic ovarian cancers according to their behaviour, histology, genetic according to Kurman and shih's original article "The origin and pathogenesis of epithelial ovarian cancer: a proposed unifying theory", type 1 and type 2 [4]. Type1 tumours are slow growing, indolent tumours and Type 2 being high grade, aggressive.

Some of the mutations associated with sporadic type1 ovarian cancers are *KRAS*, *BRAF*, *ERBB2*, *PIK3CA*, *ARID1A*, *CTNNB1* and *PTEN*. In normal cells these genes and their products will regulate the cell growth, chromatin remodelling, DNA repair, cellular proliferation and controlling of apoptosis preventing tumour development. Mutations in these genes inevitably causes increases susceptibility to development of malignancies [4].

Type 2 sporadic ovarian cancers which are high grade share the similar genetics as hereditary ovarian cancers *TP53, BRCA1 and BRCA2* [4].

3. Genetics of hereditary OC

Hereditary Breast ovarian cancer syndrome, Lynch Syndrome, Li-Fraumani, Cowden and Peutz-jeghers syndrome are some of the few of Hereditary ovarian cancer syndromes, all of which inherit in autosomal dominant pattern [5, 6]. Patients who presents at young age, multiple primaries and/or a high incidence of family history of malignancy should be considered as having hereditary OC and should be investigated for the genetic mutations. Eighty percent [80%] of this type of ovarian cancers are associated with BRCA1/2 gene mutation and minority are with *RAD51C*, *RAD51D*, *BRIP1, PALB2*, *BARD1*, *NBN* and *MRE11A*.

4. *BRCA1/2* gene structure and functions

BRCA1 and *BRCA2* genes were discovered in early nineties following extensive research on breast cancer patients and families, hence the name Breast cancer susceptibility gene [BRCA] and identified as responsible in the ovarian cancer causation as well. *BRCA1* and *BRCA2* pathogenic mutations are found in 10–15% of sporadic ovarian cancers and about 40% of Hereditary ovarian cancers [7].

These genes are tumour suppressor genes encode for tumour suppressor proteins, which will help in maintaining genomic stability. *BRCA1* and *BRCA2* are large genes contain about 100–70 Kilo bases respectively. *BRCA1* situated in long arm of chromosome 17 at 17q21 position and *BRCA2* gene is in chromosome 13 at 13q12.These 2 genes encode for different protein structures although still have got functional similarities [8]. *BRCA1* protein consists of nuclear localization sequence (NLS) and three functional domains; RING, coiled coil, and BRCT domains, whereas *BRCA2* protein has NLS, eight BRC repeats, and a DNA binding domain.

BRCA1 and *BRCA2* genes helps in repairing the double strand breakage in DNA by promoting the homologous recombination, which is a highly accurate process in the maintenance of genomic stability and regulating the cell cycle and apoptosis.

5. Action of *BRCA1* and *BRCA2* proteins in DNA double strand damage repair

Although the action of the *BRCA1* and *BRCA2* gene products in cancer causation is not fully discovered [9], their function in maintaining the genomic stability is well understood. This involves the DNA double strand break repair [DSB] which is the most deleterious type of DNA damage as no healthy DNA strand left for the repair mechanism [10]. The DSB will be repaired by 2 mechanisms in the healthy eukaryotic cells -The Homologous directed repair [HDR] pathway, which is a highly accurate system and Non-Homologous end joining [NHEJ] pathway which is prone to errors. BRCA1 and BRCA2 proteins involve in the HDR mechanism following stimulated by the cellular DNA damage response. This function is facilitated by other cellular proteins including RAD51 [11, 12], Ataxia-Telangiectasia kinase [ATM-kinase].

The following flow chart shows the mechanism of DNA DSB repair and the steps involving the BRCA1/2 proteins (**Figure 2**).

Mutation of the *BRCA1/2* genes causing loss of the encoded protein functions causes abnormal checkpoint stimulation and genomic errors in DNA repair

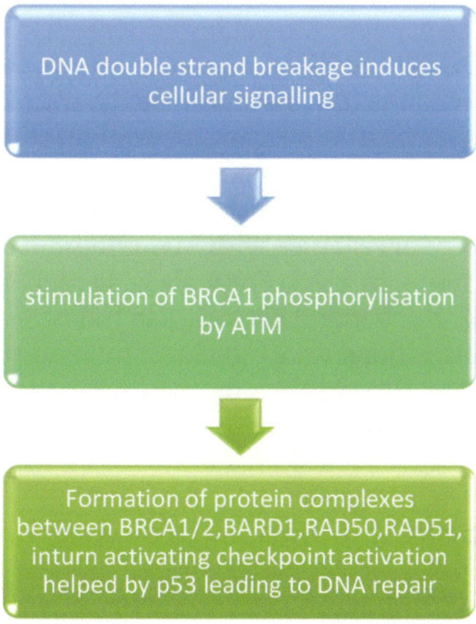

Figure 2.
Action of BRCA1/2 protein in DNA double strand break repair. Source - functions of BRCA1 *and* BRCA2 *in the biological response to DNA damage [13].*

causing cancer development through uncontrolled cellular proliferation, impaired cell apoptosis in abnormal cells.

6. Somatic vs. germline *BRCA* mutations

BRCA1/2 mutations can occur in the germline causing the hereditary susceptibility to ovarian and other types of cancers. There are *BRCA* mutations can occur in the somatic cells as well -within the tumour itself which consists of 3% of whole *BRCA* mutation found in the high grade serous ovarian cancers, without mutation in the germline. Presence of germline *BRCA* mutation gives rise to specific behaviour of the ovarian cancer, response to treatment and the prognosis. Patients with germline *BRCA* mutations will develop cancers at young age, commonly have visceral disease at presentation and shows high sensitivity to platinum-based chemotherapy and PARP inhibitors.

Clear relationship between the somatic *BRCA* mutations and the features of the response to the treatment and the clinical features are yet to be identified [14].

7. Implications of *BRCA* testing in ovarian cancer

Currently there's no proven benefit of population screening for sporadic ovarian cancer as the trial results are still pending to show reduction in the mortality and survival benefit from the early screening of asymptomatic patients in this category. However screening strategies in hereditary ovarian cancers are important for the prophylactic procedures such as bilateral Salpingo-oophorectomy which can reduce the risk of development of cancer by 79% in endometrium, fallopian tube, ovaries which has been proven by meta-analysis.

8. Testing for germline *BRCA* mutations in ovarian cancer patients

Genetic testing for germline-*BRCA1/BRCA2* mutations in epithelial ovarian cancer (EOC) was commissioned by National Health Service England in 2015 [15]. In the United Kingdom, all genetic counselling take place in Cancer Centres, and all first degree family member will be given a letter to inform them of the risk in them carrying this gene and a mean to have germline BRCA status tested on the NHS. The NHS will also provide risk reduction surgery to prophylactic Breast and Ovarian surgery once the family planning is completed and the decision made by affected family members. For those who do not wish to embark on these prophylactic surgeries, there are guidelines for surveillance with Mammograms and blood test Ca 125 for the affected gene mutation carriers. For male gene carriers, there are now early PSA surveillance available for General physician to follow.

Germline BRCA testing is done via a blood test following gaining the consent of the patient, according to the NCCP [National cancer control programme] guidelines, which is then being sent to the Cancer Molecular Diagnostics Laboratory.

9. Testing for somatic *BRCA* mutations in ovarian cancer patients

Testing for somatic *BRCA* mutation was introduced in October 2020 in UK. The samples from the previous biopsy or surgery including the ovarian cancer tissue block/slides are needed for somatic *BRCA* mutation testing. The block must be of reasonable quality, neoplastic cell content >50% included. This should be sent at room temperature with a copy of the block(s) histopathology report within 5 working days of patient registration.

Although the germline *BRCA* testing could be a straightforward blood test, the somatic BRCA mutation comes with some challenges, which are summarised below.

1. Issues with extracting high quality DNA samples from the preserved tumour samples-which needs tumour microdissection, so that a small tumour samples will not be enough for the purpose. Also poor fixation samples can cause fragmented and damaged DNA and also formalin used in fixation can cause deamination of the nucleic acids leading to sequencing errors and false mutations.

2. Analysis and interpretation of sequencing data as there is currently no standardised interpretation.

3. The stability of the somatic *BRCA* mutations can change over time due to cancer selection, resistance, treatment and within the tumour itself due to heterogeneity of the tumour cells.

For most countries the method for detecting the *BRCA* mutation still limited to one or the other due to funding issues.

10. The significance of *BRCA* mutation in HGSOC

As mentioned earlier in the chapter being positive for *BRCA* mutations when compared with the wild type, gives the ovarian cancer specific features – importantly higher response rate to platinum and other types of non-platinum chemotherapeutic agents [16] and more importantly high sensitivity to Poly(ADP-ribose) polymerase (PARP) inhibitors, which is highly important as a maintenance therapy of the patients who have responded to first line platinum based chemotherapy in improving 5 year disease free survival.

11. What are PARP inhibitors?

Poly (ADP-ribose) polymerase (*PARP*) is a protein mediated the DNA double strand break repair, which was first identified in early sixties and first PARP inhibitor was discovered in 1980 as a chemotherapy sensitizer [17].

Following figure illustrates the normal action of the PARP proteins to aid the understanding of how the PARP inhibitors work (**Figure 3**).

In 2005 and 2006, inhibiting PARP enzymes was first observed to be highly effective against cancers with homologous recombination deficiencies [19], are being utilised in the clinical setting to manage recurrent ovarian cancers. However, PARPi – Niraparib also show significant clinical benefit in patients without HR deficiencies [20]. There are currently three FDA-approved PARP inhibitors for recurrent ovarian cancer – Olaparib, Rucaparib and Niraparib.

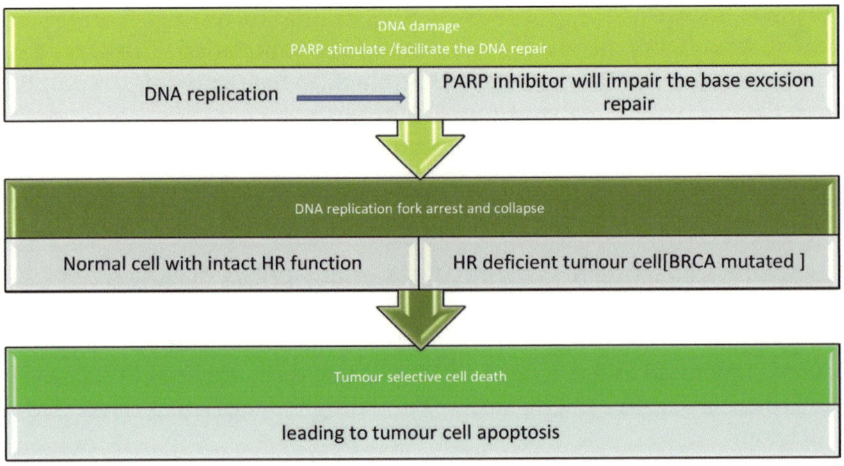

Figure 3.
Function of PARP proteins in DNA damage repair. Source: An update on PARP inhibitors—Moving to the adjuvant setting [18].

12. PARP inhibitors in the treatment of ovarian cancers

Since the discovery in 1980 s PARP inhibitors has gone through extensive scrutiny and research in the efficiency in management of the ovarian cancers.

The initial monotherapy with *PARP* inhibitors for patients with solid tumours with a germline *BRCA* mutation were published in 2009. This was a study on ovarian cancer patients with known *BRCA* mutation [21]. Other tumours included were breast, colon, melanoma, prostate, and sarcomas. In patients with known *BRCA1/2* mutations, single-agent treatment with Olaparib showed a 63% clinical benefit (including disease stabilisation).

Following this study there several other trials carried out for assessing the individual efficacy of the Olaparib, Niraparib and Rucaparib and with the outcomes of these trials Olaparib has gained the FDA approval as a first line maintenance treatment in the advanced ovarian cancer [22].

Trial name	PARPi assessed vs. other treatment agent as maintenance	Population
PRIMA/ ENGOT-OV26	Niraparib vs. Placebo	Stage III with visible residual tumour after PDS, inoperable stage III, or any stage IV ovarian cancer.
SOLO-1	Olaparib vs. Placebo	*BRCA1/2* mutated, CR or PR (≥30% decrease in tumour volume, or NED on imaging but CA-125 > ULN) to platinum-based chemotherapy (without bevacizumab)
] PAOLA-1/ ENGOT-OV25	Olaparib + bevacizumab vs. placebo + bevacizumab	Newly diagnosed stage III/IV high-grade ovarian cancer or other non-mucinous ovarian cancers with BRCA1/2 mutation, regardless of surgical outcome NED or CR or PR after first-line platinum + taxane + bevacizumab
VELIA/ GOG-3005	Veliparib + CP → veliparib vs. veliparib + CP → placebo a vs. placebo + CP → placebo	Newly diagnosed stage III/IV high-grade serous ovarian cancer in patients undergoing PDS or IDS

Key PDS - Primary debulking surgery, CR - complete response, PR - Partial response, IDS - interval debulking surgery, NED - no evidence of disease, C - Carboplatin, P - Paclitaxel.

The following is a summary of the trials on PARP inhibitors and the SOLO-1 trial being of the pivotal trials in the history of the use of PARP inhibitors [23].

13. Current UK standards for testing ovarian cancer genetics

According to current British Gynaecological Cancer Society guidelines for testing ovarian cancer genetics,

Women with High grade serous ovarian cancer or G3 endometrioid ovarian adenocarcinoma have >10% risk of an underlying BRCA mutation should be offered clinical genetics counselling and testing. (GRADE C) Recently it has been shown that ~18% (much higher in certain groups such as Ashkenazi Jews) of the population of women presenting with high grade serous or G3 endometrioid ovarian adenocarcinoma carry a germline BRCA mutation, 44% of whom have no positive family history. Every patient with a current or past histological diagnosis of HGSC or G3 endometrioid ovarian carcinoma therefore qualifies for BRCA counselling and testing, as advised by National institute for Health and Care Excellence, which should be discussed and offered.

The above guidelines and standards are supported by the evidence from the GTEOC (Genetic Testing in Epithelial Ovarian Cancer) [24] study in which the primary objective of the study was to determine the feasibility, acceptability and cost-effectiveness of screening all newly diagnosed women with EOC for *BRCA1/BRCA2* mutations by determining the mutation prevalence, calculating the cost for each gene mutation detected and assessing the psychological impact based on questionnaire responses and qualitative interviews.

This study has shown the mutation yield in unselected women diagnosed with EOC from a heterogeneous population with no founder mutations was 8% in all ages and 12% in women under 70 [25]. Unselected genetic testing in women with EOC was acceptable to patients and is potentially less resource intensive.

14. Challenges in development of universal process on screening genetic mutations in ovarian cancers

In Our Opinion, all the patients diagnosed with invasive, epithelial ovarian cancer should be offered germline genetic testing, regardless of histologic subtype, because Ovarian cancers with a *BRCA1/BRCA2* mutation are most likely to be of high-grade serous histology, although these mutations have been found in endometrioid and clear cell histologic subtypes as well. Endometrioid and clear cell ovarian cancers are also frequently associated with Lynch syndrome (germline mutations in *MLH1*, *MSH2*, *MSH6*, *PMS2*, and *EPCAM*). Additionally, nonepithelial ovarian cancers - Sertoli-Leydig cell tumours can be associated with other genetic disorders such as Peutz-Jeghers syndrome and DICER1-associated disorders and small cell carcinoma of the ovary, hypercalcaemic type has been linked to germline mutations in *SMARCA4*.

All these mutations have got clinical relevance in the management of these patients and yet to discover the treatment options and preventing the development of the other cancer types associated with the above syndromes in the future generations with genetic predisposition.

There are several identified limitations in screening these mutations including cost of testing, lack of patient and provider education regarding the importance of genetic information, and limited availability of genetic counsellors and access to genetic testing [26].

In the era of unforeseen issues with Covid-19 there are other issues with genetic testing including social distancing making the genetic counselling, consenting difficult necessitating these steps to be delivered audio-visually.

15. In summary

There are numerous types of genetic mutations causing sporadic and hereditary ovarian cancers and more to be discovered yet. These mutations cause genomic instability in turn leading to cancer causation. Having a certain type of mutation will gives rise to clinically specific type of ovarian cancer, with different response to treatment, prognosis and predictability in behaviour.

Early identification of these mutations, genetic counselling will optimise the patient outcome, prevention of the ovarian and other genetically predisposed cancers in next generations.

Developing a universal testing pathway which is cost effective, is still challenging due to various factors.

The arrival of personalising treatment with Molecular typing of Ovarian Cancer has revolutionised maintenance therapy in Ovarian Cancer that has never seen before. Not only we are routinely screening for germline and somatic BRCA mutation upfront in all newly diagnosed Ovarian Cancer, we increasingly modify our treatment paradigm by providing PARPi in DNA mismatch repair deficiency detected patients. This extends from just BRCA mutation to the other Homologous recombinant deficiency genes as delineated in **Figure 1**. In 2020, FDA approved of MEK-inhibitor, Trametinib for Low grade Ovarian Cancer. And soon to be NICE guidelines for routine screening for Microsatellite instability genes, MMR MSI in all Endometrial Cancer, in search for 40% incidence of MSI MMR deficiency.

In 2021 November, with the sentinel FDA approval for liquid biopsy testing in solid cancers, which was predominantly based on detection of BRCA genes and most HRD genes, this has solid foundation in one test for defective molecular markers in blood, hopefully well before development of Cancer, for our exciting future to come.

Author details

Shyamika Mirisse Acharige* and Chit Cheng Yeoh*
Queen Alexandra Hospital, Portsmouth, United Kingdom

*Address all correspondence to: shyamika.acharige@porthosp.nhs.uk and chitcheng.yeoh@porthosp.nhs.uk

References

[1] Jenna Lilyquist,a,b Holly LaDuca,c Eric Polley,b Brigette Tippin Davis,c Hermela Shimelis,a Chunling Hu,a Steven N. Hart,b Jill S. Dolinsky,c Fergus J. Couch,a,b and David E. Goldgar Frequency of mutations in a large series of clinically ascertained ovarian cancer cases tested on multi-gene panels compared to reference controls Science direct 2017 doi: 10.1016/j.ygyno.2017.08.030

[2] Chen S, Parmigiani G. Meta-analysis of BRCA1 and BRCA2 penetrance. Journal of Clinical Oncology 2007; 25(11):1329-1333.

[3] Kuchenbaecker KB, Hopper JL, Barnes DR, et al. Risks of breast, ovarian, and contralateral breast cancer for BRCA1 and BRCA2 mutation carriers. *JAMA* 2017; 317(23):2402-2416.[PubMed Abstract]

[4] Robert J Kurman 1, Ie-Ming Shih The origin and pathogenesis of epithelial ovarian cancer: a proposed unifying theory 2010 National Library of Medicine NIH PMID: 20154587 PMCID: PMC2841791 DOI: 10.1097/PAS.0b013e3181cf3d79

[5] Maise Al Bakir, Hani Gabra The molecular genetics of hereditary and sporadic ovarian cancer: implications for the future *British Medical Bulletin*, Volume 112, Issue 1, December 2014, Pages 57-69, https://doi.org/10.1093/bmb/ldu034 Published:02 December 2014

[6] Alexandra V. Stavropoulou,Florentia Fostira,Maroulio Pertesi,Marianthi Tsitlaidou,Gerassimos E. Voutsinas,Olga Triantafyllidou,Aristotelis Bamias,Meletios A. Dimopoulos,Eleni Timotheadou,Dimitrios Pectasides,Christos Christodoulou,George Klouvas,Christos Papadimitriou, Irene Konstantopoulou Prevalence of BRCA1 Mutations in Familial and Sporadic Greek Ovarian Cancer Cases Published: March 11, 2013 PLOS ONE https://doi.org/10.1371/journal.pone.0058182

[7] Andre jDudáš Miroslav Chovanec DNA double-strand break repair by homologous recombination Mutation research/reviews https://www.sciencedirect.com/science/journal/13835742 2004

[8] M. Moschetta, A. George, S.B. Kaye, S. Banerjee BRCA somatic mutations and epigenetic BRCA modifications in serous ovarian cancer 2016 Annals of oncology PMID: 27037296 DOI: 10.1093/annonc/mdw142

[9] Kiyotsugu Yoshida Yoshio Miki Role of BRCA1 and BRCA2 as regulators of DNA repair, transcription, and cell cycle in response to DNA damage First published: 19 August 2005 Onlinelibrary.wiley.com https://doi.org/10.1111/j.1349-7006.2004.tb02195.x

[10] Kathleen N. Moore, Mansoor Raza Mirza, Ursula A. Matulonis The poly (ADP ribose) polymerase inhibitor niraparib: Management of toxicities Gynaecologic Oncology 2018 PMID: 29397193 DOI: 10.1016/j.ygyno.2018.01.011

[11] *Robert T. Neff, Leigha Senter, Ritu Salani BRCA* mutation in ovarian cancer: testing, implications and treatment considerations First Published June 19, 2017 SAGE Journals https://doi.org/10.1177%2F1758834017714993

[12] Clinical Comissioning Policy: Genetic Testing for BRCA1 and BRCA2 2015 NHS England.

[13] U.S National Library of Medicine information on inherited diseases.

[14] Colombo N, Nicoletto M, Benedetti Panici P, et al Combination Cediranib

Plus Olaparib Improves PFS in Platinum-Resistant Ovarian Cancer. BAROCCO: A randomized phase II study of weekly paclitaxel vs cediranib-olaparib combination given with continuous or intermittent schedule in patients with recurrent platinum resistant ovarian cancer (PROC). Presented at 2019 ESMO Congress; September 27 to October 1, 2019; Barcelona, Spain. Abstract LBA58.

[15] D Chandrasekaran R Manchanda Germline and somatic genetic testing in ovarian cancer patients First published: 25 March 2018 https://doi.org/10.1111/1471-0528.15225

[16] Hualei Bu, Jingying Chen Qingshui Li Jianqing Hou Yuan Wei,Xiaohang Yang YanaMaHongsheng He Youzhong Zhang Beihua Kong BRCA mutation frequency and clinical features of ovarian cancer patients: A report from a Chinese study group https://obgyn.onlinelibrary.wiley.com/doi/abs/10.1111/jog.14090 First published: 14 August 2019 https://doi.org/10.1111/jog.14090

[17] A. Sonnenblick, E. Azambuja, M. Piccart An update on PARP inhibitors—moving to the adjuvant setting Published 2015, Nature Reviews Clinical Oncology DOI: 10.1038/nrclinonc.2014.163

[18] Ashok R. Venkitaraman Functions of BRCA1 and BRCA2 in the biological response to DNA damage Journal of Cell Science 2001 114: 3591-3598

[19] G. Bitlera Zachary L. Watsona Lindsay J. Wheelerab Kian Behbakhtab PARP inhibitors: Clinical utility and possibilities of overcoming resistance www.sciencedirect.com/science/article/pii/S009082581731363X December 2017 PMID: 29037806 PMCID: PMC5698126 DOI: 10.1016/j.ygyno.2017.10.003

[20] Caroline Helwick Three Phase III Trials Suggest Paradigm Shift with PARP Inhibitors in Ovarian Cancer 2019 The Ascopost

[21] TarraEvans, UrsulaMatulonis PARP inhibitors in ovarian cancer: evidence, experience and clinical potentialFirstPublished February3,2017 ReviewArticle FinPubmed https://doi.org/10.1177/1758834016687254

[22] Sarah A Cook 1, Anna V Tinker PARP Inhibitors and the Evolving Landscape of Ovarian Cancer Management: A Review National Library of Medicine NIH June 2019 PMID: 30895466 DOI: 10.1007/s40259-019-00347

[23] William P. Tew, MD1; Christina Lacchetti, MHSc2; Annie Ellis3,4; Kathleen Maxian, BSW5; Susana Banerjee, PhD6; Michael Bookman, MD7; PARP Inhibitors in the Management of Ovarian Cancer: ASCO Guideline DOI: 10.1200/JCO.20.01924 Journal of Clinical Oncology 38, no. 30 (October 20, 2020) 3468-3493. Published online August 13, 2020. PMID: 32790492

[24] Yvette Drew The development of PARP inhibitors in ovarian cancer: from bench to bedside December 2015 British Journal of Cancer 113(S1):S3-S9 DOI: 10.1038/bjc.2015.394

[25] Inga Plaskocinska, Hannah Shipman, james Drummond, Edward Thompson, Vanessa Buchanan, Barbara Newcombe, Charlotte Hodgkin, Elisa Barter, Paul Ridley, Rita Ng, Suzanne Miller, Adela Dann, Victoria Licence, Hayley Webb, Li Tee Tan, Margaret Daly, Sarah Ayers, Barnaby Rufford, Helena Earl, Christine Parkinson, Timothy Duncan, Mercedes Jimenez-Linan, Gurdeep S Sagoo, Stephen Abbs, Nicholas Hulbert-Williams, Paul Pharoah, Robin Crawford, James D Brenton, Marc Tischkowitz New paradigms for *BRCA1*/*BRCA2* testing in women with ovarian cancer: results

of the Genetic Testing in Epithelial Ovarian Cancer (GTEOC) study Journal of Medical Genetics 2016 http://dx.doi.org/10.1136/jmedgenet-2016-103902

[26] Zachary NashMBBSab Usha MenonMD(Res), FRCOGb Ovarian cancer screening: Current status and future directions journal homepage: www.elsevier.com/locate/ygyno December 2013 https://doi.org/10.1016/j.ygyno.2013.11.030

Chapter 3

Ovarian Cancer Tumour Biology: Genesis

Ján Varga

Abstract

Ovarian cancer (OC) is the fifth leading cause of cancer deaths among women, thus early diagnosis is of paramount importance to survival. A clear OC etiopathogenesis is not yet fully understood. Large histopathological variability predicts more initial tissue for carcinogenesis. Many connections of biologically different tissue as *locus minoris resistentiae* for carcinogenesis have been confirmed. Expansion of knowledge about OC etiopathogenesis may help to construct an algorithm for early diagnosis. Ovarian surface epithelium, ectopic Müllerian epithelium, and fallopian tubes, along with endometriosis, are significant in the process of OC development. An oxidative microenvironment caused by recurrent ovulation or arising due to a degradative process in ectopic endometrium, mainly endometriomas, play a prominent role in the development of OC.

Keywords: ovarian cancer, etiopathogenesis, ovarian surface epithelium, cortical inclusion cyst, fallopian tube, endometriosis, endosalpingiosis, ovulation, tubo-ovarian junction, ovarian carcinogenesis

1. Introduction

Although ovarian cancer (OC) is not the most common cancer, it is the fifth leading cause of cancer deaths among women [1] and accounts for 3–4% of all female cancers. Improvement of therapeutic options in OC patients has improved disease-free survival but has had no significant effect on overall survival. There is still the need for genetic profiling to identify patients who will benefit from anti-angiogenic treatment [2, 3]. Due to the typical disease characteristics, such as initially asymptomatic growth and delayed symptoms, most OC patients are diagnosed at an advanced stage. Early diagnosis at the asymptomatic stage is of paramount importance for survival. Understanding OC development pathways can help with early diagnosis and thus increase the potential of curability as well as screening programs.

2. Ovarian cancer - background

2.1 Classification

Histo-anatomy and tumour biology are main determining factors in OC classification.

Up to 90% of all OC is derived from the epithelium. The remaining 10% represents non-epithelial cancers with sex-cord stromal tumours and germ cell tumours. Epithelial OC is either mucinous (3%) or non-mucinous (97%). The most represented group, non-mucinous, includes serous OC, endometrioid ovarian cancer (EOC), clear cell ovarian cancer (CCOC), transitional cell carcinoma, and others.

The model of two different tumour types in epithelial OC is widely supported and was officially accepted by the World Health Organisation (WHO) in 2004 [4]. Type 1 OC is defined from precursor through borderline variants. These cancers usually have an indolent course and good prognosis. Type 2 OC, such as high-grade serous ovarian cancer (HGSOC), reports fast progression, aggressiveness, and poor prognosis (**Figure 1**). Ninety percent of all deaths from OC are caused by this type [5].

The most common secondary cancers are metastatic lesions in the gastrointestinal tract or breasts [6].

2.2 Carcinogenesis: basic orientation

The cells of origin for OC are well studied, although some OC may not originate in the ovaries. OC in extra-ovarian tissue can also occur. For example, mucinous OC can resemble other endocervical glands and gastro-intestinal epithelium.

EOC and CCOC often show the presence of endometriosis in their histology. Histopathological criteria can clearly define a couple of types of endometriosis with different biological potential. While benign endometriosis faces the onset of the endometriosis overthrow, atypical endometriosis is already an ongoing process. The range as well as the time interval of oxidative load significantly affect which deposit of benign endometriosis progresses. The degradation processes typically seen in ectopic endometrium are the source of oxidative stress, and close contact with the

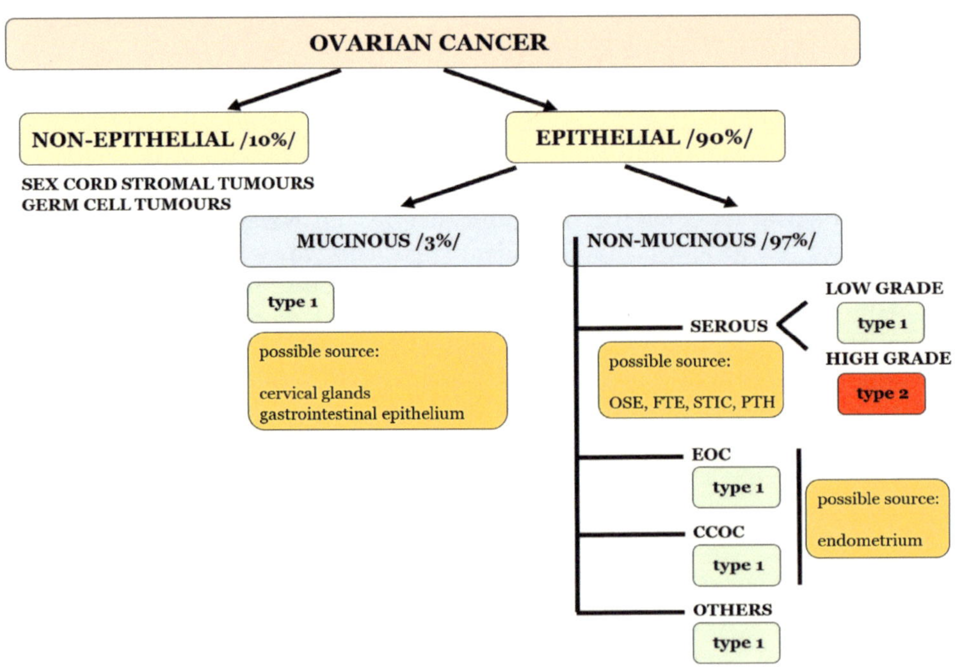

Figure 1.
Ovarian cancer classification due to histo-anatomy and tumour biology with possible initial source.

ovary potentiates this process. This explains why ovarian endometriomas have the greatest potential for progression and why there is less risk of progression in deep infiltrating endometriosis.

Serous OC can originate in the ovary as well as extra-ovarian tissue. The close relationship was observed with fallopian tube, mainly its fimbriated end. Fallopian tube epithelium (FTE) plays an important role in the development of ovarian malignancy. The precursor originating from the FTE can locally progress or, more often, adhere to the more favourable environment of the ovary. Local progression of the precursor derived from the FTE is rare. The reason for this is the inhibitory effect of the fallopian tube microenvironment on carcinogenesis when compared to the ovarian microenvironment. Oxidative stress resulting from incessant ovulation leads to accumulation of DNA changes in the FTE with subsequent exfoliation of precursors to the ovarian surface epithelium. Even more tissues for ovarian carcinogenesis with different biological potential have been recognised in the FTE. Type 1 OC, although containing oncogene alterations of RAS-PMK or PI3K-AKT, is genomically stable, for example, as in wild-type p53. Type 2 OC reports p53 mutations and pronounced genomic instability [5].

Generally, the initial tissue for OC development can be located in the ovary, ectopic Müllerian epithelium, fallopian tube, or endometrium (**Figure 1**).

Age older than 64 years is a risk factor for OC mortality and risk of disease increases significantly with advancing age. Within a genetic predisposition only limited clinically relevant mutations are currently known. Knowledge about tumour suppressor genes, *BRCA* mutations, and Lynch syndrome help to construct a preventive surgery programme for patients. An oxidative microenvironment due to incessant ovulation in the tubo-ovarian junction or degradative processes in endometriomas are considerable risk factors for DNA alterations. Thus, decreased ovulation may act as a protective factor against OC, although not every situation

Group of factors	Factor	+	—	+/−
Age	Age		•	
Genetic	Family history		•	
	BRCA mutation		•	
	Lynch syndrome		•	
Reproduction	Incessant ovulation		•	
	Menarche			•
	Menopause			•
	Parity	•		
	Lactation	•		
Hormonal	Hormonal contraceptives	•		
	Hormone replacement therapy			•
Gynaecological	Endometriosis		•	
	Pelvic inflammatory disease			•
	Fallopian tube occlusion	•		
Others	Obesity			•
	Alcohol/cigarettes/caffeine			•

Table 1.
The share of individual factors in protection (+), predisposition (−) or controversial position (+/−) in relation to the OC development.

confirms this fact (**Table 1**). The main factors influencing risk-reduction strategies are genetic predispositions, ageing, and parity.

3. Ovarian cancer: etiopathogenesis

3.1 Ovary

The infiltration of the ovaries by cancer cells even in the early stages of OC has been confirmed. Due to this fact, the initial concept was that the origin of OC is in the ovary. The ovarian surface epithelium (OSE) covers the ovary and during ovulation invagination of the OSE may occur, leading to the formation of small cystic lesions located in the ovarian cortex called cortical inclusion cysts (CICs).

The engagement of ovulation in carcinogenesis has been known for about 50 years. The oxidative stress accompanying ovulation alters the cells of the OSE. The accumulation of DNA damages arising due to the pro-inflammatory and pro-oxidative microenvironment and subsequent inability to repair them leads to the formation of pathological clone cells (**Figure 2**). In addition, women with a *BRCA* mutation and decreased ability of DNA repair are more prone to this process [7].

Incorporated CICs containing DNA-altered cells, as well as ambient pluripotent stem cells, are exposed to cyclic inflammatory activity. It has already been described that stem cell activity is silenced in cancerous OSE [8]. Thus, dysregulated pluripotency of stem cells may contribute to growth promotion and differentiation, finally leading to cancer formation [7]. Inadequate host tissue stem cell activity as the factor potentiating growth and malignant transformation in other cancers such as colorectal carcinoma has also been described [9].

The histology of certain HGSOC shows similarity to tissue developmentally derived from Müllerian ducts (**Figure 3**). One possible reason for this is that the relatively unstable, undifferentiated nature of OSE may mould the tissue of a Müllerian phenotype through the process of metaplasia [10]. Metaplastic OSE with different phenotype create after its incorporation into CIC Müllerian type of cortical inclusion cyst (mCIC), finally progressing into OC. This represents a theory of OC development from Müllerian epithelium but initially arising from metaplastic OSE. Another theory is the transport of Müllerian epithelium into the OSE from extra-ovarian localisation (e.g., ectopic Müllerian epithelium, endosalpingiosis, or fallopian tubes).

3.2 Ectopic Müllerian epithelium

As early as 1999, the theory that all epithelial OC originated initially from the ovary was challenged. As a primary source was indicated extra-ovarian müllerian epithelium (**Figure 3**). It was observed that Müllerian epithelium has more similar patterns to HGSOC than to OSE. The theory was supported by proof of the absence of ovarian tissues in primary peritoneal cancers without ovarian invasion but that were clinically and histopathologically consistent with HGSOC. Secondary Müllerian tissue as the residue of ectopic Müllerian epithelium (outside of the cervix, endometrium, or fallopian tubes) as the source of cells for carcinogenesis has been confirmed [11].

3.2.1 Endosalpingiosis

Endosalpingiosis (ES) represents an ectopic presence of FTE. When compared to endometriosis, ES shows ciliary epithelium and absence of inflammatory

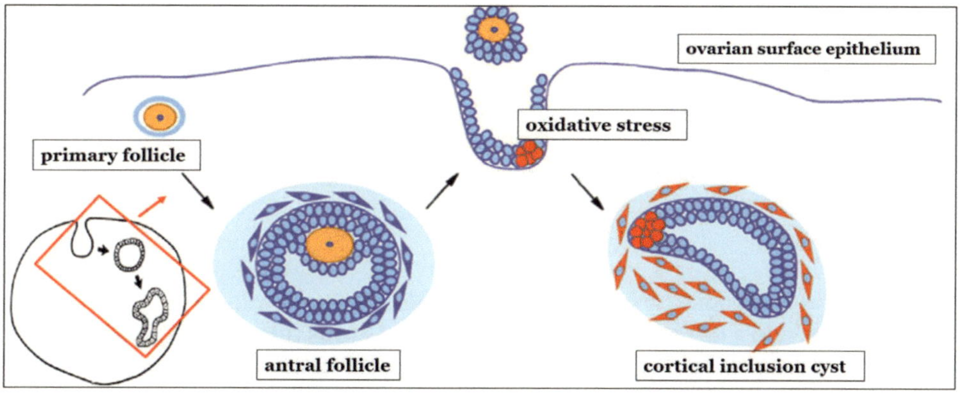

Figure 2.
Cortical inclusion cyst formation from ovarian surface epithelium under the effect of oxidative stress resulting from ovulation.

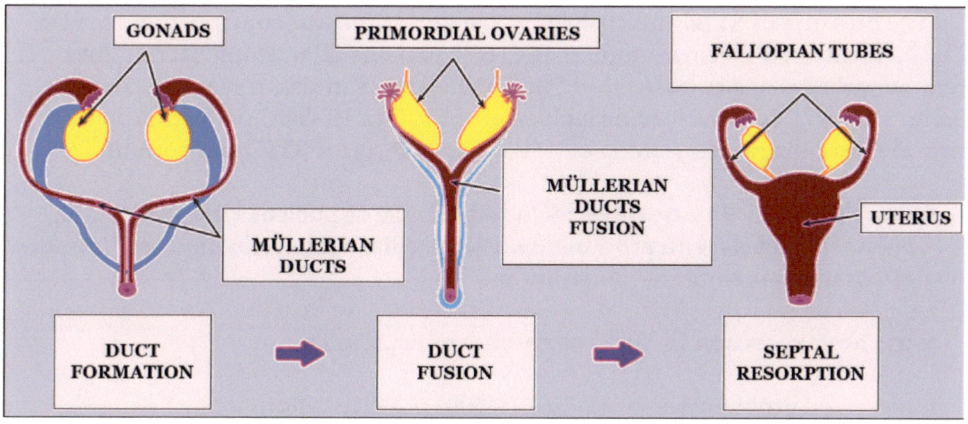

Figure 3.
The development of female genitals and role of Müllerian ducts.

reaction. In addition, there is a difference in incidence related to age among these two conditions. The discovery of fallopian tube importance in the process of ovarian carcinogenesis and subsequent implementation of sectioning and extensively examining the fimbriated end protocol (SEE-FIM) led to increased ES rates. In women aged 31–50 years, ES incidence is 37%. In menopausal women, incidence increases to 66% [12]. Endometriosis incidence rapidly decreases after menopause, whereas an opposite effect is seen in ES. This is caused by the different biology of the diseases, although both entities probably arise from dissemination of physiologically localised tissue. While endometriosis represents a hormone-dependent disease, ES probably arises from tissue detachment of FTE. Due to the hormonal attenuation after menopause, endometriosis regresses; however, increasing age increases the probability of exfoliation of FTE from fallopian tubes. Different biological potential can also be present. In ES tissues degradative processes are missing, which means less oxidative load. Thus also malignant potential of ES should be present when compare to endometriosis.

The theories of ES development discuss two possibilities. One envisages a metaplasia of pluripotent coelomic peritoneal epithelium to FTE tissue. More likely it is a process of primary dissemination of FTE. This second theory explains the presence of ES in women only and that the most common localization of ES is in the ovaries.

Relevant clinical data about ES are scarce, although recent studies show its association with gynaecological malignancies [13]. A significant relationship between ES and borderline ovarian carcinoma (BOC) has been observed. One third of serous BOC patients present with ES in their histology and incidence of ES increases to 70% in recurrent serous BOC [14]. The connection with slowly progressing cancers is likely due to low biological activity of ES.

3.3 Fallopian tube

In 2001, small dysplastic lesions similar to HGSOC containing *BRCA* mutations were discovered in a patient's fallopian tubes [15]. Serous tubal intraepithelial carcinoma (STIC) is characterised by enlarged epithelial cells with atypia of nucleoli. The distal part of the fallopian tube is the main region where STIC is seen. This is most probably due to the close connection with the ovary where ovulation with chronic inflammatory and oxidative microenvironment takes place. Immunohistochemical study of STIC showed positivity of p53 as well as γH2AX, which is a marker of double-stranded DNA breaks [16].

The presence of STIC and HGSOC at the same time was confirmed in 11–61%. The incidence of STIC in asymptomatic risky patients after prophylactic adnexectomy was reported to be 0.4%–8.5%. The incidence in risk-free patients was 0.8%–3.1% [17]. Relatively wide incidence of STIC in HGSOC patients is due to non-identical diagnostic criteria of STIC. The criteria for STIC diagnosis are:

- morphological abnormalities including change of nucleus/cytoplasm ratio, enlarged nucleus with prominent nucleoli, ciliary cells reduction, and absence of basement membrane penetration

- p53 overexpression (> 60%) or absence of expression

- increased proliferative index Ki67 (> 10% positive cells in lesion)

The knowledge of early tubal precursors increased a request for precise fallopian tubes assessment. On the other hand implementation of detailed investigation protocol uncovered more microscopic lesions with not known tasks. Apart from STIC, three other lesions need to be taken into consideration: p53 signature, secretory cell outgrowth (SCOUT), and serous intraepithelial lesion (STIL).

p53 signature represents a cluster of FTE reporting p53 positivity with Ki67 < 10%. Morphological changes are not present and therefore a diagnostic process is focused on immunohistochemical examination. It can be a bilateral and multifocal lesion; the role is not fully clarified. It can be an initial step with subsequent progression or the lesion can persist.

SCOUT is defined as a proliferation of at least 30 secretory fallopian tube cells with Bcl2 positivity as well as P53 negativity. Another feature is loss of *PAX2*, which is seen in STIC as well as in HGSOC. This predicts *PAX2* inactivity as part of carcinogenesis and SCOUT can be a step of this process. The amount of SCOUT increases with age and most likely represents a precursor of p53 lesions [18]. However, they are not reported in clinical findings due to their unclear clinical importance.

STIL contains atypia but does not reach STIC. It represents a morphological intermediate stage between p53 and STIC [18].

The process of ovarian carcinogenesis starting in the FTE under the effect of ovulation takes more than 30 years. Development of p53 signature from secretory epithelial cells of the fallopian tubes lasts approximately 10 years, and it takes another 15 years for the development of STIC, and then 5 more years for the development of HGSOC from STIC (**Figure 4**) [19].

The knowledge of FTE hypothesis as the source of OC potentiates an idea of reduction of preventive surgery range in high-risk patients. Due to the lack of information about the role of fallopian tubes on general OC incidence, the risk reduction of OC occurrence after prophylactic salpingectomy cannot be established. The omission of oophorectomy in premenopausal women prevents menopausal side effects but certain risk of OC remains.

3.3.1 STIC transport to ovaries

Although the STIC as a precursor of HGSOC is clearly defined, infiltration of the fallopian tubes was not observed in a large proportion of patients with HGSOC [20]. The reason for this is the theory of transportation of early genomically altered secretory epithelial cells from the distal part of fallopian tubes into the OSE. Implantation of tissue in the CIC of OSE leads to formation of mCIC (**Figure 5**) where the ovarian microenvironment creates better conditions for cancer progression [21].

The question of whether OC originates in the ovary or the fallopian tube is not fully answered. The microenvironment plays a crucial role. Whereas the ovary accelerates the process of cancer initiation, progression, and growth, the fallopian tubes more likely have an inhibitory effect [21]. This may explain why the precursor in case of cancer originating from the ovary cannot be detected. The process in these cancers is so rapid that precancerous lesions are often not detected. Inversely, in the fallopian tubes there is a longer time window for detecting early lesions, and after their transportation into the ovary the acceleration of the cancer is seen.

Although the conditions for progression are apparently better in the ovaries, local progression of STIC in the fallopian tubes and formation of primary fallopian tube carcinoma can occur.

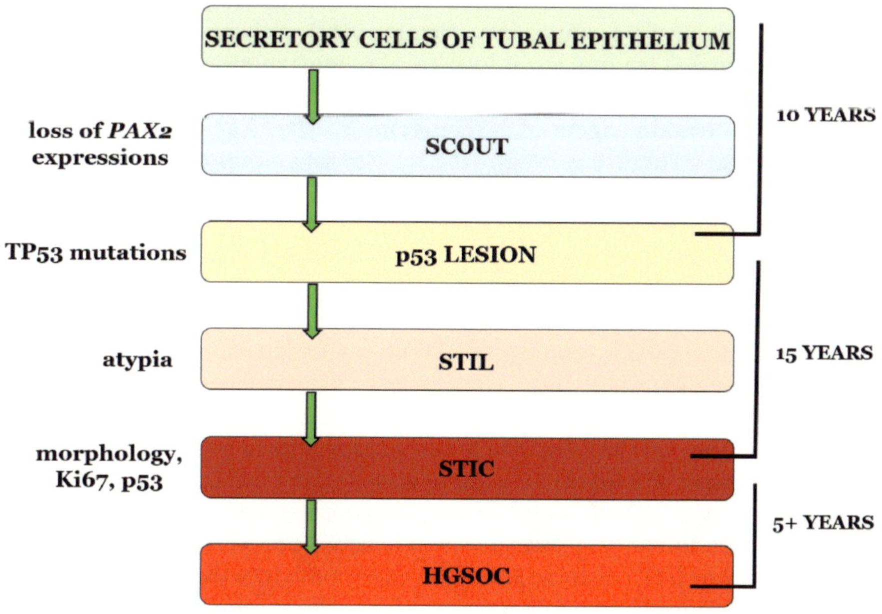

Figure 4.
The biological course of ovarian carcinogenesis starting in fallopian tube epithelium.

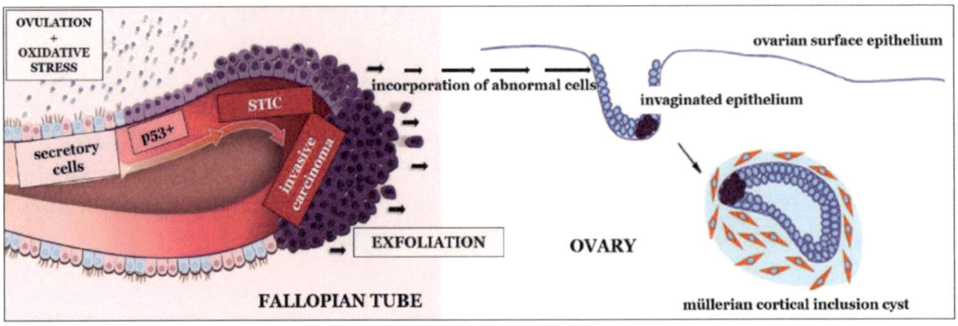

Figure 5.
The process of incorporation of fallopian tube cells into ovarian surface epithelium.

3.3.2 Papillary tubal hyperplasia

The fallopian tubes play a role in some type 1 cancers. Papillary tubal hyperplasia (PTH) represents a cluster of epithelial cells and small papillae with or without psammomatous bodies in the lumen of the fallopian tube (**Figure 6**). They float freely in tubal lumen or protrude from the epithelium into the lumen. This is a crucial difference from tubal hyperplasia. It was suggested that PTH represents the most advanced stage of tubal hyperplasia and has a significant association with some ovarian and extra-ovarian low-grade tumours. Earlier stages of tubal hyperplasia do not show such a prominent association [22].

PTH arises as the consequence of chronic inflammatory processes and can be diffuse or focal. Anatomically the most common place of appearance is the tubal ampoule. After its transport into the ovary, PTH can progress and form serous BOC and subsequently low-grade serous ovarian cancer (LGSOC). Many morphological similarities of PTH and LGSOC have been confirmed. Both contain ciliary and secretory cells as well as intraepithelial lymphocytes. Psammomatous bodies commonly present in PTH as well as LGSOC. After its transportation on peritoneal surfaces, PTH represents a precursor of ES or non-invasive implants.

Chronic inflammatory changes (i.e., chronic salpingitis or other forms of pelvic inflammatory disease) leading to architectural reconstruction of the fallopian tube induce FTE proliferation resulting in PTH. Mutation of *KRAS* or *BRAF* genes represent the main trigger of carcinogenesis. After its transportation into the ovary, the final structure is usually mCIC. Not all studies have confirmed this algorithm and significant association of PTH with LGSOC or serous BOC was not seen [23, 24]. More studies in this area are still needed.

3.3.3 Primary fallopian tube carcinoma

Primary fallopian tube carcinoma (PFTC) represents a rare entity accounting for 0.14%–1.8% of all female genital tract cancers. Nevertheless, the incidence in the last several years has increased due to the change in fallopian tube assessment. Wide implementation of the SEE-FIM protocol into clinical practice increased detection of different precursors from FTE as well as the incidence of PFTC. Unfortunately, they represent mainly asymptomatic lesions or, like in some PFTC cases, are indicated for surgery due to adnexal mass. At present, PFTC is considered to be the presence of STIC or invasion of the carcinoma into the fallopian tube mucosa or if the fallopian tube is incorporated into the tumour mass [25].

The precursor in HGSOC or high-grade serous extra-ovarian cancer is STIC with a typical p53 mutation. In case of HGSOC or extra-ovarian cancer, STIC is

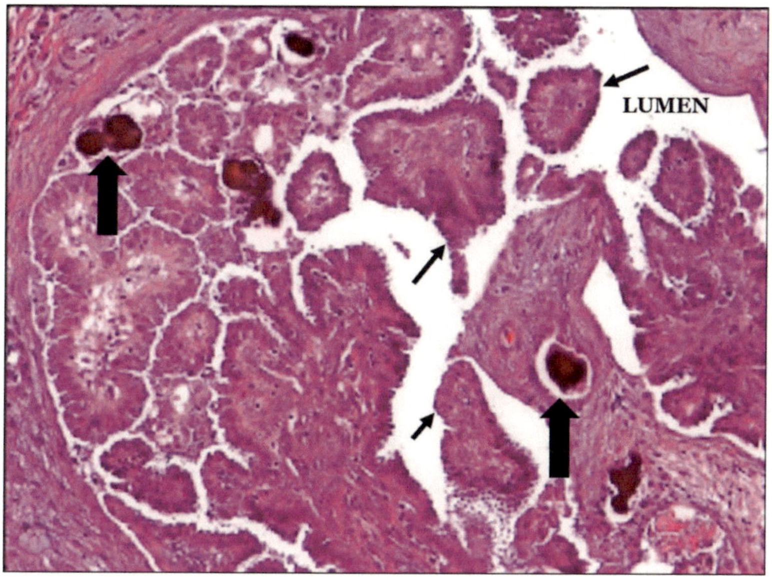

Figure 6.
Papillary tubal hyperplasia. Numerous small papillae/thin arrows/psamomatous bodies/gross arrows/.

detached from the FTE and implanted on surfaces without invasion of tissue under the basement membrane of the FTE. However, in case of PFTC a local progression of STIC with invasion into deeper structures is seen. Localisation of PFTC in the tubal lumen leads to its distension with earlier clinical symptoms. Therefore, PFTC diagnosis is done earlier than that for HGSOC. In addition, the partially closed space of tubal lumen can delay spread of disease in the abdominal cavity.

3.4 Endometriosis

Endometriosis is a clinically complex syndrome with chronic hormone-dependent inflammation and notable proliferative potential. Although endometriosis incidence is around 10%, it accounts for less than 1% of malignancies [26].

The common features of endometriosis and cancer cells have been clearly described. These include angiogenic potential of stem cells as well as their ability to evade apoptosis. Haemolysis, the process typical for endometriosis, is highly associated with oxidation. An oxidative microenvironment results in accumulation of DNA mutations and leads to, under the supervision of the immune system, either cell death or formation of pathogenic clone cells.

The similar effect like in FTE, which is for better conditions of malignization transported into ovary is also in endometriosis seen. Inflamed stroma with mutated epithelium can progress to cancer when located on the ovary. This explains why malignant overthrow is uncommon in the case of deep infiltrating endometriosis even when containing similar DNA mutations [26]. The microenvironment plays an important role in these situations as well.

Endometriosis-associated ovarian cancer (EAOC) includes mainly endometrioid ovarian cancer (EOC), clear cell ovarian cancer (CCOC), and sero-mucinous borderline ovarian cancer. Nevertheless, not every case of EAOC presents with endometriosis. EAOCs are characterised as well-differentiated tumours occurring at a younger age and initially diagnosed at an earlier stage when compared to endometriosis-free EAOC. The question which endometriotic lesion tend to progress into carcinoma remains still not completely answered.

Benign and atypical (premalignant) endometriosis can be defined using histopathological criteria. There is a significant association of atypical endometriosis (AE) with EAOC. While benign endometriosis (BE) does not contain atypia and has greater incidence, AE is less frequently seen and the atypia can be defined in two grades [27]. Cellular atypia, also called cytological atypia, defines epithelial layer changes such as hyperchromasia and pleomorphism. However, structural atypia, also called hyperplasia, deputises hyperplastic changes similar to ectopic endometrium, which includes simple or complex hyperplasia with or without cellular atypia [28]. Although plenty of studies refer to AE as tissue with cytological and structural atypia, cytological atypia are seen in cancer-free patients, whereas structural atypia are typically present in OC patients (**Figure** 7) [27].

The different potential of both types of atypia have been confirmed by studies of COX-2, Ki-67, and BAF250a. In the case of BE, immunohistochemical COX-2 positivity is significantly higher compared to that in AE. In both types of atypia in AE, rapidly higher COX-2 positivity in cytological atypia has been observed. This predicts BE as well as cytological atypia of AE into reactive changes. In Ki-67 examinations lower values in BE and cytological atypia of AE were detected. Thus, the structural atypia of AE can be concluded as the tissue with greater proliferative potential. The decrease in BAF250a was confirmed in both OC and AE patients. Comparing both types of atypia in AE, we can see lower BAF250a expressions in structural atypia patients [27].

EAOC tissue can be present with or without endometriosis. If endometriosis is confirmed, both types can be seen (BE as well as AE). In some cases even gradual transition from BE to AE and BOC can be detected. Approximately one of 10 women suffers from endometriosis and only less than 1% (0.3%–0.8%) of endometriosis patients will progress to cancer. When checked for AE incidence in endometriosis patients, 8% show atypia in their histology. The incidence of AE increases in patients with OC, whereas one-third of EAOC patients present with AE [27]. Detailed analysis of AE patients showed those with long-term history of disease, advanced stage, and older age when compared to BE patients. Current accepted criteria for AE include eosinophilic cytoplasm, large hyperchromatin or pale nuclei with moderate-to-marked pleomorphism, increased nucleus-to-cytoplasm ratio, and cell aggregation.

The endometriosis was solidly confirmed as the precursor of some OC, preferentially of certain portion of EAOC. Due to the low incidence of endometriosis

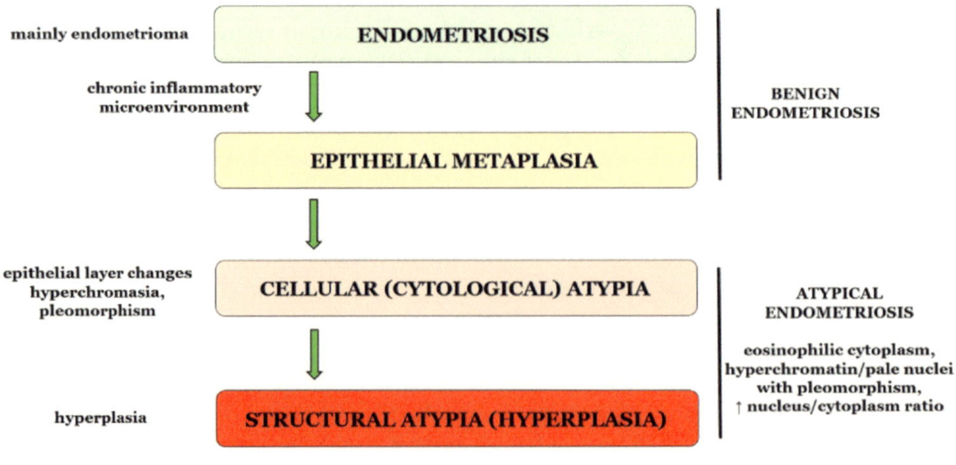

Figure 7.
The development of changes in ectopic endometrium.

Initial structure	Biological process	Final structure
OSE	Mutation + incorporation into small cyst	CIC
OSE	Metaplasia + incorporation into small cyst	mCIC
Ectopic Müllerian epithelium	Local progression transport to the ovary	Primary peritoneal cancer mCIC
ES	Transport to the ovary	Serous BOC
FTE	Transport to the ovary	mCIC
STIC	Local progression	PFTC
STIC	Transport to the ovary	HGSOC
PTH	Transport to the ovary	BOC/LGSOC
Endometriosis	Retrograde reflux/transport to tubo-ovarian junction	EOC, CCOC

Table 2.
Simplified process of ovarian carcinogenesis.

overthrow, predictive factors are not fully clarified. There is significantly greater association of endometriomas with malignancy when compared to deep infiltrating endometriosis. In those cases, the ovarian microenvironment plays a crucial role. Thus, even in endometriosis overthrow a tubo-ovarian junction is inevitably needed to ensure endometrial reflux to the ovary and then cellular progression in the endometrioma. From the clinical characteristics of OC, patients with long-term history of disease as well as large endometriomas (> 9 cm) may be defined as high-risk patients for progression and thus require more precise observation (**Table 2**) [29].

4. Conclusion

Incidence of OC is relatively low when compared to other onco-gynaecological diseases. Nevertheless, OC is the fifth leading cause of cancer deaths among women with 95% of deaths occurring in women older than 45 years.

Disease localisation in the abdominal cavity allows asymptomatic growth at the early stages. The diagnostic timing of symptomatic disease does not affect the parameters of survival. To increase survival rate, it is important to detect the disease at the early asymptomatic stage. Knowledge of disease etiopathogenesis increases the probability of detecting precancerous lesions or early-stage cancers.

The source of OC can be OSE through CIC or mCIC. Local progression is seen less frequently, whereas transport of the precursor to the ovarian surface is more common. Retrograde menstruation may be a cause of some EAOCs, mainly EOC and CCOC.

Author details

Ján Varga
Department of Gynaecology and Obstetrics, Faculty of Medicine, P.J. Šafárik University, L. Pasteur University Hospital, Košice, Slovakia

*Address all correspondence to: janko.varga@gmail.com

References

[1] Bray F, Ferlay J, Soerjomataram I, et al. Global cancer statistics 2018: GLOBOCAN estimates of incidence and mortality worldwide for 36 cancers in 185 countries. CA: A Cancer Journal for Clinicians. 2018;**68**:394-424. DOI: 10.3322/caac.21492

[2] Schmid BC, Oehler MK. Improvements in progression-free and overall survival due to the use of anti-angiogenic agents in gynecologic cancers. Current Treatment Options in Oncology. 2015;**16**:318. DOI: 10.1007/s11864-014-0318-0

[3] Tewari KS, Burger RA, Enserro D, et al. Final overall survival of a randomized trial of bevacizumab for primary treatment of ovarian cancer. Journal of Clinical Oncology. 2019;**37**: 2317-2328. DOI: 10.1200/JCO.19.01009

[4] Shih LEM, Kurman RJ. Ovarian tumorigenesis: A proposed model based on morphological and molecular genetic analysis. The American Journal of Pathology. 2004;**164**:1511-1518. DOI: 10.1016/s0002-9440(10)63708-x

[5] Kurman RJ, IeM S. The dualistic model of ovarian carcinogenesis: Revisited, revised and expanded. The American Journal of Pathology. 2016;**186**:733-747. DOI: 10.1016/j.ajpath.2015.11.011

[6] Peres LC, Cushing-Haugen KL, Anglesio M, et al. Histotype classification of ovarian carcinoma: A comparison of aproaches. Gynecologic Oncology. 2018;**151**:53-60. DOI: 10.1016/j.ygyno.2018.08.016

[7] Klotz DM, Wimberger P. Cells of origin of ovarian cancer: Ovarian surface epithelium or fallopian tube? Archives of Gynecology and Obstetrics. 2017;**296**:1055-1062. DOI: 10.1007/s00404-017-4529-z

[8] Bowen NJ, LDe W, Matyunina LV, et al. Gene expression profiling supports the hypothesis that human ovarian surface epithelia are multipotent and capable of serving as ovarian cancer initiating cells. BMC Medical Genomics. 2009;**2**:71. DOI: 10.1186/1755-8794-2-71

[9] Barker N, Ridgway RA, Es JH, et al. Crypt stem cells as the cells-of-origin of intestinal cancer. Nature. 2009;**457**:608-611. DOI: 10.1038/nature07602

[10] Kuhn E, Kurman RJ, IeM S. Ovarian cancer is an imported disease: Fact or fiction? Current Obstetrics and Gynecology Reports. 2012;**1**:1-9. DOI: 10.1007/s13669-011-0004-1

[11] Dubeau L. The cell of origin of ovarian epithelial tumors and the ovarian surface epithelium dogma: Does the emperor have no clothes? Gynecologic Oncology. 1999;**72**:437-442. DOI: 10.1006/gyno.1998.5275

[12] Sunde J, Wasickanin M, Katz TA, et al. Prevalence of endosalpingiosis and other benign gynecologic lesions. PLoS One. 2020;**15**:e0232487. DOI: 10.1371/journal.pone.0232487

[13] Hermens M, Altena AM, Bulten J, et al. Increased association of ovarian cancer in women with histological proven endosalpingiosis. Cancer Epidemiology. 2020;**65**:101700. DOI: 10.1016/j.canep.2020.101700

[14] Chui MH, Xing D, Zeppernick F, et al. Clinicopathologic and molecular features of paired cases of metachronous ovarian serous borderline tumor and subsequent serous carcinoma. The American Journal of Surgical Pathology. 2019;**43**:1462-1472. DOI: 10.1097/PAS.0000000000001325

[15] Piek JM, van Diest PJ, Zweemer RP, et al. Dysplastic changes in prophylactically removed fallopian

tubes of women predisposed to developing ovarian cancer. The Journal of Pathology. 2001;**195**:451-456. DOI: 10.1002/path.1000

[16] Kobayashi H, Iwai K, Niiro E, et al. The conceptual advances of carcinogenic sequence model in high-grade serous ovarian cancer. Biomedical Reports. 2017;**7**:209-213. DOI: 10.3892/br.2017.955

[17] Chen F, Gaitskell K, Garcia MJ, et al. Serous tubal intraepithelial carcinomas associated with high-grade serous ovarian carcinomas: A systematic review. BJOG. 2017;**124**:872-878. DOI: 10.1111/1471-0528.14543

[18] Nakamura M, Obata T, Daikoku T, et al. The association and significance of p53 in gynecologic cancers: The potential of targeted therapy. International Journal of Molecular Sciences. 2019;**20**:5482. DOI: 10.3390/ijms20215482

[19] Wu NYY, Fang C, Huang HS, et al. Natural history of ovarian high-grade serous carcinoma from time effects of ovulation inhibition and progesterone clearance of p53-defective lesions. Modern Pathology. 2020;**33**:29-37. DOI: 10.1038/s41379-019-0370-1

[20] Bowtell DD, Böhm S, Ahmed AA, et al. Rethinking ovarian cancer II: Reducing mortality from high-grade serous ovarian cancer. Nature Reviews. Cancer. 2015;**15**:668-679. DOI: 10.1038/nrc4019

[21] Karnezis AN, Cho KR, Gilks CB, et al. The disparate origins of ovarian cancers: Pathogenesis and prevention strategies. Nature Reviews. Cancer. 2017;**17**:65-74. DOI: 10.1038/nrc.2016.113

[22] Kurman RJ, Russell V, Junge J, et al. Papillary tubal hyperplasia: The putative precursor of ovarian atypical proliferative (borderline) serous tumors, noninvasive implants, and endosalpingiosis. The American Journal of Surgical Pathology. 2011;**35**:1605-1614. DOI: 10.1097/PAS.0b013e318229449f

[23] Wolsky RJ, Price MA, Zaloudek CJ, et al. Mucosal proliferations in completely examined fallopian tubes accompanying ovarian low-grade serous tumors: Neoplastic precursor lesions or normal variants of benign mucosa? International Journal of Gynecological Pathology. 2018;**37**:262-274. DOI: 10.1097/PGP.0000000000000410

[24] Horn LC, Angermann K, Hentschel B, et al. Frequency of papillary tubal hyperplasia (PTH), salpingoliths and transition from adenoma to borderline ovarian tumors (BOT): A systematic analysis of 74 BOT with different histologic types. Pathology, Research and Practice. 2017;**213**:305-309. DOI: 10.1016/j.prp.2017.02.001

[25] Singh N, Gilks CB, Hirschowitz L, et al. Primary site assignment in tuboovarian highgrade serous carcinoma: Consensus statement on unifying practice worldwide. Gynecologic Oncology. 2016;**141**:195-198. DOI: 10.1016/j.ygyno.2015.10.022

[26] Anglesio MS, Papadopoulos N, Ayhan A, et al. Cancer associated mutations in endometriosis without cancer. The New England Journal of Medicine. 2017;**376**:1835-1848. DOI: 10.1056/NEJMoa1614814

[27] Niguez Sevilla I, Machado Linde F, Marín Sánchez MDP, et al. Prognostic importance of atypical endometriosis with architectural hyperplasia versus cytologic atypia in endometriosis associated ovarian cancer. Journal of Gynecologic Oncology. 2019. DOI: 10.3802/jgo.2019.30.e63

[28] Tanase Y, Kawaguchi R, Uchiyama T, et al. Long-term follow up

after surgical management for atypical endometriosis: A series of nine cases. Case Reports in Oncology. 2019;**12**: 76-83. DOI: 10.1159/000496178

[29] Tanase Y, Furukawa N, Kobayashi H, et al. Malignant transformation from endometriosis to atypical endometriosis and finally to endometrioid adenocarcinoma within 10 years. Case Reports in Oncology. 2013;**6**:480-484. DOI: 10.1159/000355282

Chapter 4

Epigenetic Events in Ovarian Cancer

Yanisa Rattanapan and Takol Chareonsirisuthigul

Abstract

Epigenetic aberrations are now well established in the development and progression of ovarian cancer, including DNA methylation, histone modifications, and microRNA dysregulation, and their progressive accumulation is correlated with the progression of the stage grade of disease. Epigenetic aberrations are relatively stable, linked to various subtypes of the disease, and present in circulating serum, representing promising diagnostic, prognostic, and pharmacodynamic biomarkers. Unlike DNA mutations and deletions, aberrant gene-repressive epigenetic changes, including DNA methylation inhibitors or histone-modifying enzymes, are theoretically reversible by epigenetic therapies. While no action against solid tumors, including ovarian cancer, has been shown in epigenetic monotherapies, preclinical studies indicate that they may be successful when used in conjunction with one another or with conventional chemotherapy, and combinatorial epigenetic therapy regiments are being investigated in cancer clinical trials. Improved interventions against this debilitating malignancy will provide a greater understanding of epigenetics' role in ovarian cancer.

Keywords: ovarian cancer, epigenetic, miRNA, DNA methylation, histone modification

1. Introduction

Among gynecological malignancies, ovarian cancer, a molecularly heterogeneous condition associated with poorest prognosis. The highest mortality rates are associated with ovarian cancer, reflecting the third most prevalent cancer in female carcinomas of the gynecologic system. While it accounts for just 3% of all female cancers, the worldwide annual prevalence of ovarian cancer is 220,000, with 21,750 reported new cases and 13,940 estimated deaths annually [1]. Specific diagnosis in more than 70% of OC cases is a potent factor for high fatality rates at an advanced disease stage and carries a poor prognosis with current therapies. In ovarian cancer, the median age of disease diagnosis is 60 years and its lifetime incidence is one in seventy with estimated lifetime mortality of one in ninety-five [2, 3]. Epithelial ovarian cancer (EOC) accounts for 90% of all types of OC cases distinguished at histopathological, clinical, and molecular levels by heterogeneity. The precise cause of the malignancy of the ovaries is still unclear. Significant risk factors associated with OC have been identified as a strong family history of either ovarian or breast cancer. More than one-fifth (approximately 23%) of ovarian carcinomas have inherited susceptibility and have BRCA1 and BRCA2 tumor suppressor gene mutations [4].

Rapid growth, unspecific clinical symptoms at the early stage of the disease, and the absence of earlier diagnosis methods make it challenging to diagnose promptly due to lack of effective screening. As a result, when the tumor has spread beyond the pelvis and is unlikely to be entirely removed by surgery, EOC is usually diagnosed at an advanced stage (FIGO III/IV). Long-term survival rates are poor (10–30 percent for women with disseminated malignancies. However, an ovarian cancer diagnosis at the localized level is considerable curable (over 95 percent five-year survival rate; [5]). Therefore, it is needed to explore cost effective and sensitive screening program for early detections and biomarkers to predict disease behaviors and responses to therapies. In identifying promising biomarkers of clinical utility for early diagnosis of OC, a better understanding of the EOC genome portrait would benefit.

Altered epigenetic states are closely associated with tumorigenesis of the ovaries. Epigenetics is characterized as a heritable alteration in gene expression without the DNA sequence itself being altered and involves DNA methylation, histone modification, nucleosome repositioning, and micro-RNAs (miRNAs) posttranscriptional gene regulation [6, 7]. Cancer vulnerability is inherited, but most of this inheritability remains unknown. Epigenetic changes in the parental germ line that do not require transmission of genetic variants from parent to offspring may mediate such missing heritability. DNA methylation, the addition of a methyl moiety to the cytosine-5 location within the sense of a CpG dinucleotide, mediated by DNA methyltransferases (DNMTs), is the most studied epigenetic shift [6]. While most CpG sites are methylated in the human genome, CpG-dense regions known as CpG islands (often gene-associated) are usually unmethylated in normal tissue. Also, histone proteins associated with DNA are subject to extensive modifications that mediate the assembly of chromatin that is transcriptionally permissive or restrictive (i.e., open or closed). DNA methylation and histone modifications are now recognized to be closely related [6]. The complete epigenetic state corresponding to a particular cell phenotype (e.g., DNA methylation, histone modification, and miRNA expression) is now referred to as the epigenome [8]. Though repressive epigenetic changes (including DNA methylation) control genes in normal tissues (e.g., imprinted genes and inactivation of female X-chromosomes), they are dramatically altered in cancer [6, 9]. Global DNA hypomethylation and localized hypermethylation of promoter-associated CpG islands occur primarily in cancer cells, with the latter acting as a replacement for point mutations or deletions to induce transcriptional silencing of tumor suppressor genes [6].

2. DNA methylation in ovarian cancer

The substantial shortcomings of the therapies examined above in the treatment of ovarian cancer have set the stage for the use, either alone or in combination with other therapies, of novel epigenetic therapies to treat this disease. By adding a methyl group to stimulate regions of DNA to silence gene expression, the epigenetic alteration of DNA methylation controls gene expression. This mechanism is critical during sensitive cellular processes, such as embryonic development, inactivation of X-chromosomes, and genomic imprinting. The organ's normal development and maturation are determined by a precise balance of active and silenced genes [10]. On the other hand, cancer promotes global hypermethylation of CpG islands associated with promoters, which are typically unmethylated in normal tissue, silencing genes essential for cellular homeostases, such as genes suppress tumors. To promote tumorigenesis, aberrant DNA methylation and structural chromatin changes will alter gene expression [11]. A repressive and tightly woven chromatin structure is caused by DNA methylation, which can minimize gene expression in DNA repair, apoptosis, differentiation, drug resistance, angiogenesis, and metastasis. In cancer, gene promoters' hypermethylation causes the genes involved in cell cycle control, including BRCA1, CDKN2A, RASSF1A, LOTI, DAPK, ICAM-l, PALB2, RAD51C, and BRIP1 to be downregulated. Therefore, substantial loss of CpG hypermethylation in ovarian cancer is correlated with cancer cell growth inhibition [12].

In ovarian cancers, hypermethylation of particular gene promoters has been established. Compared to non-neoplastic tissues, promoter hypermethylation of tumor suppressors BRCA1 and RASSF1A were significantly higher in ovarian cancers [13]. This hypermethylation silences expression to suppress BRCA1 activity, driving genomic instability in ovarian cancers, analogous to the mutations in BRCA1 discussed earlier. RASSF1A encodes a protein controlling the cell cycle; silencing this gene promotes cell-cycle progression and unregulated cell development. Compared to benign cases, tissues from patients with serous and non-serous EOC display significantly higher RASSF1A promoter methylation. [14]. In clear-cell ovarian cancer, hypermethylation is also observed. 22 separate CpG loci associated with nine genes (VWA1, FOXP1, FGFRL1, LINC00340, KCNH2, ANK1, ATXN2, NDRG21 and SLC16A11) were hypermethylated. Inversely associated with tumor gene expression, multiple loci methylation, most notably KCNH22 (HERG, a potassium channel). Loss of KCNH2 (HERG) expression by methylation may be a good prognostic marker, provided that overexpression of the Eag family members of the potassium channel promotes increased proliferation and results in poor prognosis [15]. However, superficial cell carcinomas also suppress methylation of the gene encoding the HNF1B transcription factor, while this gene is methylated in high-grade serous ovarian cancers [16]. In invasive carcinomas, Makarla et al. found hypermethylation of eight cancer-related genes (p16, RARβ, E-cadherin, H-cadherin, APC, GSTP1, MGMT, and RASSF1A) was significantly higher compared to non-invasive cancers and benign cystadenomas [17].

3. Histone modification in ovarian cancer

Chromatin modifying enzymes are altered in ovarian cancers beyond DNA methylation. High levels of H3K9 methyltransferase G9a, which adds histone methyl groups (H3K9) to promote the compact structure of chromatin and silence genes, have been associated with late-stage high-grade and serous ovarian cancer, as well as shorter survival in patients with ovarian cancer [18]. Genes marked by the chromatin modifications of activating H3K4me3 and silencing H3K27me3 are identified as "poised" or bivalent; these are not transcribed into embryonic stem cells but resolved as differentiated stem cells into active and transcribed (H3K4me3) or silenced and not transcribed (H3K27me3). In 499 high-grade serous ovarian cancers, compared to eight normal fallopian tube samples, these bivalent chromatin loci were silenced and included genes in the PI3K and TGF-beta signaling pathways. Stem-like cells of ovarian cancer and chemo-resistant cells of ovarian cancer have demonstrated increased silencing of these genes [19]. As previously mentioned, the gene encoding the ARID1A chromatin remodeler is mutated in over 50 percent of ovarian clear cell carcinomas. In a mouse model of ovarian cancer, Bitler et al. showed inhibiting EZH2 methyltransferase, which adds the H3K27me3 mark to silence gene expression, induced regression of ARID1A-mutated tumors. This occurred via PIK3IPI upregulation, an ARID1A and EZH2 target increased by EZH2 inhibition and inhibits PI3K/Akt oncogenic signaling [20].

4. MicroRNA dysregulation in ovarian cancer

The most recently discovered epigenetic miRNAs represent ovarian tumors have recently become a phenomenon, and it was found to substantially up-regulate miR-199a, miR-200a, miR-200a, miR-214, and down-regulate miR-100 and, precisely, miR-100 and miR-214 to target the tumor suppressor, miR-214 was shown to PTEN and is associated with resistance to platinum [21, 22]. Let-7 miRNA family as one of the regulator of the MYCN pathway that linking to the platinum-resistant trait. It was recently discovered that miRNA let-7i was a tumor substantially down-regulated suppressor in platinum-resistant ovarian tumors, and restored let-7i gain-of-function chemoresistant ovarian cancer drug sensitivity cells, thus representing a biomarker and therapeutic candidate goal [23]. MiR-429, miR-200a, and miR-200b, respectively a single primary transcript was found to be clustered on epithelial-to-mesenchymal transition-regulated (EMT, a metastatic phenotype) ZEB1/SIP1 repressor, with negative regulation of miR-200a and miR-200b ZEB1/SIP1 and the development of a loop of double-negative feedback [24]. In another study, 27 miRNAs were substantially correlated with chemotherapy response, indicating a chemotherapy response miRNA (similar to DNA methylation) represent potential biomarkers for ovarian prognosis and diagnosis [25]. Regarding the regulation of miRNA genes, a group of six chromosomes, 19 miRNAs clustered on chromosome 19, and seven clusters were up-regulated on chromosome 14, DNMT-inhibitor decitabine inhibitor, showing that miRNAs can be controlled by DNA methylation [26]. What's more, an overall, collective tumor—MiRNAs' suppressive effect has been suggested by Drosha and Dicer down-regulation, involving two enzymes in the processing of miRNA, being significantly connected with an early stage of ovarian cancer and poor prognosis [27, 28].

5. Epigenetic biomarkers for ovarian cancer

As mentioned above, the development of ovarian cancer is well characterized by a range of combinatorial epigenetic aberrations distinct from this malignancy, including but not limited to RASSF1A, DAPK, H-Sulf-1, BRCA1, and HOXA10 DNA methylation. As a result, these methylated DNA sequences represent potential diagnostic, staging, prognostic, and therapy response monitoring (predictive biomarkers) biomarkers [29]. DNA methylation biomarkers have several advantages over other types of biomarkers, such as proteins, gene expression, and DNA mutations, including their stability, ability to amplify (thus greatly enhancing detection sensitivity), relatively low cost of the assessment, and restriction to small DNA regions (CpG islands) [30]. It also acts as a biomarker to predict response to platinum-based chemotherapy regimen and the poly-ADP ribose polymerase inhibitor (PARPi). In the future, DNA methylation tests of resected ovarian tumors are highly likely to be used to customize care individually, similar to the recently discovered predictive markers of non-small cell lung cancer in stage I [31]. While single-gene methylation evaluation lacks adequate specificity for ovarian cancer diagnosis, it is believed that multiple methylation biomarker panels will achieve the precision needed for widespread population screening [30, 32]. To that end, a panel of 112 methylated DNA markers was found to correlate progression-free survival with ovarian cancer [33].

6. Clinical trials of epigenetic therapeutic in ovarian cancer

DNA methylation inhibitor and HDAC inhibitor are cancer therapeutics, begins primarily as a treatment for hematological disorders in the early 2000s. The FDA approved 5-Azacytidine (AZA) and 5-aza-2′-deoxycytidine (decitabine) for myelodysplastic syndrome (MDS) in 2004 and 2006, while the HDAC suberoylanilide hydroxamic acid (SAHA) inhibitor was approved in 2006 for the treatment of persistent or cutaneous T cell lymphoma [34]. Epigenetic therapy was initially performed in a clinical trial. It was setting either alone or with the standard in combination care to resensitize either the tumor to anticancer treatment or avoid therapy resistance production. Ultimately, these medications have been tested against resilient OC tumors, like both SAHA and AZA clinical trials, ovarian cancer, which is platinum-resistant. Although there are no antitumors, the behavior was detected after SAHA treatment, and AZA demonstrated the partial reaction. Still, it was correlated with significant adverse effects such as tiredness and myelosuppression [35]. The HDAC inhibitor, in a related analysis Belinostat, was given to platinum-resistant patients with ovarian tumors. Still, they have similarly caused significant adverse reaction events such as thrombocytopenia, neutropenia, and vomiting, leading to the end of the analysis with no clinical advantage over conventional therapy [34]. Similarly, in a phase I study, the vorinostat pan-HDACi carboplatin or gemcitabine was administered despite the extreme hematological toxicities caused and caused observed partial response, leading to the termination of the study [36].

7. Future prospects

Exponential advancement in DNA methylation-based biomarker growth has been observed over the last decade. A variety of cfDNA and tissue-dependent screening assays have paved their way into clinics due to the consistency of DNA and methylation patterns. Several tests for early detection of colon, lung, and prostate cancer are commercial success based on DNA methylation biomarkers. New technologies that enable the rapid identification of methylation signatures directly from the blood can promote sample-to-respond solutions, allowing molecular diagnostics for the next-generation point of care. Besides, ongoing work on liquid biopsies together with the latest advanced technologies such as digital PCR, bisulfite sequencing, methyl immune precipitation coupled with next-generation sequencing, and methylation arrays together with advanced statistical data analysis will mitigate the complicated problems of non-invasive system creation by overcoming the existing challenges to precision medicine.

8. Conclusion

Ovarian cancer causes substantial morbidity and mortality. Owing to unspecific signs at the early stage of the disease, their appearance at an advanced stage, and poor survival, the difficulty of promptly diagnosing ovarian cancer at its early stage remains difficult. Improved methods of detection are, therefore, urgently needed. This chapter identifies the possible clinical usefulness of epigenetic signatures such as DNA methylation, modifications of histones, and microRNA dysregulation, which play an essential role in ovarian carcinogenesis and its use in the development of diagnosis, prognosis, and biomarkers for prediction. New treatment options separate from conventional treatment options chemotherapy that benefits from developments in the understanding of ovarian cancer pathophysiology to enhance performance, they are required. Recent work has shown that mutations in epigenetic regulator-encoding genes are mutated in ovarian cancer, driving tumorigenesis and drug resistance. Several of these modifiers of epigenetics for ovarian cancer treatment have emerged as promising drug targets.

Author details

Yanisa Rattanapan[1] and Takol Chareonsirisuthigul[2]*

1 School of Allied Health Sciences, Walailak University, Nakhon Si Thammarat, Thailand

2 Department of Pathology, Faculty of Medicine Ramathibodi Hospital, Mahidol University, Bangkok, Thailand

*Address all correspondence to: toptakol@gmail.com

References

[1] Siegel RL, Miller KD, Jemal A. Cancer statistics, 2020. CA Cancer J Clin. 2020;70(1):7-30. doi:10.3322/caac.21590

[2] Cannistra SA. Cancer of the ovary [published correction appears in N Engl J Med. 2005 Jan 6;352(1):104]. N Engl J Med. 2004;351(24):2519-2529. doi:10.1056/NEJMra041842

[3] Howe HL, Wu X, Ries LA, et al. Annual report to the nation on the status of cancer, 1975-2003, featuring cancer among U.S. Hispanic/Latino populations. Cancer. 2006;107(8):1711-1742. doi:10.1002/cncr.22193

[4] Ramus SJ, Harrington PA, Pye C, et al. Contribution of BRCA1 and BRCA2 mutations to inherited ovarian cancer. Hum Mutat. 2007;28(12):1207-1215. doi:10.1002/humu.20599

[5] Siegel R, Ward E, Brawley O, Jemal A. Cancer statistics, 2011: the impact of eliminating socioeconomic and racial disparities on premature cancer deaths. CA Cancer J Clin. 2011;61(4):212-236. doi:10.3322/caac.20121

[6] Jones PA, Baylin SB. The epigenomics of cancer. Cell. 2007;128(4):683-692. doi:10.1016/j.cell.2007.01.029

[7] Lopez J, Percharde M, Coley HM, Webb A, Crook T. The context and potential of epigenetics in oncology. Br J Cancer. 2009;100(4):571-577. doi:10.1038/sj.bjc.6604930

[8] Bernstein BE, Meissner A, Lander ES. The mammalian epigenome. Cell. 2007 Feb 23;128(4):669-81. doi: 10.1016/j.cell.2007.01.033. PMID: 17320505.

[9] Esteller M. Epigenetics in cancer. N Engl J Med. 2008;358(11):1148-1159. doi:10.1056/NEJMra072067

[10] Jones PA, Issa J-PJ, Baylin S. Targeting the cancer epigenome for therapy. Nat Rev Genet. 2016;15(17(10)):630-41.

[11] Nervi C, De Marinis E, Codacci-Pisanelli G. Epigenetic treatment of solid tumours: a review of clinical trials. Clin Epigenetics. 2015;7:127. Published 2015 Dec 10. doi:10.1186/s13148-015-0157-2

[12] Ahluwalia A, Yan P, Hurteau JA, et al. DNA methylation and ovarian cancer. I. Analysis of CpG island hypermethylation in human ovarian cancer using differential methylation hybridization. Gynecol Oncol. 2001;82(2):261-268. doi:10.1006/gyno.2001.6291

[13] Ibanez de Caceres I, Battagli C, Esteller M, et al. Tumor cell-specific BRCA1 and RASSF1A hypermethylation in serum, plasma, and peritoneal fluid from ovarian cancer patients. Cancer Res. 2004;64(18):6476-6481. doi:10.1158/0008-5472.CAN-04-1529

[14] Rattanapan Y, Korkiatsakul V, Kongruang A, et al. EGFL7 and RASSF1 promoter hypermethylation in epithelial ovarian cancer. Cancer Genet. 2018;224-225:37-40. doi:10.1016/j.cancergen.2018.04.117

[15] Cicek MS, Koestler DC, Fridley BL, et al. Epigenome-wide ovarian cancer analysis identifies a methylation profile differentiating clear-cell histology with epigenetic silencing of the HERG K+ channel. Hum Mol Genet. 2013;22(15):3038-3047. doi:10.1093/hmg/ddt160

[16] Shen H, Fridley BL, Song H, et al. Epigenetic analysis leads to identification of HNF1B as a subtype-specific susceptibility gene for ovarian cancer. Nat Commun. 2013;4:1628. doi:10.1038/ncomms2629

[17] Makarla PB, Saboorian MH, Ashfaq R, et al. Promoter hypermethylation profile of ovarian epithelial neoplasms. Clin Cancer Res. 2005;11(15):5365-5369. doi:10.1158/1078-0432.CCR-04-2455

[18] Hua KT, Wang MY, Chen MW, et al. The H3K9 methyltransferase G9a is a marker of aggressive ovarian cancer that promotes peritoneal metastasis. Mol Cancer. 2014;13:189. Published 2014 Aug 12. doi:10.1186/1476-4598-13-189

[19] Chapman-Rothe N, Curry E, Zeller C, et al. Chromatin H3K27me3/H3K4me3 histone marks define gene sets in high-grade serous ovarian cancer that distinguish malignant, tumour-sustaining and chemo-resistant ovarian tumour cells. Oncogene. 2013;32(38):4586-4592. doi:10.1038/onc.2012.477

[20] Bitler BG, Aird KM, Garipov A, et al. Synthetic lethality by targeting EZH2 methyltransferase activity in ARID1A-mutated cancers. Nat Med. 2015;21(3):231-238. doi:10.1038/nm.3799

[21] Iorio MV, Visone R, Di Leva G, et al. MicroRNA signatures in human ovarian cancer. Cancer Res. 2007;67(18):8699-8707. doi:10.1158/0008-5472.CAN-07-1936

[22] Yang H, Kong W, He L, et al. MicroRNA expression profiling in human ovarian cancer: miR-214 induces cell survival and cisplatin resistance by targeting PTEN [published correction appears in Cancer Res. 2008 Mar 1;68(5):1609]. Cancer Res. 2008;68(2):425-433. doi:10.1158/0008-5472.CAN-07-2488

[23] Yang N, Kaur S, Volinia S, et al. MicroRNA microarray identifies Let-7i as a novel biomarker and therapeutic target in human epithelial ovarian cancer. Cancer Res. 2008;68(24):10307-10314. doi:10.1158/0008-5472.CAN-08-1954

[24] Bracken CP, Gregory PA, Kolesnikoff N, et al. A double-negative feedback loop between ZEB1-SIP1 and the microRNA-200 family regulates epithelial-mesenchymal transition. Cancer Res. 2008;68(19):7846-7854. doi:10.1158/0008-5472.CAN-08-1942

[25] Boren T, Xiong Y, Hakam A, et al. MicroRNAs and their target messenger RNAs associated with ovarian cancer response to chemotherapy. Gynecol Oncol. 2009;113(2):249-255. doi:10.1016/j.ygyno.2009.01.014

[26] Zhang L, Volinia S, Bonome T, et al. Genomic and epigenetic alterations deregulate microRNA expression in human epithelial ovarian cancer. Proc Natl Acad Sci U S A. 2008;105(19):7004-7009. doi:10.1073/pnas.0801615105

[27] Merritt WM, Lin YG, Han LY, et al. Dicer, Drosha, and outcomes in patients with ovarian cancer [published correction appears in N Engl J Med. 2010 Nov 4;363(19):1877]. N Engl J Med. 2008;359(25):2641-2650. doi:10.1056/NEJMoa0803785

[28] Rattanapan Y, Korkiatsakul V, Kongruang A, Siriboonpiputtana T, Rerkamnuaychoke B, Chareonsirisuthigul T. MicroRNA Expression Profiling of Epithelial Ovarian Cancer Identifies New Markers of Tumor Subtype [published online ahead of print, 2020 Jul 22]. Microrna. 2020;10.2174/2211536609666200722125737. doi:10.2174/2211536609666200722125737

[29] Balch C, Huang TH, Brown R, Nephew KP. The epigenetics of ovarian cancer drug resistance and resensitization. Am J Obstet Gynecol. 2004;191(5):1552-1572. doi:10.1016/j.ajog.2004.05.025

[30] Laird PW. The power and the promise of DNA methylation markers. Nat Rev Cancer. 2003;3(4):253-266. doi:10.1038/nrc1045

[31] Brock MV, Hooker CM, Ota-Machida E, et al. DNA methylation markers and early recurrence in stage I lung cancer. N Engl J Med. 2008;358(11):1118-1128. doi:10.1056/NEJMoa0706550

[32] Balch C, Montgomery JS, Paik HI, Kim S, Kim S, Huang TH, Nephew KP 2005 New anti-cancer strategies: epigenetic therapies and biomarkers. Front Biosci 10:1897-1931

[33] Wei SH, Balch C, Paik HH, et al. Prognostic DNA methylation biomarkers in ovarian cancer. Clin Cancer Res. 2006;12(9):2788-2794. doi:10.1158/1078-0432.CCR-05-1551

[34] Nervi C, De Marinis E, Codacci-Pisanelli G. Epigenetic treatment of solid tumours: a review of clinical trials. Clin Epigenetics. 2015;7:127. Published 2015 Dec 10. doi:10.1186/s13148-015-0157-2

[35] Fu S, Hu W, Iyer R, et al. Phase 1b-2a study to reverse platinum resistance through use of a hypomethylating agent, azacitidine, in patients with platinum-resistant or platinum-refractory epithelial ovarian cancer. Cancer. 2011;117(8):1661-1669. doi:10.1002/cncr.25701

[36] Matulonis UA, Oza AM, Ho TW, Ledermann JA. Intermediate clinical endpoints: a bridge between progression-free survival and overall survival in ovarian cancer trials. Cancer. 2015;121(11):1737-1746. doi:10.1002/cncr.29082

Chapter 5

Genetics and Mutational Landscape of Ovarian Sex Cord-Stromal Tumors

Trang Nguyen, Trang Minh Tran, Yee Shen Choo, Maria Alexiadis, Peter J. Fuller and Simon Chu

Abstract

Ovarian sex cord-stromal tumors (SCST) are uncommon tumors accounting for approximately 8% of all ovarian malignancies. By far, the most common are granulosa cell tumors (GCT) which represent approximately 90% of SCST. SCST are also found in the hereditary syndromes: Peutz-Jeghers syndrome, Ollier disease and Maffucci syndrome, and DICER1 syndrome. Key genomic and genetic events contributing to their pathogenesis have been the focus of recent studies. Most of the genomic studies have been limited to GCT which have identified a number of recurring chromosomal abnormalities (monosomy and trisomy), although their contribution to pathogenesis remains unclear. Recurrent DICER1 mutations are reported in non-hereditary cases of Sertoli cell and Sertoli–Leydig cell tumors (SLCT), while recurrent somatic mutations in both the juvenile (jGCT) and adult forms of GCT (aGCT) have also been reported. Approximately 30% of jGCT contain a somatic mutation in the *gsp* oncogene, while a further 60% have activating mutations or duplications in the *AKT* gene. For aGCT, a well characterized mutation in the FOXL2 transcription factor (FOXL2 C134W) is found in the majority of tumors (primary and recurrent), arguably defining the disease. A further mutation in the human telomerase promoter appears to be an important driver for recurrent disease in aGCT. However, despite several studies involving next generation sequencing, the molecular events that determine the stage, behavior and prognosis of aGCT still remain to be determined. Further, there is a need for these studies to be expanded to other SCST in order to identify potential targets for personalized medicine.

Keywords: ovarian cancer, ovary, sex cord stromal tumor, Granulosa cell tumor, FOXL2 C134W, TERT, Sertoli-Leydig cell tumor, DICER1 mutation, transcriptomics, Whole Exome Sequencing

1. Introduction

Ovarian sex cord-stromal tumors (SCST) are a clinically significant group of uncommon neoplasms that represent approximately 8% of ovarian cancers. They are thought to arise primarily from the gonadal sex-cord (granulosa and Sertoli cells) and/or gonadal stromal cells (theca cells) [1]. Malignant ovarian tumors are a group of morphologically, genetically and functionally distinct diseases, but associated with the same organ, the ovary. Epithelial ovarian cancers (EOC)

- A. Granulosa-stromal cell tumors
  - 1. Granulosa cell tumor
    - a. Adult granulosa cell tumor
    - b. Juvenile granulosa cell tumor
  - 2. Tumors in the thecoma-fibroma group
    - a. Thecoma
      - i. typical
      - ii. luteinized
    - b. Fibroma
    - c. Unclassified
- B. Sertoli–Leydig cell tumors
  - 1. Well-differentiated
    - a. Sertoli cell tumor
    - b. Sertoli cell tumor with lipid storage
    - c. Sertoli–Leydig cell tumor (tubular adenoma with Leydig cells)
  - 2. Moderately differentiated
  - 3. Poorly differentiated (sarcomatoid)
  - 4. Retiform with heterologous elements
- C. Gynandroblastoma
- D. Unclassified

[a]*Adapted from Scully [1] and the 2014 WHO classification [3].*

Table 1.
Histological classification of ovarian sex cord-stromal tumors[a].

represent the majority of ovarian cancers (accounting for 85–90%), the other two primary classifications are the SCST and the rarer germ cell tumors [2]. Ovarian SCST are primarily classified histologically as granulosa cell tumors (GCT), Sertoli stromal tumors and SCST of mixed or unclassified cell type, theca-fibroma. In the most recent World Health Organization (WHO) classification of female reproductive tract tumors, SCSTs are separated into pure stromal, pure sex cord and mixed SCST [3] with the sub-classifications of these groups as shown in **Table 1**. GCT are the most common accounting for approximately 90% of all malignant SCST. The clinical and molecular features of GCT has been extensively reviewed by Jamieson and Fuller [2]. Although recurrent and advanced stage GCT are associated with a very high mortality [2], they remain a relatively neglected subset of tumors. The high mortality rate of advanced disease has not been helped by the tendency to group these ovarian cancers with EOC, and apply treatment regimens that are based on therapeutic approaches for EOC, rather than tailoring treatment to the specific SCST [2]. Thus, understanding the genetics and hence the biology of these distinct tumors has an immediacy beyond just understanding tumor biology, with targeted therapeutics urgently needed for women with SCST. In this review we will provide an overview of studies that explore insights into the genetics and genomics of these tumors, with the aim to seek to identify key unanswered questions.

2. Ovarian SCST: clinical, histology and functional aspects

2.1 Granulosa cell tumors

Granulosa cell tumors (GCT) of the ovary are the most common type of SCST, accounting for approximately 5% of all ovarian cancers [4]. GCT are subdivided into two types: the more common adult (aGCT) and the rarer juvenile (jGCT) form. The jGCT subtype represents approximately 5% of all GCT. The two subtypes have different etiologies, and classification for either are not based on age alone as either tumor type can occur at any age. GCT arise from the granulosa cells (GC) of the ovarian follicle, and exhibit many features of normal GC, including expression of the follicle stimulating hormone (FSH) receptor gene, estrogen synthesis, ERβ expression, inhibin subunit expression with synthesis of biologically active inhibin, and anti-Müllerian hormone (AMH) expression [2]. Their presentation may include endocrine manifestations such as features of estrogen excess in prepubertal girls and postmenopausal women. The gonadal peptides inhibin and anti- Müllerian hormone (AMH) can be used in diagnosis and more specifically as tumor markers [2]. Studies from our laboratory as well as those of others have examined gene expression and signaling pathways involved in GC development, and have provided compelling support that not only are GC the cell type of origin for GCT, but that GCT also have consistent features with proliferating GC of the early antral follicle [5].

GCT are classified as low-grade malignancies, that are commonly detected at an early stage, providing a relatively favorable prognosis due to their overt clinical symptoms and indolent course. However, GCT have an unusual propensity for fatal late relapse, ~80% of women with aggressive or recurrent tumors will succumb to the disease [6]. At present, there are no standard methods for predicting relapse, no efficacious targeted therapies (aside from surgery) and no comprehensive understanding of the exact etiology of this disease.

2.2 Fibromas

Ovarian fibromas are the most common benign solid ovarian tumors, they represent 4% of all ovarian tumors. They are well-circumscribed masses that encompass spindle-shaped fibroblastic cells and abundant collagen bundles [1]. Ovarian fibromas can occur at any age but usually after menopause and rarely before 30 years old. The most common recommended treatment is surgery [7, 8]. However, preoperative diagnosis is often difficult due to their solid nature and the lack of specific clinical signs which can result in misdiagnosis as uterine myoma [8, 9]. Ovarian fibromas can also be associated with hydrothorax and ascites causing Meigs' syndrome, a rare condition which is usually misdiagnosed as a malignant myoma [9, 10].

2.3 Thecomas

Ovarian thecoma was first described by Loeffer and Priesel in 1932 who observed that these tumors resembled thecal cells, lutein cells and fibroblasts [11]. Thecoma accounts for 0.5% - 1% of all ovarian cancers. It occurs in mostly postmenopausal women with a mean age of 59 years with only 10% of patients younger than 30 years [12]. Thecomas can be divided into two main types; typical or luteinized, which are thecomas that contain steroid-type cells resembling luteinized theca and stromal cells [12]. The most common symptom experienced by patients is postmenopausal bleeding [13]. The tumors range in size from small to solid masses larger than 15cm [12]. Burnandt *et al.*, found that thecoma tumors were all unilateral; the tumors are well circumscribed and rarely encapsulated, and are often described as yellow-tan, yellow-white or grayish white with no evidence of hemorrhage or necrosis [13].

2.4 Sertoli–Leydig cell tumors

Sertoli–Leydig cell tumors (SLCT) also called androblastomas and arrhenoblastomas, exhibit cellular and molecular markers consistent with a dysgenesis of the ovarian stromal cells, reminiscent of disorders of gonadal dysgenesis [14]. They are rare, accounting for less than 0.5% of all ovarian cancers [3] and can occur in women of all age groups, but they are more often encountered in women under 40 years of age [15]. Patients usually present with symptoms related to androgen excess but can also present with estrogenic manifestations or have an asymptomatic clinical profile. SLCT are typically unilateral tumors and over 97% are diagnosed at Stage 1 [3, 15]. The prognosis is correlated with the degree of differentiation and stage of the tumor with the five year survival rate of well differentiated SLCT being ~100% [3]. In contrast to GCT, patients with SLCT relapse early, approximately two to three years following initial diagnosis [16]. Many SLCT are associated with somatic or germline mutations in a gene encoding an RNase III endoribonuclease, DICER1, which is involved in the generation of microRNAs (miRNAs) that modulate gene expression at the post-transcriptional level [17–20]. Some studies have reported that 60% of SLCT harbor a DICER1 mutation [21], whereas others have reported that up to 97% of SLCT are DICER1 related [22]. It has been suggested that up to 100% of moderately and poorly differentiated SLCT have DICER1 mutations [17]. A whole exome sequencing study of 17 Chinese patients found somatic mutations in CDC27 (52.6%), DICER1 (21.1%) and MUC22 (21.1%) [23]. Germline and somatic mutations of DICER1 were higher in patients who were younger than 18 years than those in older patients [23].

Taking into consideration that the majority of patients presenting with SLCT are premenopausal with well differentiated tumors at an early stage, fertility sparing surgery with the removal of the affected ovary is recommended [21]. More aggressive surgery and chemotherapy is considered in patients with advanced stage or stage 1 patients with the presence of risk factors such as intermediate and poorly differentiated tumors, heterologous elements, increased mitotic rate, rupture or spillage of the tumor or presence of metastatic tumor [16].

2.5 Gynandroblastomas

The term gynandroblastoma was coined in 1930 by Robert Meyer, who deemed them as an extremely rare variant of SCST comprising of both ovarian (granulosa cell) and testicular (Sertoli cell) histological features [24]. These low-grade hormonally active tumors may also exhibit morphological evidence of stromal theca cells and luteinized cells resembling Leydig cells [24]. Since their first description, only a further 29 cases have been documented [25]. Based on the exceedingly low prevalence of gynandroblastomas, it appears they have a relatively benign disease course [26].

Currently, molecular insights into the histogenesis and pathogenesis of gynandroblastomas are lacking, but it has been postulated that they originate from a single progenitor cell that undergoes differentiation into both female and male elements [27]. This tumor type also shares many clinicopathologic features with other SCST including GCT and SLCT, as previously reported by Jang et al. [26]. Patients typically present with hormonal dysfunction with either estrogenic or androgenic symptoms [28].

The diagnostic criteria for this tumor type stipulate that either Sertoli-Leydig or granulosa cells should comprise at least 10% of the entire tumor mass [29]. There are several sex cord-stromal cell related immunohistochemical markers that exists to facilitate differential diagnoses including inhibin, calretinin, SF1 and CD56, however these are not specific to gynandroblastomas [29]. Other useful diagnostic markers include MART-1/melan-A [30] (specific to Sertoli-Leydig cell and steroid cell tumors), and the cell regulatory protein 14–3-3 sigma [28] (specific to GCT and steroid cell tumors). Further characterization of the molecular pathways mediating the development of gynandroblastomas as well as comprehensive histologic and genetic studies are required.

3. Hereditary syndromes associated with ovarian SCST

3.1 Peutz-Jeghers syndrome

Peutz-Jeghers syndrome (PJS) is associated with ovarian SCST that have histological appearance that is intermediate between GCT and SLCT [31]. The majority of cases are caused by autosomal dominant germ line mutations in the *STK11/LKB1* (serine/threonine kinase 11/liver kinase B1) gene on chromosome 19p13.3 [32, 33]. It carries a lifetime risk of 21% [32].

LKB1 activates AMP kinase (and its 13 superfamily members), regulating multiple biological processes such as cell polarity, cell cycle arrest, embryo development, apoptosis, and bioenergetics metabolism. LKB1 has become recognized as a critical tumor-suppressor gene that is frequently mutated in a broad spectrum of human cancers. As a tumor suppressor, a number of studies have shown the contributions of the genetic loss of LKB1 to tumorigenesis. The role of LKB1 in controlling cell metabolism through AMPK signaling has been widely documented. The LKB1-AMPK axis controls lipid and glucose metabolism, and acts as a negative regulator of the Warburg effect with the consequence of suppressing tumor growth [34]. Patients with PJS present with gastrointestinal hamartomata, polyposis and both benign and malignant tumors of various organs together with pigmentation of the lips, buccal mucosa and digits [35]. Neither loss of heterozygosity (LOH) at chromosome 19p13.3 nor mutations in the *LKB1* gene have been observed in sporadic ovarian SCST [36, 37].

3.2 Ollier disease and Maffucci syndrome

Ollier disease (OD) and Maffucci syndrome (MS) are both subtypes of enchondromatosis and are considered rare nonhereditary skeletal disorders [38–44], with an estimated prevalence of 1 in 100,000 individuals [45]. They are characterized by multiple enchondromas (benign cartilaginous tumors) and when accompanied with additional subcutaneous soft tissue hemangioma, the condition is referred to as MS [45, 46]. Both disorders can lead to swollen extremities, joint deformities, limitations in joint mobility, scoliosis, and other bone anomalies [47].

OD and MS have been linked to ovarian jGCT, the first reported case of this association dates to 1972 [48], and since that time, a further 16 additional cases have been documented [49, 50]. In 2011 Amary *et al.* demonstrated that >90% tumor patient samples with OD/MS harbored somatic missense mutations in the isocitrate dehydrogenase (IDH) 1 and 2 genes, 65% of which encodes a R132C amino acid substitution on exon 4 [51, 52]. The mutant IDH gene produces the potential 'oncometabolite' 2-hydroxyglutarate (2-HG) which induces histone hypermethylation [45, 51, 53]. The role of either the mutant IDH variant or 2-HG in the pathogenesis of OD/MS needs to be further explored, however they may represent an early post-zygotic event which has implications in tumorigenesis [51, 54].

4. Genomic changes in ovarian SCST

As previously mentioned, studies of changes at a genomic level in ovarian SCST have largely been restricted to aGCT. In contrast to EOC, GCT have a relatively stable karyotype [55]. Cytogenetic analysis [56] and comparative genomic hybridization (CGH) [57] studies have revealed trisomy of chromosomes 12 and 14 in approximately one third of aGCT cases and a similar percentage of monosomy of chromosome 22 [56, 57]. Between 5% and 20% of aGCT are aneuploid, however, neither the karyotype nor ploidy provides prognostic information [56, 58–60]. Mutations of lesser frequency have been observed at other loci, again providing no prognostic significance.

In a study by Caburet *et al.*, who applied CGH to a panel of aGCT, as well as collating data from a total of 94 aGCT from previous studies [61], they observed that a total of 64 tumors had large-scale chromosomal changes. Supernumerary chromosomes 8, 9, 12 and 14 were reported, with the latter being very common (25 of 64). Partial or complete loss of chromosomes 1p, 13p, 16, 11 and 22, with monosomy 22 were also very common (36 of 64). There was co-occurrence of chromosomal alterations although there was only a statistically significant non-random association for +14 with −22 and + 7 with −16q. Further, Caburet *et al.* combined transcriptomic data from a previous study [62], seeking to identify gene copy number changes that may reflect putative driver changes in the pathogenesis of aGCT [61]. Twenty genes were identified from the regions of chromosomal imbalance with a plausible, pathological role across nine chromosomes (1, 5, 11, 12, 14–17, 22) including the *AKT1* gene being the most frequently amplified (6 of 10 tumors) and the nuclear receptor, rev-erbAα being the second most frequent (5 of 10 GCT). The latter is consistent with the findings of our previous study examining gene expression of all 48 nuclear receptors in aGCT [63]. Caburet *et al.* also sought to identify recurrent 'broken' genes (the presence of a mapping breakpoint within the genes in two or more tumors). They observed that five genes fitted this criterion on 5 different chromosomes. The authors [61] speculated on the potential of these genes in driving the pathogenesis of GCT, while recognizing the limitation of the study where the correlation set comprised of only ten aGCT, nine of which were stage one disease [61].

For other SCSTs, reports of cytogenetic analyses are extremely scarce. A recent clinical case report describes three patients, from two unrelated families, with 14q32 deletions encompassing the DICER1 locus. Two of these patients have a history of DICER1-related tumors, including a 15-year-old female with a SLCT [64]. For thecoma-fibromas, a report by Streblow *et al.* found that trisomy 12 is a non-random chromosomal abnormality, while gain of chromosome 9 and loss of chromosome 4 and/or 9 were features of fibromas [65]. Loss of chromosome 9 copy number in a subset of the fibromas analyzed is noteworthy because of the association of ovarian fibromas and Gorlin-Goltz syndrome or nevoid basal cell carcinoma [66]. Gorlin-Goltz syndrome is an autosomal dominant disorder featuring distinctive congenital malformations and a predisposition to a variety of benign and malignant neoplasms, including ovarian fibroma [67]. The gene for Gorlin-Goltz syndrome, PTCH1, has been localized to 9q22.3 and is characterized as a tumor suppressor gene encoding for a transmembrane protein that functions as a receptor for sonic hedgehog [68]. LOH of one chromosome 9 homolog in three non-syndromic ovarian fibromas suggests a somatic role of the *PTCH1* tumor suppressor gene in these neoplasms. Additional studies of sporadic and syndromic ovarian tumors of the thecoma-fibroma group using other approaches may expose an even higher frequency of *PTCH1* loss or mutation.

4.1 Somatic genetics of jGCT

Juvenile GCT (jGCT), as with aGCT, exhibit macroscopically a mixture of solid and cystic components with hemorrhagic areas. Thus, it is difficult to differentiate jGCT and aGCT by radiologic and morphologic findings. However, their histology differs from aGCT with a follicular or diffuse pattern of larger luteinized cells [69]. JGCT follicles have various sizes and shapes containing basophilic secretions. The cells have rich eosinophilic and/or vacuolated cytoplasm (indicating luteinization) and indistinct cell borders. They contain round, hyperchromatic or markedly bizarre nuclei which lack the nuclear grooving characteristic of aGCT [2, 69]. Unlike aGCT, Call- Exner bodies are not a feature of jGCT. The mitotic rate is high with marked nuclear atypia [2, 26]. Although the histologic appearances are therefore more 'aggressive' than for aGCT, the prognosis is generally better. The distinction between aGCT *vs* jGCT is therefore primarily based on the histology.

This by itself can create diagnostic dilemmas, however, these are increasingly being resolved by the use of the molecular markers, which are discussed below [70–72].

The gene expression profile of GCT are similar to an FSH-primed proliferating preovulatory GC [5]. FSH stimulation of GC growth is mediated by the FSH receptor, a G-protein-coupled, seven-transmembrane domain receptor. We and others have hypothesized that activation of these pathways, perhaps through activating mutations in these signaling molecules of the FSH signaling pathway, may play a role in the pathogenesis of GCT as is common in other endocrine tumors [2]. Despite extensive investigations, this does not appear to be the case for aGCT. However, mutations were found in the *gsp* oncogene in approximately 30% of jGCT [73]. The activating mutations at position 201 of the stimulatory alpha-subunit of the heterotrimeric G-protein ($G\alpha_s$), which couples with seven-transmembrane domain receptors such as the FSH receptor, have been reported as somatic mutations in pituitary, thyroid and adrenal tumors as well as being the inherited mutation in the McCune–Albright syndrome [74]. In jGCT, the mutation is either R201C or R201H, and reported to be associated with a poorer prognosis [73].

In addition, it has been postulated that as the FSH receptor signals through the oncoprotein AKT, that mutations in this signaling pathway may contribute to the pathogenesis of jGCT [75]. Indeed, in one study, >60% of jGCT had an in-frame duplication of the plekstrin-homology domain leading to activation of AKT1. Other AKT1 point mutations of uncertain significance were also observed in jGCT. It was speculated that the resulting mutated AKT1 proteins are hyperactive with increased membrane association of AKT1, resulting in constitutive FOXO3 repression [75]. A subsequent study using transcriptomic analyses found that the changes in gene expression in these tumors may reflect a limited set of transcription factors altered by AKT1 activation [76].

4.2 Somatic genetics of aGCT

Many cancers develop from somatic mutations in driver genes that occur sporadically during replication or as a result of environmental factors and are not inherited. It is therefore important for the development of new therapeutic techniques to identify and consider how somatic mutations accumulate in caner genomes. In 2009, Shah *et al.* described a somatic missense mutation in the *FOXL2* gene that was found in >97% of aGCT examined [55]. Their approach utilized whole transcriptome paired-end RNA-sequencing (RNA-Seq) to analyze four aGCT. They identified a somatic missense mutation in codon 134 (402C → G) that results in the substitution of a highly conserved cysteine residue by tryptophan. Numerous studies, including our own (reviewed in Ref. [2]), have confirmed this finding [55]. Both heterozygosity and hemi-homozygosity of this mutation are also reported [2, 55]. The mutation is unique to aGCT and has not been observed in jGCT [2]. The rare exceptions to this rule appear either to be mixed tumors in which elements are in fact of GC origin or the occasional tumor which truly is 'the exception to the rule' [70].

The presence of the FOXL2 C134W mutation provides a clear distinction between jGCT and aGCT. In jGCT, FOXL2 expression is low or absent [70, 77], whereas in aGCT expression levels in tumors bearing the mutation are generally consistent with levels seen in the normal ovary [70]. FOXL2 expression in heterozygous tumors appears equivalent for the wild-type and mutant FOXL2 alleles. In jGCT, low or absent expression of FOXL2 is associated with aggressive disease and carries a poor prognosis. The presence of the FOXL2 C134W mutation provides a molecular diagnosis of aGCT which has proven helpful in resolving the diagnosis of aGCT in histologically ambiguous or problematic cases [70–72].

FOXL2 plays a fundamental and essential role in ovarian development; its biology has been extensively studied [78–80]. It is a member of the forkhead box (FOX) family of evolutionarily conserved transcription factors. The C134W mutation is predicted to lie close to, but not in the DNA-binding domain [55]. Despite an extensive understanding of the biology of FOXL2 [78–80], the mechanisms of the tumorigenesis mediated by this somatic mutation in aGCT remain to be clearly established. *In vitro* evidence indicates that it impacts both steroidogenesis and apoptosis in GC [79]. In addition, post-translational modifications (sumoylation, phosphorylation, acetylation and ubiquitinylation) may also play a critical role in the modulation of FOXL2 function [78, 79]. Kim *et al.* (45) reported increased phosphorylation of FOXL2 as a result of the C134W mutation, subsequently leading its ubiquitinylation and degradation. The mutation would likely impact on critical protein–protein interactions of FOXL2, but these remain to be clearly elucidated. Caburet *et al.* argues that FOXL2 is a tumor suppressor gene with loss-of-function being associated with malignancy, as is seen in jGCT, and therefore the C134W mutation compromises function rather than being associated with activation or gain of function [78]. Conversely, others have argued that FOXL2 may act as a tumor suppressor gene in jGCT but the FOXL2 C134W mutation may be oncogenic in aGCT [80]. It's role is likely to be more complex than a simple loss-of-function, as one would speculate that other inactivating mutations in the FOXL2 gene would have been identified in aGCT [2]. It may be reminiscent of the DICER1 mutation in SLCT where one facet of DICER function is selectively lost [81]. It is also curious that aGCT express the wild-type FOXL2 allele at equivalent levels to the mutant allele, a scenario which arguably affirms that the mutant FOXL2 must be 'dominant negative' if there is suppression of function.

Although the majority of aGCT are stage 1 tumors and cured by surgical resection, those who have advanced stage disease or recurrent disease carry a poor prognosis [2]. As the FOXL2 C134W mutation is present in the vast majority of all aGCT, it does not explain differences in stage or behavior. It may be, as with certain inherited mutations, e.g., the ret. proto-oncogene in medullary thyroid cancer [82], that the transition from 'hyperplasia' induced by the somatic mutation to frank malignancy requires a second independent hit. Evidence to date indicates that this second event may be less specific than the first. In the case of aGCT, the genomic changes described above may for instance reflect the 'second hit' that results in aggressive clonal expansion. The subsequent somatic mutations that presumably drive tumorigenesis, recurrence, aggressive behavior, transcoelomic spread and metastatic disease still remain to be fully elucidated.

4.3 The GCT transcriptome

Evidence provided by recent transcriptomic studies have elucidated the genes whose expression has been modified, in some instances, may reflect genomic rearrangements. Gene expression microarray was used by Benayoun *et al.* comparing 10 aGCT with two GC samples acquired during *in vitro* fertilization (IVF) egg retrieval [62]. In principle, IVF provides a ready source of 'normal' tissue to be used as a control, however, the limitation of this control is that the GC are collected after IVF cycles involving a hyperstimulation regimen with gonadotropin, and hence the GC being partially luteinized at the time of collection [5]. Thus, these controls do not reflect GCs from the proliferative phase [5]. The authors identified genes involved in cell proliferation and a decrease in expression of genes that promote apoptosis [62]. Interestingly, the group showed modulation of genes that are known to be FOXL2 targets. Genes typically down-regulated by FOXL2 but increased in this context, were those associated with tumorigenicity. Conversely, genes usually upregulated by FOXL2 and associated with apoptosis were down-regulated. Hence, it was suggested that the FOXL2 C134W mutation causes a partial loss-of-function suggesting it is a tumor suppressor gene. This notion is consistent with jGCT also lacking FOXL2 expression as previously mentioned [78].

Our laboratory has generated transcriptomic profiles between a cohort of six stage 1 and six stage 3 aGCT patients using a gene microarray approach to reveal significant differential gene expression between early and advanced stages. All of the aGCT samples were sequenced and also found to be heterozygous for the FOXL2 C134W mutation [83]. A total of 16 genes were reported as highly abundant in the advanced aGCT, with a further 8 genes found to be more highly expressed in the stage 1 aGCT (p value <0.05, >2fold-change). Curiously, two genes associated with malignancy were found to be highly expressed in the advanced stage aGCT, a member of the cytokine family called CXCL14 (chemokine C-X-C-motif ligand 14), and a multifunctional secretion protein called MFAP5 (microfibrillar-associated protein 5 transcript variant 1), which were 40- and 26-fold higher, respectively. Of the genes whose expression was high in the stage 1 aGCT, INSL3 (insulin-like 3 transcript variant 2) gene expression was 75-fold higher in stage 1 aGCT and provided robust discrimination of the two groups [83]. Whether INSL3 inhibits tumorigenesis or whether the diminished expression in advanced stage disease is simply a marker of de-differentiation of the tumor remains to be determined. Applying Gene Set Enrichment Analysis (GSEA) to these data sets [83] showed increased expression of genes on chromosome 7p15 in the stage 3 aGCT, which is consistent with the report of Lin *et al.* [57] found using CGH, gain of chromosome region 7p15-p21 in some aGCT samples.

4.4 The genomic landscape of GCT

Aside from the identification of the FOXL2 C134W mutation in GCT, there have been several studies that have aimed to identify genomic alterations through sequencing candidate genes and known oncogenes [2]. Genes commonly mutated in other malignancies such as p53, PI3K, RAS and BRAF, are not a feature in GCT, and thus, putative 'second-hit' mutations still remain to be identified. But specific. The approach taken by The Cancer Genome Atlas project (TCGA) where a defined cohort of tumors are subjected to a full suite of genomic analyses [84] has yet to be applied to aGCT or indeed to other ovarian SCST.

The critical challenge to be addressed as a precursor to both improved prognostication (predicting recurrence) and identification of GCT-specific therapeutic targets (to address the high mortality of advanced disease) is to identify the molecular drivers of GCT pathogenesis beyond the aetiologic FOXL2 mutation.

In our own whole exome sequencing (WES) study, DNA from 22 fresh frozen, FOXL2 C134W mutation-positive GCT (14 stage 1 and 8 stage 3) was sequenced [85]. The analysis identified on average 64 coding and essential splice-site variants in each tumor, however recurrent mutations were not identified in individual genes or in related genes. The genes that were identified to contain truncating (stop, gain or frameshift) mutations, essential splice site mutations, non-synonymous mutations and stop/loss mutations in the stage I (970 variants) and recurrent (434 variants) tumors, were subject to variant effect pathway analysis. The canonical pathways identified were linked to DNA replication and/or repair as might be expected in malignancy; and to signaling through the epidermal growth factor receptor (EGFR) family. We also identified a high frequency of a TERT promoter mutation (see below).

Hillman *et al.* [86] reported a comparable outcome for adult GCT subjected to WES [86], in a study that focused on truncating mutations of the histone lysine methyltransferase gene KMT2D (also known as MLL2) as a recurrent somatic event. They reported these mono-allelic KMT2D-truncating variants to be more frequent in recurrent (23%) compared with primary (3%) GCT when an expanded GCT cohort was examined. KMT2D is a tumor suppressor gene that is the target of frequent inactivating mutations in several tumor types, including medulloblastoma and lymphoma. Interestingly, these mutations did not correlate with loss of protein as determined by immunohistochemistry (IHC). We found heterozygous KMT2D frameshift variants in only three (2x stage 3) of 22 GCT in our cohort [85] and Zehir *et al.* (see below) reported two frameshift variants in 11 GCT [87]. Hillman et al. [86] did not determine the TERT promoter mutation status of their GCT cohort.

Zehir and colleagues determined the mutational landscape in tumors from 10,000 patients using their targeted MSK-IMPACT panel of 341 cancer associated genes; within this study, there were 11 FOXL2 mutation–positive GCT (two primary and nine "metastasis") [87]. They identified mutations in 17 (5%) of the 341 cancer-associated genes on the array in these GCT samples; in only four of these genes was the mutation also found in our WES study [85].

In a recent study by Pilsworth *et al.*, the authors used a combination of whole genome sequencing and targeted sequencing [88], and reported a similar frequency of KMT2D inactivating mutations as that of the Hillman *et al.* study [86] (10.8% compared to 13.9%). The difference between the two studies however was that in this study, there was no association of the KMT2D mutation with recurrence [88]. This is consistent with another published study [89] which also showed no association of this gene mutation with recurrent disease. The low frequency of this mutation in these studies as well as our own, suggests that they may be pathogenic driver mutation in only a subset of aGCT. Additional inactivating mutations were also identified in low frequency, including the candidate tumor suppressor gene WNK2 and a newly discovered protein called NLRC5, which has been linked to the regulation of cancer immune evasion [88].

In another study, TP53 mutations were identified in 9.1% of patients, with higher tumor mutational burden and mitotic activity [90]. These findings suggest that tumors harboring TP53 mutations may be a high-grade subgroup of aGCT. It is noteworthy however, that other studies have not observed mutations in TP53 at similar frequencies [2, 88].

Indeed, the lack of overlap in the mutational variants identified in these various studies is curious. Also, somewhat surprising is the very limited number of recurrent mutations in specific genes, given that, by many criteria [83, 91], including the pathognomonic mutation in the FOXL2 gene [70], GCT are remarkably homogenous. It is conceivable that the lack of clear driver mutations may indicate that the key drivers are: 1) as in other cancers, including endocrine cancers, gene fusion events (splice-variants and translocations) which contribute the "second hit"; or that in ~40% of GCT, TERT mutations are an important tumorigenic event with perhaps loss of KMT2D in a small subset.

4.5 TERT promoter mutation

Our WES study [85] confirmed the report, from Pilsworth et al., of a telomerase gene (TERT) promoter mutation [92]. The TERT gene encodes the catalytic subunit of telomerase; TERT transcriptional regulation is the limiting step in telomerase activity. Elongation and/or preservation of telomere length is regarded as a hallmark of cancer. Two hot-spot mutations in the telomerase promoter, -124C > T and -146C > T are commonly found in specific cancers: melanoma, glioblastoma, bladder cancer and thyroid cancer, but not in common epithelial cancers, such as breast and prostate [87]. Our analysis using targeted PCR identified 11 of 26 (i.e., 42%)

of the GCT in our analysis to be heterozygous for the -124C > T TERT promoter mutation - a frequency that matches the above cancers [87]. 29% of the stage 1 GCT were heterozygous for the mutation, while 67% of the stage 3 GCT contained the mutation [85]. The -124C > T mutation is also present in the aGCT-derived KGN cell line [85]. There are *in vitro* data that the two promoter mutations are not equivalent [93], suggesting that in GCT there is a tumorigenic advantage only for the -124C > T promoter mutation.

Increased telomerase activity appears also to be associated with cell proliferation independent of telomere lengthening [94]. TERT has been reported to interact with major oncogenic signaling pathways including c-MYC, NFκB, and Wnt/β-catenin. Of these, activation of NFκB signaling has been reported in the KGN cell line [91, 95] and p65 nuclear localization has been reported in GCT [96], although previous studies [85, 86, 88, 90] have not identified mutations in these pathways.

It has been noted that melanoma, glioma, and papillary thyroid and bladder carcinomas, all of which have a high frequency of TERT promoter mutations, are characterized by activation through BRAF or EGFR mutation of the MAPK signaling pathway [97]. This association is intriguing given this high frequency of the TERT promoter mutation in GCT and the suggestion from pathway analysis of the WES study linking one of the canonical pathways to signaling through the EGFR family [85]. The high incidence of the TERT promoter mutation in GCT, together with the correlation of the presence of this mutation with stage, suggests that the presence of the TERT promoter mutation, as in other tumors, may be of prognostic and/or pathogenic significance, and acquired during tumor progression after the initial FOXL2 driver mutation.

4.6 DICER1 syndrome

DICER1 syndrome is a rare inherited disorder that increases the risk of a variety of cancerous and non-cancerous tumors that occur in the lungs, kidneys, ovaries and thyroid. DICER1 syndrome results from germ-line mutations in the *DICER1* gene, located on chromosome 14, position q32.13, encodes an RNase III endoribonuclease which plays a critical role in processing micro(mi)RNA to their mature forms. DICER1 contains two highly conserved RNase III domains (RNaseIIIa and RNaseIIIb) which forms a catalytic dimer, creating a single processing center for dsRNA cleavage, with each RNase III domain cleaving one strand of the dsRNA resulting in miRNA named by their prime end origin (3p/5p miRNA) [98]. Germ line and somatic mutations in the *DICER1* gene have been described in ovarian SCST, predominantly for SLCT. DICER1 mutations were initially reported to cause familial pleuro-pulmonary blastoma, but have been subsequently found in a variety of tumors, including ovarian SLCT and in association with benign thyroid pathologies [20]. The mutations occur in approximately 60% of ovarian SLCT of which 80% are the p.E1705K mutation [19, 20]. DICER1 mutations are also seen in gynandroblastomas. They have not been associated with GCT or, testicular stromal tumors [19, 20, 72]. The functional consequence of DICER1 mutations is there is a bias caused by the mutated DICER toward processing of the RNasIIIa strand of the miRNA duplex [19, 81]. Thus, there is a selective reduction in RNaseIIIb activity and retention of RNaseIIIa activity, resulting in an excess of 3p-miRNA and a depletion of 5p-miRNA [19, 81, 98]. One copy of the altered gene is sufficient to cause an increased risk of developing tumors. Although a mutation in the DICER1 gene can infer an increased chance of developing SLCT, many individuals who carry a mutation in the DICER1gene do not necessarily develop tumors [99]. The therapeutic or diagnostic value of these mutations for SLCT warrants further investigations.

5.The 'miRNA-ome' and other non-coding RNAs

A pathogenic role for miRNA in SCST can be indicated by the identification of aberrant miRNA processing in SLCT and gynandroblastomas. However, studies of the 'miRNA-ome' have been limited. Rosario *et al.* profiled miRNA expression and regulation in the KGN and COV434 cell lines [100]. They observed that COV434 cells preferentially expressed miR-17 family members whereas the KGN cells preferentially expressed members of the let-7 miRNA gene family [100]. There has not however, been any systematic studies in GCT or, to our knowledge, for other SCST.

Long non-coding (lnc) RNA's have also been implicated in oncogenesis [101]. Evidence indicates that lncRNA can produce short peptides from small open reading frames (smORFs) which can regulate biological processes [102]. The status of both lncRNA, and indeed, smORFs remains to be investigated in SCST.

6. GCT-derived cell lines

The human KGN and COV434 cell lines, have been thought to be derived from GCT, and are extensively used in studies of GCT as well as to model normal GC function. Both cell lines exhibit some features that are reminiscent of normal proliferating GC, including a functional FSH receptor and aromatase activity. Jamieson *et al.* analyzed the FOXL2 status of both cell lines [70], concluding the COV434 cells lack FOXL2 expression and indeed the C134W mutation, lending to the assumption that they are derived from a jGCT [70]. In contrast, the KGN cell line (established from a metastatic aGCT), expresses FOXL2 and is heterozygous for the FOXL2 mutation, which is consistent with it being derived from an aGCT [70]. Both cell lines were established from patients with advanced aggressive disease.

Both KGN and COV434 cell lines are notable for constitutive activity of the NFκB and Braf/ERK signaling pathways [91, 95, 103]. A molecular study using a transcriptomic approach conducted by Rosario *et al.* was used to identify potential targets of FOXL2 in KGN and COV434 cells [104]. They observed that many of the genes regulated by wild-type FOXL2 were also regulated by the mutant FOXL2, notably genes involved in the transforming growth factor-beta (TGF-β) signaling pathway. Their analysis also highlighted the significant differences between the COV434 and the KGN gene-expression profiles [104]. In our transcriptomic analysis of aGCT [83], we observed over 3000 entities that differed greater than twofold (p value of <0.05) when 12 aGCT were compared with the KGN cells. This was in stark contrast to only 24 differentially expressed genes observed when comparing the stages 1 and 3 aGCT. Thus, although the two cell lines are valuable tools in the analysis of signaling pathways in the context of both GCT and indeed GC, they do not assist in the genomic and/or genetic analysis of aGCT.

The classification of COV434 as a GCT-derived cell line has been questioned. Recent studies show that this cell line was likely derived from a small-cell carcinoma of the ovary hypercalcemic-type (SCCOHT) [105–107]. The cell of origin of these tumors is unknown, with reports postulating they are likely derived from the germ cells [108]. Recent advances in molecular genetics have indicated that SCCOHT can be regarded as an ovarian malignant teratoid/rhabdoid tumor (MRT) [109]. SCCOHT are characterized by the loss of both SMARCA2 and SMARCA4, which are also not expressed in COV434 cells [105, 107]. Moreover, the lack of expression of RUNX2 and high expression of RUNX3 in COV434 suggests that these cells do not represent primary jGCT [106]. Noticeably, the study of Karnezis *et al.* indicates that COV434 cell line has all morphological, immunohistochemical, genetic and clinical characteristics of SCCOHT [107]. They also noted that the level of serum calcium in mice increases when transplanting with COV434 [107].

7. Animal models of ovarian SCST

A number of mouse models in which GCT arise have been reported, however none truly recapitulate the human disease [2, 110]. Liu *et al.* have described the development of GCT in mice with conditional inactivation of FOXO1/3 in GC [110]. The development of these tumors was accelerated with perturbation of the multi-functional tumor suppressor gene PTEN. An examination of PTEN and FOXO1/3 expression in five primary human aGCT samples found low expression for each [110], leading them to conclude that this mouse model, in contrast to others, shares some characteristics with aGCT. Arguably however, involvement of PTEN in the model, is more consistent with activation of PI3K/AKT which is more of a feature of jGCT. It should be noted that neither mutation, over-expression of PIK3CA or PIK3R1, nor loss of expression of PTEN, has been reported in aGCT [111]. Work from Lague *et al.* has provided evidence in mouse models for a synergistic effect of the Wnt/β-catenin and PI3K/AKT pathways in the formation of GCT, which is of interest given the potential role for AKT1 mutations in jGCT [112]. Wnt/β-catenin signaling pathway has well established roles in ovarian development and in GC function [2]. Although dysregulation of Wnt/β-catenin signaling has been identified in many human cancers, there is no evidence for activation of this pathway in human GCT [113, 114], which contrasts to equine GCT where there is clear evidence of Wnt/β-catenin signaling activation [113]. Increased ovarian R-spondin1 signaling, which modulates Wnt signaling is associated with GC-like tumors [115]. Gao *et al.* targeted expression of a constitutively activated TGF-β receptor to GC and found GCT that were associated with elevated inhibin and estrogen levels [116] as is seen in human GCT which perhaps more closely recapitulates the clinical situation than earlier models in which inhibin gene deletion resulted in GCT (see below) [117]. One of the downstream consequences of this activation is again, increased AKT signaling. The knockout of the inhibin α subunit (shared by both inhibin A and B) causes the development of SCST in mice of both sexes as early as four weeks [117–119]. In these inhibin α null mice, FSH levels has increased by two to three fold which correspond to inhibin's physiological function to suppress FSH [118]. However, a double knockout of inhibin α and FSH unexpectedly showed development of gonadal tumors in the mice; the tumors developed after 12 weeks of age [117–121]. The inhibin α knockout led to increasing levels of activin which induce the activation of SMAD2/3 signaling pathway in GC [117, 121]. The study of Madh3 (SMAD3-null) and inhibin α double knockout mice demonstrated slow progression of tumor growth; SMAD 3 is thus important for tumor progression [121–123].

8. Treatment strategies for SCST

The uncommon nature of SCST limits the ability to develop targeted therapies and evaluate them in well-powered clinical trials. A recent search of clinicaltrials.gov showed only 11 trials that are either active of recruiting involving SCSTs, with only five completed results described. The application of new sequencing technologies may lead to the discovery of novel driver genes that lead to these rare ovarian cancers. However, as discussed above, these have so far been elusive from the limited studies performed to date.

8.1 Treatment of GCT

Surgical treatment is the mainstay for peri-and postmenopausal women diagnosed with aGCT, with total abdominal hysterectomy (TAH), bilateral salpingo-oophorectomy (BSO) and full staging surgery thought to be the most appropriate initial treatment [124]. Randomized trials of adjuvant chemotherapy are not available, and for patients with poor prognosis, adjuvant platinum-based chemotherapy is generally considered either alone or in combination with doxorubicin and cyclophosphamide (CAP) [125, 126], vinblastine and bleomycin (PVB) [127], etoposide or etoposide and bleomycin (BEP) [128, 129]. The use of these treatment regimens is often based on those employed for epithelial ovarian cancer and in the main have proven to be of limited benefit [130].

Hormone treatment has shown promise in the treatment of advanced GCT based on their frequent estrogen dependence [2, 131, 132]. A systematic review of hormonal therapy for GCT revealed a pooled response rate of 71% and aromatase inhibitors (AI) were identified by far the most effective agents [131]. In a more recent study, the use of AI in 25 cases with known outcomes, the response rate to AIs was 48% (12/25) and the clinical benefit rate was 76% (19/25) [132]. Although these numbers are limited, they indicate the use of AIs as a potential alternative to chemotherapy, although the mechanisms involved in GCT sensitivity to AIs remains undefined. Other forms of hormone therapy have also previously shown promise with reports of prolonged remission (14–42 months) documented in patients with extensive disease treated with high doses of medroxyprogestroneacetate [133, 134].

The expression of vascular endothelial growth factor (VEGF) appears persistent with most GCT, with almost all tumors (93%) showing positive VEGF immunostaining in one study [135, 136]. The use of the anti-VEGF-A monoclonal antibody, bevacizumab, was shown to cause apoptosis in GCT-derived cells *in vitro* [136]. Extending this to a small retrospective study showed promising activity with bevacizumab in 8 women with recurrent GCT [137]. There was one complete response in an overall response rate of 38%, with the clinical benefit rate being 63%. Bevacizumab is also effective in treating ascites in recurrent GCT, reflecting the role of tumor-derived VEGF in the formation of cancer-related ascites [138]. This led to a prospective phase II clinical trial of bevacizumab in relapsed aGCT which reported a 16.7% response rate and median progression free survival of 9.3 months (95% CI 4.1–15 months) in the 36 patients recruited [139].

Tyrosine kinases are well recognized as being fundamental to many growth factor signaling pathways in both normal and malignant cells. The advent of specific inhibitors of tyrosine kinases (TKI) has focused attention on the potential of TK as therapeutic targets. In view of the evidence of activation of cell signaling in GCT and a case report of a recurrent GCT responding to the TKI, imatinib (Gleevec), our group demonstrated that the GCT-derived cell lines were inhibited by imatinib and indeed by the newer more potent analog, nilotinib, but at concentrations higher than those required for the targeted receptor kinases [140]. The AP-1 signaling pathway is also constitutively activated in GCT [95]. We tested a TKI, sorafenib (Nexavar, Bayer), which has high affinity for Raf-1 and Braf, in addition to the above-mentioned TK, and found that this TKI elicits a dose dependent inhibition of both cellular proliferation and viability in both cell lines at concentrations equivalent to that seen in other systems [141]. A commercially available Raf-1 kinase inhibitor was also examined and found to have no effect on cell proliferation and viability in both cell lines, thus implicating Braf in the activated AP-1 signaling [141]. Based on these data, clinical investigation of sorafenib or possibly a more potent BRAF inhibitor, such as vemurafenib or dabrafenib, may be warranted.

Little is known about the immune response in SCST. Expression of the immune checkpoint protein, programmed death-ligand 1 (PD-L1) has been reported only in abstract form, and present in ~75% of SCSTs [142], however, immunotherapy has not been reported in a clinical trial for these tumors. A more recent study by Pierini et al., suggests that tumor infiltrating lymphocytes (TILS) are the main immune population in GCT [143], and that after *ex vivo* expansion of TILS isolated from 11 GCT patients, showed they vigorously reacted against autologous tumors (100% patients) and against FOXL2 peptides (57.1% of patients). This suggests that FOXL2 immune targeting can produce substantial long-term clinical benefits and lay a foundation for future trials testing immunotherapeutic approaches toward GCT [143].

Based on several studies, there is also the potential for more targeted therapies that arise from identifying the molecular mechanisms that contribute to the pathogenesis of GCT. The NFκB signaling pathway is often involved in cancer development; activated NFκB increases the expression of genes involved in cell proliferation, metastasis, angiogenesis and anti-apoptosis [144]. Apoptosis is directed by activated caspases. The Inhibitors of Apoptosis (IAP) proteins suppress apoptosis through the inhibition of the caspases. The cellular IAP1 (cIAP1 or BIRC2), cellular IAP2 (cIAP2 or BIRC3) and X chromosome-linked IAP (XIAP or BIRC4) are the main IAPs with known roles in apoptosis and cancer [145–147]. XIAP is the best characterized and also the most potent caspase inhibitor, blocking both intrinsic and extrinsic apoptotic signals by directly inhibiting caspases-3, −7 and − 923. cIAP1 and cIAP2 have less potent roles in opposing these pathways as they do not directly bind caspases, however they can indirectly cause caspase cleavage [145–147]. Inhibition of cIAPs and XIAP causes cells to become more receptive to both intra- and extracellular apoptotic signals [148]. XIAP is predominantly regulated by an endogenous mitochondrial protein called second mitochondria-derived activator of caspases (Smac), which is released during apoptosis, and interacts with XIAP through conserved amino acid residues in the BIR3 domain of XIAP to antagonize XIAP-mediated caspase inhibition [149].

Due to its elevated expression and prominent ability to inhibit cell death, XIAP is an attractive therapeutic target for anti-cancer treatment [145–147]. Smac-mimetics (SM) bind directly to XIAP with high affinity to prevent caspase binding, thus neutralizing XIAPs pro-oncogenic function. A number of Smac-mimetics have demonstrated good anti-cancer activity in preclinical studies, and several have already passed primary phase clinical trials, suggesting that these compounds are well tolerated [146]. Though XIAP, IAP or pan-IAP inhibitors have shown some efficacy as single agents, the majority of studies have shown more promise when used in a rational drug combination strategy [146]. We have shown *in vitro* and using GCT explants in culture, that targeting XIAP as a combination therapy with activation of the peroxisome proliferator-activated receptor-gamma protein (PPARγ) provides a novel and specific therapeutic strategy for GCT [150, 151]. It remains to be determined the effectiveness of this combination approach in *in vivo* studies.

9. Conclusions

Recent genetic discoveries have provided profound insights into the molecular pathogenesis of ovarian SCST. As with other uncommon tumor types, insight from research of SCST will potentially be prismatic; that is, it will help clarify molecular mechanisms involved in oncogenesis. In SLCT, the discovery of DICER1 mutations highlight both the complexity and asymmetry of miRNA processing, while also supporting the potential for 'non-coding' RNA in playing a critical role in malignant cancers. In the case of jGCT, the presence of the recurring mutations in the *gsp* oncogene and in AKT1, highlights the critical role of the cyclic AMP/protein kinase A and PI3kinase/AKT signaling pathways in hormone-mediated cell proliferation, as well as when constitutively activated, in malignancy. We and others have demonstrated that the FOXL2 C134W mutation found in aGCT would appear to be pathognomonic, however, the precise mechanism of this mutation still remains some-what controversial, despite being discovered over a decade ago. For other SCST, gene alterations and mutations appear restricted to their syndromic context. The above findings have provided insights into the biology of the respective genes involved in the pathogenesis, and to the role they play in sex-cord stromal cell development. The prognostic significance and therapeutic potential of these findings are of critical interest to those women afflicted with these malignancies. What is also very clear is that these tumors are uniquely different to the EOC, which in the context of the age of 'precision' medicine, each tumor type must be treated with a tumor-, and/or a mutation-specific approach. As an example, for the more common aGCT tumor type, advanced stage disease carries a poor prognosis, and yet, options beyond the FOXL2 mutation are still to be identified. Targeting the FOXL2 mutation is likely to be difficult. Hence further targets are potentially needed in order to treat this disease with a more targeted approach. It is clear that other genetic or genomic changes must determine late recurrence or an advanced stage. With a multi-omics approach involving the application of whole genome sequencing, whole-exome sequencing, RNA-seq as well as interrogation of the miRNA-ome, critical driver mutations for GCT or the other SCST will likely be identified, with the hope that these are 'actionable' mutations, and thus leading to more precision targeted therapy.

Acknowledgements

This work is supported by grants-in-aid from the RIVKIN, US Department of Defense (OC170256), Australian Government Medical Research Future Fund (MRFF #1199749), Cancer Council Victoria; the Ovarian Cancer Research Foundation (S.C.); the Granulosa Cell Tumor of the Ovary Foundation; the National Health & Medical Research Council of Australia through a Project Grant (#1058334). The Hudson Institute is supported by the Victorian Government's Operational Infrastructure Scheme.

Author details

Trang Nguyen, Trang Minh Tran, Yee Shen Choo, Maria Alexiadis, Peter J. Fuller and Simon Chu*
Hudson Institute of Medical Research, Clayton, Victoria, Australia

*Address all correspondence to: simon.chu@hudson.org.au

References

[1] Scully, R.E., *Classification of human ovarian tumors.* Environ Health Perspect, 1987. **73**: p. 15-25.

[2] Jamieson, S. and P.J. Fuller, *Molecular pathogenesis of granulosa cell tumors of the ovary.* Endocr Rev, 2012. **33**(1): p. 109-144.

[3] Kurman RJ, C.M., Herrington CS, Young RH., *WHO Classification of Tumours of Female Reproductive Organs.* 4th ed Lyon: WHO Press, 2014.

[4] Schumer, S.T. and S.A. Cannistra, *Granulosa cell tumor of the ovary.* J Clin Oncol, 2003. **21**(6): p. 1180-1189.

[5] Chu, S., et al., *FSH-regulated gene expression profiles in ovarian tumours and normal ovaries.* Mol Hum Reprod, 2002. **8**(5): p. 426-433.

[6] Amsterdam, A. and N. Selvaraj, *Control of differentiation, transformation, and apoptosis in granulosa cells by oncogenes, oncoviruses, and tumor suppressor genes.* Endocr Rev, 1997. **18**(4): p. 435-461.

[7] Kitajima, K., Y. Kaji, and K. Sugimura, *Usual and unusual MRI findings of ovarian fibroma: Correlation with pathologic findings.* Magn Reson Med Sci, 2008. **7**(1): p. 43-48.

[8] Parwate, N.S., et al., *Ovarian fibroma: A Clinico-pathological study of 23 cases with review of literature.* J Obstet Gynaecol India, 2016. **66**(6): p. 460-465.

[9] Leung, S.W. and P.M. Yuen, *Ovarian fibroma: A review on the clinical characteristics, diagnostic difficulties, and management options of 23 cases.* Gynecol Obstet Invest, 2006. **62**(1): p. 1-6.

[10] Kim, S.G., Kim, Y.S., Lee, H.J. , *A giant fibroma associated with Meigs' syndrome misdiagnosed as a giant myoma: A case report.* European Journal of Gynaecological Oncology, 2020. **41**(1): p. 134-137.

[11] Li, X., et al., *Imaging features and pathologic characteristics of ovarian thecoma.* J Comput Assist Tomogr, 2012. **36**(1): p. 46-53.

[12] Nocito, A.L., et al., *Ovarian thecoma: Clinicopathological analysis of 50 cases.* Ann Diagn Pathol, 2008. **12**(1): p. 12-16.

[13] Burandt, E. and R.H. Young, *Thecoma of the ovary: A report of 70 cases emphasizing aspects of its histopathology different from those often portrayed and its differential diagnosis.* Am J Surg Pathol, 2014. **38**(8): p. 1023-1032.

[14] Schultz, K.A., et al., *Ovarian sex cord-stromal tumors.* J Oncol Pract, 2016. **12**(10): p. 940-946.

[15] Durmus, Y., et al., *Sertoli-Leydig cell tumor of the ovary: Analysis of a single institution database and review of the literature.* J Obstet Gynaecol Res, 2019. **45**(7): p. 1311-1318.

[16] Nasioudis, D., et al., *Ovarian Sertoli-Leydig and granulosa cell tumor: Comparison of epidemiology and survival outcomes.* Arch Gynecol Obstet, 2020. **302**(2): p. 481-486.

[17] de Kock, L., et al., *DICER1 mutations are consistently present in moderately and poorly differentiated Sertoli-Leydig cell tumors.* Am J Surg Pathol, 2017. **41**(9): p. 1178-1187.

[18] Rabban, J.T., A.N. Karnezis, and W.P. Devine, *Practical roles for molecular diagnostic testing in ovarian adult granulosa cell tumour, Sertoli-Leydig cell tumour, microcystic stromal tumour and their mimics.* Histopathology, 2020. **76**(1): p. 11-24.

[19] Conlon, N., et al., *A survey of DICER1 hotspot mutations in ovarian and testicular sex cord-stromal tumors.* Mod Pathol, 2015. **28**(12): p. 1603-12.

[20] Heravi-Moussavi, A., et al., *Recurrent somatic DICER1 mutations in nonepithelial ovarian cancers.* N Engl J Med, 2012. **366**(3): p. 234-242.

[21] Lim, D. and E. Oliva, *Ovarian sex cord-stromal tumours: An update in recent molecular advances.* Pathology, 2018. **50**(2): p. 178-189.

[22] Schultz, K.A.P., et al., *DICER1-related Sertoli-Leydig cell tumor and gynandroblastoma: Clinical and genetic findings from the international ovarian and testicular stromal tumor registry.* Gynecol Oncol, 2017. **147**(3): p. 521-527.

[23] Yuan, Z., et al., *Clinical characteristics and mutation analyses of ovarian Sertoli-Leydig cell tumors.* Oncologist, 2020. **25**(9): p. e1396-e1405.

[24] McCluggage, W.G., et al., *Gynandroblastoma of ovary with juvenile granulosa cell component and heterologous intestinal type glands.* Histopathology, 1996. **29**(3): p. 253-257.

[25] Hwang, S., et al., *Ovarian Gynandroblastoma with a Juvenile Granulosa Cell Tumor Component in a Postmenopausal Woman.* Diagnostics (Basel), 2020. **10**(8).

[26] Jang, N.R., et al., *Ovarian Gynandroblastoma with a juvenile granulosa cell tumor component in a postmenopausal woman: A case report and literature review.* J Pathol Transl Med, 2018. **52**(5): p. 344-348.

[27] Oparka, R., et al., *The C134W (402 C>G) FOXL2 mutation is absent in ovarian gynandroblastoma: Insights into the genesis of an unusual tumour.* Histopathology, 2012. **60**(5): p. 838-842.

[28] Chivukula, M., et al., *Recurrent gynandroblastoma of ovary-a case report: A molecular and immunohistochemical analysis.* Int J Gynecol Pathol, 2007. **26**(1): p. 30-33.

[29] Wilberger, A. and B. Yang, *Gynandroblastoma with juvenile granulosa cell tumor and concurrent renal cell carcinoma: A case report and review of literature.* Int J Surg Pathol, 2015. **23**(5): p. 393-398.

[30] Zhao, C., et al., *Identification of the most sensitive and robust immunohistochemical markers in different categories of ovarian sex cord-stromal tumors.* Am J Surg Pathol, 2009. **33**(3): p. 354-366.

[31] Young, R.H., et al., *Ovarian sex cord tumor with annular tubules: Review of 74 cases including 27 with Peutz-Jeghers syndrome and four with adenoma malignum of the cervix.* Cancer, 1982. **50**(7): p. 1384-1402.

[32] Hemminki, A., et al., *A serine/threonine kinase gene defective in Peutz-Jeghers syndrome.* Nature, 1998. **391**(6663): p. 184-187.

[33] Hemminki, A., et al., *Localization of a susceptibility locus for Peutz-Jeghers syndrome to 19p using comparative genomic hybridization and targeted linkage analysis.* Nat Genet, 1997. **15**(1): p. 87-90.

[34] Shackelford, D.B. and R.J. Shaw, *The LKB1-AMPK pathway: Metabolism and growth control in tumour suppression.* Nat Rev Cancer, 2009. **9**(8): p. 563-575.

[35] Yoo, L.I., D.C. Chung, and J. Yuan, *LKB1--a master tumour suppressor of the small intestine and beyond.* Nat Rev Cancer, 2002. **2**(7): p. 529-535.

[36] Kato, N., et al., *The STK11/LKB1 Peutz-Jegher gene is not involved in the pathogenesis of sporadic sex cord-stromal tumors, although loss of heterozygosity at*

19p13.3 indicates other gene alteration in these tumors. Hum Pathol, 2004. **35**(9): p. 1101-1104.

[37] Wang, Z.J., et al., *Allele loss and mutation screen at the Peutz-Jeghers (LKB1) locus (19p13.3) in sporadic ovarian tumours.* Br J Cancer, 1999. **80**(1-2): p. 70-72.

[38] Clement, P.B., R.H. Young, and R.E. Scully, *Clinical syndromes associated with tumors of the female genital tract.* Semin Diagn Pathol, 1991. **8**(4): p. 204-233.

[39] Gell, J.S., et al., *Juvenile granulosa cell tumor in a 13-year-old girl with enchondromatosis (Ollier's disease): A case report.* J Pediatr Adolesc Gynecol, 1998. **11**(3): p. 147-150.

[40] Leyva-Carmona, M., M.A. Vazquez-Lopez, and F. Lendinez-Molinos, *Ovarian juvenile granulosa cell tumors in infants.* J Pediatr Hematol Oncol, 2009. **31**(4): p. 304-306.

[41] Rietveld, L., et al., *First case of juvenile granulosa cell tumor in an adult with Ollier disease.* Int J Gynecol Pathol, 2009. **28**(5): p. 464-467.

[42] Tamimi, H.K. and J.W. Bolen, *Enchondromatosis (Ollier's disease) and ovarian juvenile granulosa cell tumor.* Cancer, 1984. **53**(7): p. 1605-1608.

[43] Tanaka, Y., et al., *Ovarian juvenile granulosa cell tumor associated with Maffucci's syndrome.* Am J Clin Pathol, 1992. **97**(4): p. 523-527.

[44] Young, R.H., G.R. Dickersin, and R.E. Scully, *Juvenile granulosa cell tumor of the ovary. A clinicopathological analysis of 125 cases.* Am J Surg Pathol, 1984. **8**(8): p. 575-596.

[45] Goudie, C., et al., *Paediatric ovarian tumours and their associated cancer susceptibility syndromes.* J Med Genet, 2018. **55**(1): p. 1-10.

[46] Pansuriya, T.C., H.M. Kroon, and J.V. Bovee, *Enchondromatosis: Insights on the different subtypes.* Int J Clin Exp Pathol, 2010. **3**(6): p. 557-569.

[47] Kumar, A., et al., *Ollier disease: Pathogenesis, diagnosis, and management.* Orthopedics, 2015. **38**(6): p. e497-e506.

[48] Grenet, P., et al., *[Dyschondroplasia and ovarian tumor].* Ann Pediatr (Paris), 1972. **19**(11): p. 759-64.

[49] Jalaeefar, A., et al., *Granulosa cell tumor of the ovary accompanying with Ollier's disease: First case of contralateral presentations.* J Obstet Gynaecol India, 2020. **70**(1): p. 81-85.

[50] Xu, H.S., E. Zhong, and J. Rotman, *Juvenile granulosa cell tumor associated with Maffucci syndrome in pregnancy: A case report.* Clin Imaging, 2019. **56**: p. 77-80.

[51] Amary, M.F., et al., *Ollier disease and Maffucci syndrome are caused by somatic mosaic mutations of IDH1 and IDH2.* Nat Genet, 2011. **43**(12): p. 1262-1265.

[52] Pansuriya, T.C., et al., *Somatic mosaic IDH1 and IDH2 mutations are associated with enchondroma and spindle cell hemangioma in Ollier disease and Maffucci syndrome.* Nat Genet, 2011. **43**(12): p. 1256-1261.

[53] Jin, Y., et al., *Mutant IDH1 dysregulates the differentiation of mesenchymal stem cells in association with gene-specific histone modifications to cartilage- and bone-related genes.* PLoS One, 2015. **10**(7): p. e0131998.

[54] Verdegaal, S.H., et al., *Incidence, predictive factors, and prognosis of chondrosarcoma in patients with Ollier disease and Maffucci syndrome: An international multicenter study of 161 patients.* Oncologist, 2011. **16**(12): p. 1771-1779.

[55] Shah, S.P., et al., *Mutation of FOXL2 in granulosa-cell tumors of the ovary.* N Engl J Med, 2009. **360**(26): p. 2719-2729.

[56] Mayr, D., et al., *Characteristic pattern of genetic aberrations in ovarian granulosa cell tumors.* Mod Pathol, 2002. **15**(9): p. 951-957.

[57] Lin, Y.S., et al., *Molecular cytogenetics of ovarian granulosa cell tumors by comparative genomic hybridization.* Gynecol Oncol, 2005. **97**(1): p. 68-73.

[58] King, L.A., et al., *Mitotic count, nuclear atypia, and immunohistochemical determination of Ki-67, c-myc, p21-ras, c-erbB2, and p53 expression in granulosa cell tumors of the ovary: Mitotic count and Ki-67 are indicators of poor prognosis.* Gynecol Oncol, 1996. **61**(2): p. 227-232.

[59] Miller, B.E., et al., *Parameters of differentiation and proliferation in adult granulosa cell tumors of the ovary.* Cancer Detect Prev, 2001. **25**(1): p. 48-54.

[60] Villella, J., et al., *Clinical and pathological predictive factors in women with adult-type granulosa cell tumor of the ovary.* Int J Gynecol Pathol, 2007. **26**(2): p. 154-159.

[61] Caburet, S., et al., *Combined comparative genomic hybridization and transcriptomic analyses of ovarian granulosa cell tumors point to novel candidate driver genes.* BMC Cancer, 2015. **15**: p. 251.

[62] Benayoun, B.A., et al., *Adult ovarian granulosa cell tumor transcriptomics: Prevalence of FOXL2 target genes misregulation gives insights into the pathogenic mechanism of the p.Cys134Trp somatic mutation.* Oncogene, 2013. **32**(22): p. 2739-2746.

[63] Alexiadis, M., et al., *Nuclear receptor profiling of ovarian granulosa cell tumors.* Horm Cancer, 2011. **2**(3): p. 157-169.

[64] Herriges, J.C., et al., *Identification of two 14q32 deletions involving DICER1 associated with the development of DICER1-related tumors.* Eur J Med Genet, 2019. **62**(1): p. 9-14.

[65] Streblow, R.C., et al., *Imbalances of chromosomes 4, 9, and 12 are recurrent in the thecoma-fibroma group of ovarian stromal tumors.* Cancer Genet Cytogenet, 2007. **178**(2): p. 135-140.

[66] Gailani, M.R., et al., *Developmental defects in Gorlin syndrome related to a putative tumor suppressor gene on chromosome 9.* Cell, 1992. **69**(1): p. 111-117.

[67] Tsuji, T., L. Catasus, and J. Prat, *Is loss of heterozygosity at 9q22.3 (PTCH gene) and 19p13.3 (STK11 gene) involved in the pathogenesis of ovarian stromal tumors?* Hum Pathol, 2005. **36**(7): p. 792-796.

[68] Chen, Y. and G. Struhl, *Dual roles for patched in sequestering and transducing hedgehog.* Cell, 1996. **87**(3): p. 553-563.

[69] Kalfa, N., et al., *[Juvenile granulosa-cell tumor: clinical and molecular expression].* Gynecol Obstet Fertil, 2009. **37**(1): p. 33-44.

[70] Jamieson, S., et al., *The FOXL2 C134W mutation is characteristic of adult granulosa cell tumors of the ovary.* Mod Pathol, 2010. **23**(11): p. 1477-1485.

[71] Rosario, R., et al., *Adult granulosa cell tumours (GCT): Clinicopathological outcomes including FOXL2 mutational status and expression.* Gynecol Oncol, 2013. **131**(2): p. 325-329.

[72] Stewart, C.J., et al., *An immunohistochemical and molecular analysis of problematic and unclassified ovarian sex cord-stromal tumors.* Hum Pathol, 2013. **44**(12): p. 2774-2781.

[73] Kalfa, N., et al., *Activating mutations of the stimulatory g protein in juvenile ovarian granulosa cell tumors: A new prognostic factor?* J Clin Endocrinol Metab, 2006. **91**(5): p. 1842-1847.

[74] Salpea, P. and C.A. Stratakis, *Carney complex and McCune Albright syndrome: An overview of clinical manifestations and human molecular genetics*. Mol Cell Endocrinol, 2014. **386**(1-2): p. 85-91.

[75] Bessiere, L., et al., *A hot-spot of In-frame duplications activates the Oncoprotein AKT1 in juvenile granulosa cell tumors*. EBioMedicine, 2015. **2**(5): p. 421-431.

[76] Auguste, A., et al., *Molecular analyses of juvenile granulosa cell tumors bearing AKT1 mutations provide insights into tumor biology and therapeutic leads*. Hum Mol Genet, 2015. **24**(23): p. 6687-6698.

[77] Kalfa, N., et al., *Extinction of FOXL2 expression in aggressive ovarian granulosa cell tumors in children*. Fertil Steril, 2007. **87**(4): p. 896-901.

[78] Caburet, S., et al., *The transcription factor FOXL2: at the crossroads of ovarian physiology and pathology*. Mol Cell Endocrinol, 2012. **356**(1-2): p. 55-64.

[79] Leung, D.T.H., P.J. Fuller, and S. Chu, *Impact of FOXL2 mutations on signaling in ovarian granulosa cell tumors*. Int J Biochem Cell Biol, 2016. **72**: p. 51-54.

[80] Rosario, R., P.A. Cohen, and A.N. Shelling, *The role of FOXL2 in the pathogenesis of adult ovarian granulosa cell tumours*. Gynecol Oncol, 2014. **133**(2): p. 382-387.

[81] Wang, Y., et al., *The oncogenic roles of DICER1 RNase IIIb domain mutations in ovarian Sertoli-Leydig cell tumors*. Neoplasia, 2015. **17**(8): p. 650-660.

[82] Wells, S.A., Jr., et al., *Revised American Thyroid Association guidelines for the management of medullary thyroid carcinoma*. Thyroid, 2015. **25**(6): p. 567-610.

[83] Alexiadis, M., et al., *Transcriptomic analysis of stage 1 versus advanced adult granulosa cell tumors*. Oncotarget, 2016. **7**(12): p. 14207-14219.

[84] Cancer Genome Atlas Research, N., *Integrated genomic analyses of ovarian carcinoma*. Nature, 2011. **474**(7353): p. 609-15.

[85] Alexiadis, M., et al., *Mutational landscape of ovarian adult granulosa cell tumors from whole exome and targeted TERT promoter sequencing*. Mol Cancer Res, 2019. **17**(1): p. 177-185.

[86] Hillman, R.T., et al., *KMT2D/MLL2 inactivation is associated with recurrence in adult-type granulosa cell tumors of the ovary*. Nat Commun, 2018. **9**(1): p. 2496.

[87] Zehir, A., et al., *Mutational landscape of metastatic cancer revealed from prospective clinical sequencing of 10,000 patients*. Nat Med, 2017. **23**(6): p. 703-713.

[88] Pilsworth, J.A., et al., *Adult-Type Granulosa Cell Tumor of the Ovary: A FOXL2-Centric Disease*. J Pathol Clin Res, 2021.

[89] Da Cruz Paula, A., et al., *Genomic profiling of primary and recurrent adult granulosa cell tumors of the ovary*. Mod Pathol, 2020. **33**(8): p. 1606-1617.

[90] Roze, J., et al., *Whole Genome Analysis of Ovarian Granulosa Cell Tumors Reveals Tumor Heterogeneity and a High-Grade TP53-Specific Subgroup*. Cancers (Basel), 2020. **12**(5).

[91] Jamieson, S. and P.J. Fuller, *Characterization of the inhibitor of kappaB kinase (IKK) complex in*

granulosa cell tumors of the ovary and granulosa cell tumor-derived cell lines. Horm Cancer, 2013. **4**(5): p. 277-292.

[92] Pilsworth, J.A., et al., *TERT promoter mutation in adult granulosa cell tumor of the ovary.* Mod Pathol, 2018.

[93] Li, Y., et al., *Non-canonical NF-kappaB signalling and ETS1/2 cooperatively drive C250T mutant TERT promoter activation.* Nat Cell Biol, 2015. **17**(10): p. 1327-1338.

[94] Pestana, A., et al., *TERT biology and function in cancer: Beyond immortalisation.* J Mol Endocrinol, 2017. **58**(2): p. R129-R146.

[95] Chu, S., et al., *Transrepression of estrogen receptor beta signaling by nuclear factor-kappab in ovarian granulosa cells.* Mol Endocrinol, 2004. **18**(8): p. 1919-1928.

[96] Bilandzic, M., et al., *Betaglycan alters NFkappaB-TGFbeta2 cross talk to reduce survival of human granulosa tumor cells.* Mol Endocrinol, 2013. **27**(3): p. 466-479.

[97] Bell, R.J., et al., *Understanding TERT promoter mutations: A common path to immortality.* Mol Cancer Res, 2016. **14**(4): p. 315-323.

[98] Vedanayagam, J., et al., *Cancer-associated mutations in DICER1 RNase IIIa and IIIb domains exert similar effects on miRNA biogenesis.* Nat Commun, 2019. **10**(1): p. 3682.

[99] Robertson, J.C., C.L. Jorcyk, and J.T. Oxford, *DICER1 Syndrome: DICER1 Mutations in Rare Cancers.* Cancers (Basel), 2018. **10**(5).

[100] Rosario, R., C. Blenkiron, and A.N. Shelling, *Comparative study of microRNA regulation on FOXL2 between adult-type and juvenile-type granulosa cell tumours in vitro.* Gynecol Oncol, 2013. **129**(1): p. 209-215.

[101] McCleland, M.L., et al., *CCAT1 is an enhancer-templated RNA that predicts BET sensitivity in colorectal cancer.* J Clin Invest, 2016. **126**(2): p. 639-652.

[102] Saghatelian, A. and J.P. Couso, *Discovery and characterization of smORF-encoded bioactive polypeptides.* Nat Chem Biol, 2015. **11**(12): p. 909-916.

[103] Steinmetz, R., et al., *Mechanisms regulating the constitutive activation of the extracellular signal-regulated kinase (ERK) signaling pathway in ovarian cancer and the effect of ribonucleic acid interference for ERK1/2 on cancer cell proliferation.* Mol Endocrinol, 2004. **18**(10): p. 2570-2582.

[104] Rosario, R., et al., *The transcriptional targets of mutant FOXL2 in granulosa cell tumours.* PLoS One, 2012. 7(9): p. e46270.

[105] Chan-Penebre, E., et al., *Selective killing of SMARCA2- and SMARCA4-deficient small cell carcinoma of the ovary, hypercalcemic type cells by inhibition of EZH2: In vitro and In vivo preclinical models.* Mol Cancer Ther, 2017. **16**(5): p. 850-860.

[106] Chen, H., et al., *RUNX3 Promotes the Tumorigenic Phenotype in KGN, a Human Granulosa Cell Tumor-Derived Cell Line.* Int J Mol Sci, 2019. **20**(14).

[107] Karnezis, A.N., et al., *Re-assigning the histologic identities of COV434 and TOV-112D ovarian cancer cell lines.* Gynecol Oncol, 2021. **160**(2): p. 568-578.

[108] Ulbright, T.M., et al., *Poorly differentiated (small cell) carcinoma of the ovary in young women: Evidence supporting a germ cell origin.* Hum Pathol, 1987. **18**(2): p. 175-184.

[109] Foulkes, W.D., et al., *No small surprise - small cell carcinoma of the ovary, hypercalcaemic type, is a malignant*

rhabdoid tumour. J Pathol, 2014. **233**(3): p. 209-214.

[110] Liu, Z., et al., *FOXO1/3 and PTEN depletion in granulosa cells promotes ovarian granulosa cell tumor development.* Mol Endocrinol, 2015. **29**(7): p. 1006-1024.

[111] Bittinger, S., M. Alexiadis, and P.J. Fuller, *Expression status and mutational analysis of the PTEN and P13K subunit genes in ovarian granulosa cell tumors.* Int J Gynecol Cancer, 2009. **19**(3): p. 339-342.

[112] Lague, M.N., et al., *Synergistic effects of Pten loss and WNT/CTNNB1 signaling pathway activation in ovarian granulosa cell tumor development and progression.* Carcinogenesis, 2008. **29**(11): p. 2062-2072.

[113] Boerboom, D., et al., *Misregulated Wnt/beta-catenin signaling leads to ovarian granulosa cell tumor development.* Cancer Res, 2005. **65**(20): p. 9206-9215.

[114] Ohishi, Y., et al., *Nuclear localization of E-cadherin but not beta-catenin in human ovarian granulosa cell tumours and normal ovarian follicles and ovarian stroma.* Histopathology, 2011. **58**(3): p. 423-432.

[115] De Cian, M.C., et al., *Amplification of R-spondin1 signaling induces granulosa cell fate defects and cancers in mouse adult ovary.* Oncogene, 2017. **36**(2): p. 208-218.

[116] Gao, Y., et al., *Constitutively active transforming growth factor beta receptor 1 in the mouse ovary promotes tumorigenesis.* Oncotarget, 2016. **7**(27): p. 40904-40918.

[117] Matzuk, M.M., et al., *Alpha-inhibin is a tumour-suppressor gene with gonadal specificity in mice.* Nature, 1992. **360**(6402): p. 313-319.

[118] Kumar, T.R., Y. Wang, and M.M. Matzuk, *Gonadotropins are essential modifier factors for gonadal tumor development in inhibin-deficient mice.* Endocrinology, 1996. **137**(10): p. 4210-4216.

[119] Matzuk, M.M., et al., *Development of cancer cachexia-like syndrome and adrenal tumors in inhibin-deficient mice.* Proc Natl Acad Sci U S A, 1994. **91**(19): p. 8817-8821.

[120] Makanji, Y., et al., *Inhibin at 90: From discovery to clinical application, a historical review.* Endocr Rev, 2014. **35**(5): p. 747-794.

[121] Kim, S.Y., *Insights into granulosa cell tumors using spontaneous or genetically engineered mouse models.* Clin Exp Reprod Med, 2016. **43**(1): p. 1-8.

[122] Li, Q., et al., *SMAD3 regulates gonadal tumorigenesis.* Mol Endocrinol, 2007. **21**(10): p. 2472-2486.

[123] Looyenga, B.D. and G.D. Hammer, *Genetic removal of Smad3 from inhibin-null mice attenuates tumor progression by uncoupling extracellular mitogenic signals from the cell cycle machinery.* Mol Endocrinol, 2007. **21**(10): p. 2440-2457.

[124] Kottarathil, V.D., et al., *Recent advances in granulosa cell tumor ovary: A review.* Indian J Surg Oncol, 2013. **4**(1): p. 37-47.

[125] Pectasides, D., N. Alevizakos, and A.E. Athanassiou, *Cisplatin-containing regimen in advanced or recurrent granulosa cell tumours of the ovary.* Ann Oncol, 1992. **3**(4): p. 316-318.

[126] Uygun, K., et al., *Clinical parameters and treatment results in recurrent granulosa cell tumor of the ovary.* Gynecol Oncol, 2003. **88**(3): p. 400-3.

[127] Zambetti, M., et al., *Cis-platinum/vinblastine/bleomycin combination chemotherapy in advanced or recurrent granulosa cell tumors of the ovary.* Gynecol Oncol, 1990. **36**(3): p. 317-320.

[128] Homesley, H.D., et al., *Bleomycin, etoposide, and cisplatin combination therapy of ovarian granulosa cell tumors and other stromal malignancies: A gynecologic Oncology group study.* Gynecol Oncol, 1999. **72**(2): p. 131-137.

[129] Pautier, P., et al., *Combination of bleomycin, etoposide, and cisplatin for the treatment of advanced ovarian granulosa cell tumors.* Int J Gynecol Cancer, 2008. **18**(3): p. 446-452.

[130] Seagle, B.L., et al., *Ovarian granulosa cell tumor: A National Cancer Database study.* Gynecol Oncol, 2017. **146**(2): p. 285-291.

[131] van Meurs, H.S., et al., *Hormone therapy in ovarian granulosa cell tumors: A systematic review.* Gynecol Oncol, 2014. **134**(1): p. 196-205.

[132] Yang, A.D., Curtin, J. & Muggia, F., *Ovarian adult-type granulosa cell tumor: Focusing on endocrine-based therapies.* Int J Endocr Oncol, 2018. **5**(2): p. IJE08.

[133] Isaacs, R., G. Forgeson, and S. Allan, *Progestagens for granulosa cell tumours of the ovary.* Br J Cancer, 1992. **65**(1): p. 140.

[134] Malik, S.T. and M.L. Slevin, *Medroxyprogesterone acetate (MPA) in advanced granulosa cell tumours of the ovary--a new therapeutic approach?* Br J Cancer, 1991. **63**(3): p. 410-411.

[135] Farkkila, A., et al., *Vascular endothelial growth factor (VEGF) and its receptor VEGFR-2 are highly expressed in ovarian granulosa cell tumors.* Eur J Endocrinol, 2011. **164**(1): p. 115-122.

[136] Farkkila, A., et al., *Serum vascular endothelial growth factor a (VEGF) is elevated in patients with ovarian granulosa cell tumor (GCT), and VEGF inhibition by bevacizumab induces apoptosis in GCT in vitro.* J Clin Endocrinol Metab, 2011. **96**(12): p. E1973-E1981.

[137] Tao, X., et al., *Anti-angiogenesis therapy with bevacizumab for patients with ovarian granulosa cell tumors.* Gynecol Oncol, 2009. **114**(3): p. 431-436.

[138] Kesterson, J.P., P. Mhawech-Fauceglia, and S. Lele, *The use of bevacizumab in refractory ovarian granulosa-cell carcinoma with symptomatic relief of ascites: A case report.* Gynecol Oncol, 2008. **111**(3): p. 527-529.

[139] Brown, J., et al., *Efficacy and safety of bevacizumab in recurrent sex cord-stromal ovarian tumors: Results of a phase 2 trial of the gynecologic Oncology group.* Cancer, 2014. **120**(3): p. 344-351.

[140] Chu, S., M. Alexiadis, and P.J. Fuller, *Expression, mutational analysis and in vitro response of imatinib mesylate and nilotinib target genes in ovarian granulosa cell tumors.* Gynecol Oncol, 2008. **108**(1): p. 182-190.

[141] Jamieson, S. and P.J. Fuller, *Tyrosine kinase inhibitors as potential therapeutic agents in the treatment of granulosa cell tumors of the ovary.* Int J Gynecol Cancer, 2015. **25**(7): p. 1224-1231.

[142] T.J., H., et al., *PD-1, PD-L1 expression in 1599 gynecological cancers: Implications for immunotherapy.* Gynexol. Oncol., 2015. **137**: p. 204-205.

[143] Pierini, S., et al., *Ovarian granulosa cell tumor characterization identifies FOXL2 as an immunotherapeutic target.* JCI Insight, 2020. **5**(16).

[144] Baldwin, A.S., Jr., *The NF-kappa B and I kappa B proteins: New discoveries and insights.* Annu Rev Immunol, 1996. **14**: p. 649-683.

[145] Fulda, S., *Smac mimetics as IAP antagonists.* Semin Cell Dev Biol, 2015. **39**: p. 132-138.

[146] Fulda, S., *Smac mimetics to therapeutically target IAP proteins in Cancer.* Int Rev Cell Mol Biol, 2017. **330**: p. 157-169.

[147] Fulda, S. and D. Vucic, *Targeting IAP proteins for therapeutic intervention in cancer.* Nat Rev Drug Discov, 2012. **11**(2): p. 109-124.

[148] Berthelet, J. and L. Dubrez, *Regulation of apoptosis by inhibitors of apoptosis (IAPs).* Cells, 2013. **2**(1): p. 163-187.

[149] Vaux, D.L. and J. Silke, *IAPs, RINGs and ubiquitylation.* Nat Rev Mol Cell Biol, 2005. **6**(4): p. 287-297.

[150] Leung, D.T.H., et al., *Combined PPARgamma activation and XIAP inhibition as a potential therapeutic strategy for ovarian granulosa cell tumors.* Mol Cancer Ther, 2019. **18**(2): p. 364-375.

[151] Leung, D.T.H., et al., *Targeting XIAP and PPARgamma in granulosa cell tumors alters metabolic signaling.* J Proteome Res, 2019.

Section 2

Ovarian Cancer Surgical Updates

Chapter 6

The Role of Ultra-Radical Surgery in the Management of Advanced Ovarian Cancer: State or Art

Felicia Elena Buruiana, Lamiese Ismail, Federico Ferrari and Hooman Soleymani Majd

Abstract

The ovarian cancer, also known as "silent killer", has remained the most lethal gynaecological malignancy. The single independent risk factor linked with improved survival is maximum cytoreductive effort resulting in no macroscopic residual disease. This could be gained through ultra-radical surgery which demands tackling significant tumour burden in pelvis, lower and upper abdomen which usually constitutes bowel resection, liver mobilisation, ancillary cholecystectomy, extensive peritonectomy, diaphragmatic resection, splenectomy, resection of enlarged pelvic, paraaortic, and rarely cardio-phrenic lymph nodes in order to achieve optimal debulking. The above can be achieved through a holistic approach to patient's care, meticulous patient selection, and full engagement of the family. The decision needs to be carefully balanced after obtaining an informed consent, and an appreciation of the impact of such surgery on the quality of life against the survival benefit. This chapter will describe the complexity and surgical challenges in the management of advanced ovarian cancer.

Keywords: ovarian cancer, stage III and IV, cytoreductive surgery, ultraradical surgery, residual disease, holistic approach, quality of life

1. Introduction

The most common gynaecological cancer treated in women is uterine cancer, however the number of women who die from ovarian cancer is much higher [1]. Ovarian cancer has remained the most lethal cancer treated by gynaecological oncological surgeons and is often referred to as the "silent killer".

Ovarian cancer is the 7th most common cancer, and 8th most common cause of death from cancer in women in the world [2]. World Ovarian Cancer Coalition 2018 estimated that by 2035, the incidence of ovarian cancer will increase to 371, 000 per year. It is currently around 239, 000 cases annually [2]. The crude incidence is 23 to 30 in 100 000 women and most women present with advanced disease and little prospect of cure; the five-year survival rate for all stages of ovarian cancer is just over 40% and has remained quite low [3].

The treatment for patients with ovarian cancer is debulking surgery and platinum-based chemotherapy. The amount of residual disease after surgery is the most important prognostic factor for survival [4–11] and a recent phase III clinical trial [9]

confirmed this finding. Debulking surgery is a multi-visceral operation involving the pelvis, lower and upper abdomen, aiming at a complete resection (CR) of all visible disease to a microscopic cellular level [8–11]. This is also called cytoreductive surgery.

We present the latest surgical developments in ultra-radical surgery for the management of advanced ovarian cancer.

2. Evolution of gynaecological oncology surgery

Gynaecological oncological surgery has a rather interesting evolution. This is evident in the management of uterine and vulval cancers, where there has been transition to less aggressive surgery. In vulval cancer the utilisation of sentinel node biopsy plays a major role to reduce the morbidity associated with lymphadenectomy, whilst the application of minimal access surgery in the management of uterine cancer, has ensured faster surgical recovery and significantly shortened length of hospital stay. In contrast, the surgical approach to ovarian cancer has gone through an inverse transition in the last twenty years and despite all efforts to optimise

Carcinoma of the Ovary
Stage I: Tumour confined to ovaries
IA. Tumour limited to 1 ovary, capsule intact, no tumour on surface, negative washings
IB. Tumour involves both ovaries otherwise like IA
IC. Tumour limited to 1 or both ovaries
IC1. Surgical spill
IC2. Capsule rupture before surgery or tumour on ovarian surface
IC3. Malignant cells in the ascites or peritoneal washings
Stage II: Tumour involves 1 or both ovaries with pelvic extension (below the pelvic brim) or primary peritoneal cancer
IIA. Extension and/or implant on uterus and/or fallopian tubes
IIB. Extension to other pelvic intraperitoneal tissues
Stage III: Tumour involves 1 or both ovaries, confirmed spread to extra-pelvic peritoneum and/or metastasis to the retroperitoneal lymph nodes
IIIA. Positive retroperitoneal lymph nodes and/or microscopic metastasis beyond the pelvis
IIIA1. Positive retroperitoneal lymph nodes only
IIIA1(i). Metastasis ≤10 mm
IIIA1(ii). Metastasis >10 mm
IIIA2. Microscopic, extra-pelvic (above the brim) peritoneal involvement ± positive retroperitoneal lymph nodes
IIIB. Macroscopic, extra-pelvic, peritoneal metastasis ≤2 cm ± positive retroperitoneal lymph nodes. Includes extension to capsule of liver/spleen.
IIIC. Macroscopic, extra-pelvic, peritoneal metastasis >2 cm ± positive retroperitoneal lymph nodes. Includes extension to capsule of liver/spleen.
Stage IV: Distant metastasis excluding peritoneal metastasis
IVA. Pleural effusion with positive cytology
IVB. Hepatic and/or splenic parenchymal metastasis, metastasis to extra-abdominal organs (including inguinal lymph nodes and lymph nodes outside of the abdominal cavity)

Table 1.
Ovarian cancer staging (Society of Gynaecologic Oncology).

medical management throughout the introduction of targeted therapies, surgery has remained the mainstay of treatment and has progressively more radical [12].

In ovarian cancer, a midline laparotomy is usually performed to fully access anatomical structures in the pelvis and intra-abdominal cavity. With a midline laparotomy the patient will have a longer hospital stay, as opposed to laparoscopy, or robotic surgery.

Minimally invasive surgery can be performed when the disease is confined to the primary site (stage I ovarian cancer). In widespread disease, total hysterectomy with bilateral salpingo-oophorectomy, infracolic omentectomy and systematic pelvic/para-aortic lymphadenectomy are required in order to determine the need for adjuvant treatment and complete full surgical staging. However, the latter does not regularly apply to ovarian cancer since 80% of patients with ovarian cancer present with advanced disease (stages III and IV) Advanced disease implies a short time for management and treatment; as usually the cancer has spread to the upper abdomen, mandating multi-visceral resection.

Before effective treatment can be offered for ovarian cancer, the disease needs to be correctly staged. This can be achieved by means of radiological modalities or exploratory laparoscopy, or a combination of both. Ovarian cancer staging is presented in **Table 1** [13].

3. Ovarian cancer treatment

3.1 Background

Historically the treatment of ovarian cancer was primary debulking surgery followed by chemotherapy, whenever it was deemed to be feasible.

When to perform the debulking surgery in advanced ovarian cancer (AOC) has been the cause of debate and controversy for almost a decade [14]. The supporters of primary debulking surgery (PDS) advocate significantly better overall survival (OS) and progression-free survival (PFS) rates, whilst the opponents argue higher surgical morbidity and often fatal disease [14–17]. It is well recognised that for each 10% increase in maximal cytoreduction, there is an associated 5.5% increase in median survival [14, 18, 19]. However, in the vast majority of cases, complete debulking is associated with multivisceral resection which requires extensive surgical expertise, training and infrastructural support.

Neoadjuvant chemotherapy (NACT) and interval debulking surgery (IDS) have been considered as means to reduce surgical morbidity.

In 2010, Vergote et al. conducted a phase III randomised control trial (EORTC) [9] where neoadjuvant chemotherapy followed by interval debulking surgery (IDS) was compared with upfront primary debulking surgery (PDS) followed by adjuvant chemotherapy. This trial demonstrated that survival in both arms was similar (29 and 30 months, respectively), however there was less morbidity in patients who had chemotherapy first, mainly in those cases deemed difficult to operate [9]. The same findings were corroborated by the CHORUS phase III randomised controlled trial [20] that was used as a benchmark to justify the role of neoadjuvant chemotherapy in patients who were not candidates for upfront surgery. The survival remained 22 and 24 months, respectively. There have been many debates since the publication of these two RCTs, with regards to survival outcome and the need for a more radical surgical approach, in order to achieve complete cytoreduction.

The Trial on Radical Upfront Surgery in Advanced Ovarian Cancer (TRUST) will hopefully enlighten the adequate management of patients with AOC and will also establish predictive and prognostic biomarkers of operability and survival, as well as identify valid fragility scores for vulnerable patients, with the aim of obtaining a more individualised surgical approach [14, 21].

Radical procedures to resect advanced ovarian cancer have been reported since 1965 [22]. In the late 70's the "peritoneal compartment" concept was developed, with the introduction of en-bloc resection of pelvic organs and the surrounding peritoneum [23]. The logic of en-bloc resection is based on the notion of ovarian cancer as a peritoneal disease, where the peritoneum acts as a dissemination conduit but also limiting the spread. In fact, it is less frequent to see dissemination to the retroperitoneal organs. The en-bloc resection aims at seeking dissection planes within healthy tissue, minimising tumour manipulation and avoiding cutting through cancer tissue. Rapid tumour growth is usually supported by significant angiogenesis, primarily at the tumour periphery. As a result, there is a distortion of normal anatomy and findings of aberrant vascularisation. Therefore, a surgical technique that finds cleavage planes beyond the tumour growth is likely to reduce blood loss.

Visceral-Peritoneal Debulking (VPD) is offered to patients with stage III–IV ovarian cancer [24]. VPD applies the concept of en-bloc resection to all abdominal quadrants.

Maximal cytoreductive surgery aims at total macroscopic tumour clearance combined with platinum-based chemotherapy, these being the cornerstone of modern primary epithelial ovarian cancer (EOC) management [25]. Numerous prospective and retrospective series have demonstrated a strong positive association between total macroscopic tumour clearance rates and survival [25, 26]. A study comparing a surgical population, with a population who received chemotherapy alone (in 2 different cancer centres) showed that 43.8% of patients who had surgery died versus 86% of patients in the chemotherapy group [25].

Cytoreductive surgery is a standard part of national and international guidelines [25, 27, 28], hence surgical management with maximal therapeutic effort is the aim of treatment, even for patients with a higher tumour load, as survival of the patients has been clearly demonstrated [25].

3.2 Patient selection

The mainstay of treatment is a holistic approach to the patient's care. The patient needs to fully understand the benefits, risks and alternatives to surgery. Consent for this procedure needs to be carefully considered and fully informed.

3.3 Clinical assessment

The patient needs to be assessed with regards to their ability to walk and carry out ordinary activities independently, which includes climbing a flight of stairs. The advice of the anaesthetist is valuable, and cardiopulmonary exercise testing (CPET) may also be required to determine the anaerobic threshold of the patient prior to major surgery [24].

Demographic characteristics which have to be considered when selecting patients are age, previous abdominal surgery, ASA score, presence of ascites, preoperative Ca125, preoperative level of haemoglobin, albumin, FIGO stage, histological cancer type [29].

The triage process of patients for debulking includes:

a. a suitable WHO Performance Status (PS) at the preoperative assessment.

b. absence of lung or multiple parenchymal liver metastases on the CT scan.

c. exploratory laparoscopy did not demonstrate small bowel serosal disease or porta hepatis encasement [30].

Liu et al. [31, 32] reported that more than a quarter of women with advanced ovarian cancer treated with neoadjuvant chemotherapy (NACT) do not ever undergo cytoreductive surgery. Significant risk factors contributing to the inability to undergo surgery were advanced age, low albumin levels, frailty scores and extensive disease of predominantly high-grade serous histology. The main reasons identified were extent of disease not amenable to surgery or lack of response to NACT, patient co-morbidities preventing surgery and extent of disease. The patients who did not have debulking surgery, had an over 3-fold increase in mortality of any cause, compared to those who had surgery at some point [31, 32].

In patients with advanced disease, there is a strong rationale to personalise the surgical treatment and implement predictive and prognostic scores [31]. The aim is to allocate the right treatment to the right patient, in order to avoid unnecessary iatrogenic damage [31].

Appreciation of potential impact on the quality of life (QoL) has to be thoroughly assessed and balanced against survival benefit.

3.4 Investigations

A pre-operative CT scan for the thorax, abdomen and pelvis with contrast is essential. The patients with disease progression with lung metastasis or three or more liver segments involvement should be triaged for neo-adjuvant chemotherapy strategy [24]. Tozzi et al. has shown that exploratory laparoscopy added to the CT scan could potentially identify porta hepatis peritoneal disease [33] as well as small bowel serosal involvement. Several advantages of the exploratory laparoscopy have been reported, amongst which a correct diagnosis based on the histology of the tissue biopsy, accurate evaluation of the spread of the disease, including the spread of small military disease, a better selection of the patients for ultra-radical surgery and a better planning of resources in view of the surgery [34]. The authors concluded that this combination of investigations is of a high reliability, and encouraged surgical outcomes [33, 34].

3.5 Diagnostic laparoscopy

Following confirmation of suitability for surgery based on the CT scan, it is recommended to consider an exploratory laparoscopy to rule out diffuse small bowel serosa deposits and porta hepatis encasement [24]. There are controversies around this approach, however it has been demonstrated [24] that the use of Palmer's point and Hasson's technique to enter the abdomen is an easy and safe technique. This is a short procedure, very informative, allowing a thorough assessment of the intraabdominal cavity, and helps in avoiding a laparotomy if the chances of no residual disease are unlikely.

3.6 Systematic abdominal exploration

A systematic approach is required, and this is performed by assessing in systematic manner.

a. In the *upper abdomen* the diaphragm, liver, with its Glisson's capsule, falciform ligament, ligamentum teres, Morison's pouch, the stomach, lesser omentum also known as gastro-hepatic ligament, spleen, tail of pancreas, porta hepatis also known as hepato-dudenal ligament, foramen of Winslow, and the coeliac trunk needs to be assessed. The latter two can be examined by palpation at laparotomy only, and this represents a limiting factor.

b. In the *mid abdomen* the omentum is fully assessed, the ileocaecal junction is identified and small bowel is run u to the point of DJ junction (duodeno-jeoujenal junction), as well as the root of the small bowel mesentery and the small bowel serosa. If the small bowel serosa is extensively affected requiring removal of a large part of the small bowel in order to achieve R0 (leaving a small bowel of less than 150 cm), a debulking procedure should be abandoned.

c. The *lower abdomen (pelvis)* - a thorough assessment looks at the extent of the disease in the pelvis starting with spread to the uterine body, fallopian tubes, round ligaments and sigmoid, with further assessment of the pouch of Douglas and the bladder peritoneum.

After all these assessments the conclusion can be withdrawn as whether the surgery will be beneficial and results in no residual disease. This often requires an intra-operative multi-disciplinary consultation between two senior gynaecological oncologist.

4. Surgical procedure

4.1 Preoperatively

A close collaboration and clear communication with the anaesthetist and the other members of the team are hugely important, as the preparation of the patient is paramount. The patient is positioned in Lloyd Davis with attention to avoiding common peroneal nerve injury/femoral nerve neuropraxia or lower limb compartment syndrome. The use of the correct retractor (i.e. Greys, Bookwalter) will also help in gaining an optimal access to the pelvis, but also to the right and left upper quadrants.

4.2 Intraoperatively

A midline laparotomy is always required in order to allow a good access to all the pelvic and intraabdominal areas mentioned above. An understanding about the radicality of the procedure is further required, and this is highlighted in **Table 2** [35].

The majority of ovarian cancers present in advanced stages and are treated by debulking surgery and platinum-based chemotherapy. The disease starts in the pelvis, involving the ovaries, tubes, the uterus, and the bowel and then spreads to the upper abdomen. Once established that an R0 is feasible the procedure starts in the pelvis.

In the case all pelvic organs are matted, a technique is needed to remove the tumour with cancer free margins. To achieve the least residual disease, multivisceral pelvic and upper abdominal surgery is often necessary [36–39].

Ten steps of the en-bloc resection of the pelvis (**Figure 2**) are described below [24]:

1. Access to the retroperitoneal space: isolation of the ureter, ligation of the infundibulo-pelvic ligament.

2. Resection of sigmoid.

Classification	Groups	Criteria
NICE	Standard	Total abdominal hysterectomy, bilateral salpingo-oophorectomy, omentectomy (**Figure 1**), pelvic and/or para-aortic lymphadenectomy, bowel surgery outside the definition of 'ultra-radical' (localised colonic resection, non-multiple bowel resection)
	Ultraradical	Diaphragmatic stripping, extensive peritoneal stripping, multiple resections of the bowel (excluding localised colonic resection), liver resection, partial gastrectomy, cholecystectomy, splenectomy
Pomel	Standard	Hysterectomy, bilateral salpingo-oophorectomy, pelvic peritonectomy, total omentectomy, appendicectomy, pelvic and/or para-aortic lymphadenectomy
	Radical	Recto-sigmoid resection
	Supra-radical	Diaphragmatic stripping, liver resection, cholecystectomy, splenectomy, any digestive resection excluding recto-sigmoid resection

Table 2.
Description of surgical radicality.

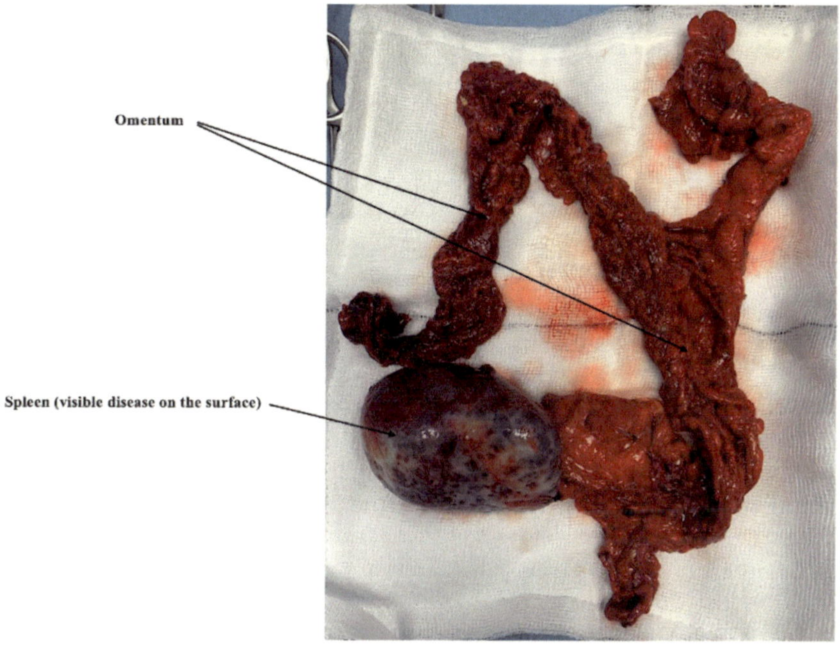

Figure 1.
Total omentectomy.

3. Mobilisation of the sigmoid from the sacrum by coagulation and resection of the meso-sigmoid

4. Access to the pre-sacral space.

5. Mobilisation of the bladder peritoneum with access to the vesico-vaginal space.

6. Colpotomy of the anterior vaginal wall.

7. Retrograde resection of the parametria.

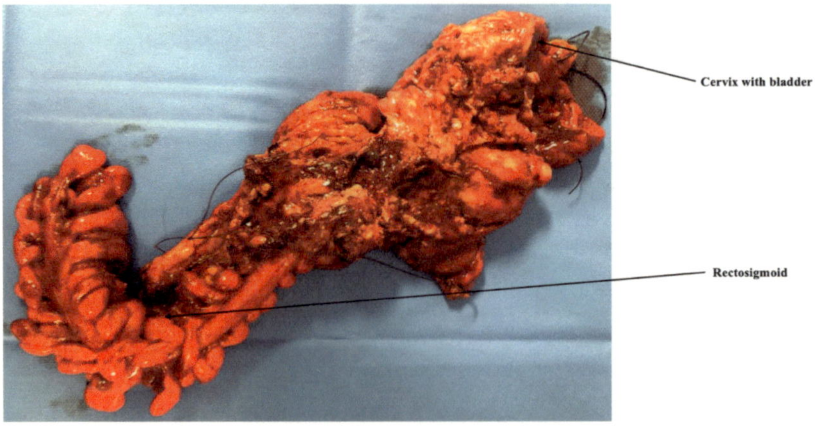

Figure 2.
En-bloc modified posterior pelvic exenteration-including bladder, pelvic, peri-ureteric peritoneum, uterus, cervix, tubes, ovaries and rectosigmoid.

8. Colpotomy of the posterior vaginal wall, access to the recto-vaginal septum.

9. Dissection, coagulation and division of the meso-rectum.

10. Resection of rectum ± anastomosis.

A particular attention needs to be given to bowel resection. Recto-sigmoid resection (RSR) is the most commonly non-gynaecologic procedure performed. It can be associated with early postoperative complications, most severe being the break-down of the anastomosis or anastomotic leak [36, 40, 41].

The literature reports 0.8% - 6.8% risk of anastomotic leak in patients who underwent bowel resection during debulking surgery for ovarian cancer [36]. Therefore, sigmoid rectum resection is sometimes accompanied by a diverting loop ileostomy (DLI) with the aim to reduce the anastomotic leak. This is not without complications, and although it is typically intended to be reversible, the non-reversal rate of ileostomy is 9.5–35% in the colorectal literature [36, 42–46].

RSR is the resection of any large bowel segment from the pelvic brim to the anal canal. The decision to undertake RSR is made at the time of surgery and was usually part of an en-bloc resection of the pelvis [36, 47].

DLI is a loop of small bowel, 10–15 cm proximal to the ileocaecal junction, used to divert the faecal stream and protect the colorectal anastomosis. The indications for DLI are [29, 33]:

- multiple bowel resections.
- RSR < 6 cm from anal verge.
- non-tension free anastomosis.
- poor tissue quality.
- air spillage through the anastomosis at trans-anal air test.

DLI reversal was planned at the end of the chemotherapy and if the patient has three months disease-free interval verified on CT scan. The morbidity of DLI is very challenging, and more for patients who are metabolically deranged, older age, low albumin level, fluid imbalance. DLI morbidity can delay chemotherapy due to dehydration. The optimal timing for reversal remains unclear, usually 6–8 weeks postoperatively [36]. End-colostomy is easier to manage than an end-ileostomy [36, 48], hence for the patients presenting with risk factors for non-reversal, a careful consideration should be given to the type of bowel diversion performed during debulking surgery [36, 47].

According to a study performed by Tozzi et al. [47] patients in IDS had a slightly higher rate of bowel diversion compared to patients in PDS group (46% vs. 26.5%). Also, patients in IDS were more likely to receive bowel diversion due to impaired tissue quality (44.8% vs. none) while patients in PDS were more likely to receive a bowel diversion when receiving multiple bowel resections (92.3% vs. 34.5%) [47].

Bowel resection has to be limited to what is required, as multiple bowel resections will increase the morbidity [29], as already mentioned above. The tumour must be excised whilst the blood supply is avoided. In order to safely do this, a technique is to dim the theatre light, assess the blood supply and identify the right colic, middle colic, left colic. Once the bowel resection is performed, further assessment for potential ischaemic changes is required.

It is possible to perform small bowel mesenteric peritonectomy or excision of the mesocolon without the need to perform full bowel resection.

After the disease in the pelvis has been tackled the procedure continues in the upper abdomen. To achieve complete resection, extensive upper abdominal procedures are warranted. Strong evidence suggests that upper abdominal procedures improve the survival rates regardless of the time of the debulking [33, 49–55].

The upper abdomen is divided in right and left quadrant and a systematic approach is required. The assessment starts with the mobilisation of the liver (**Figures 3–5**), dividing the falciform ligament, the coronary ligaments in order to assess the posterior aspect of the liver.

Diaphragmatic peritonectomy (**Figures 6** and 7) with or without pleurectomy, partial liver resection, cholecystectomy, splenectomy with or without distal pancreatectomy and resection of the tumour at the porta hepatis (PH) may be required in order to achieve complete resection [33].

Diaphragmatic assessment for cancer invasion is paramount. One of the key dilemmas is to decide which patient would benefit from full diaphragmatic resection, as opposed to peritonectomy only [56, 57]. Tozzi et al. performed a study on

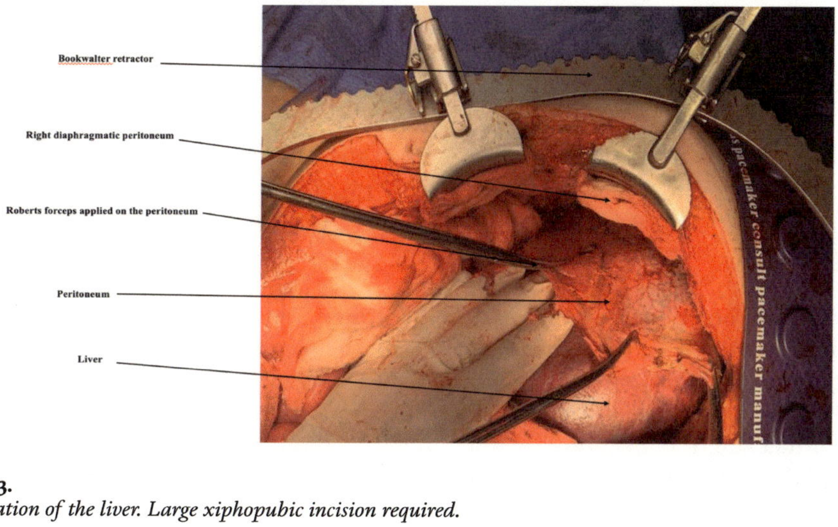

Figure 3.
Mobilisation of the liver. Large xiphopubic incision required.

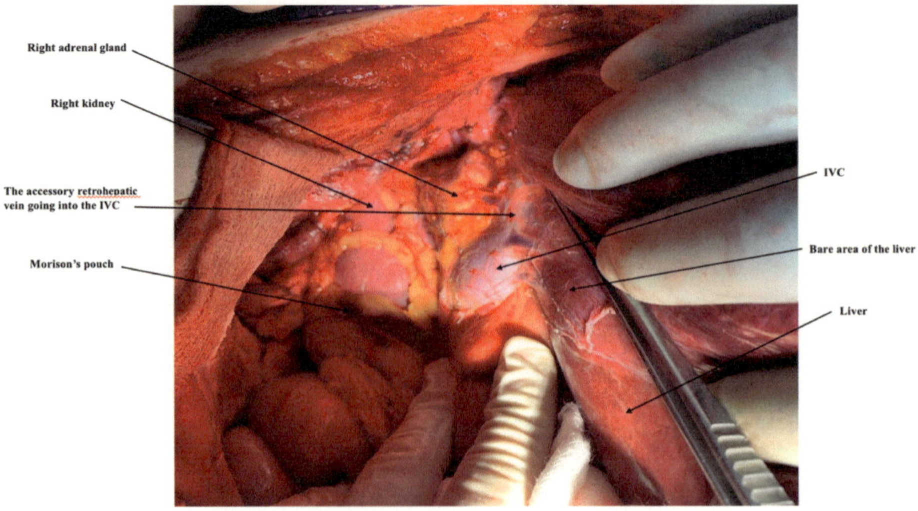

Figure 4.
Type III liver mobilisation exposing retrohepatic space.

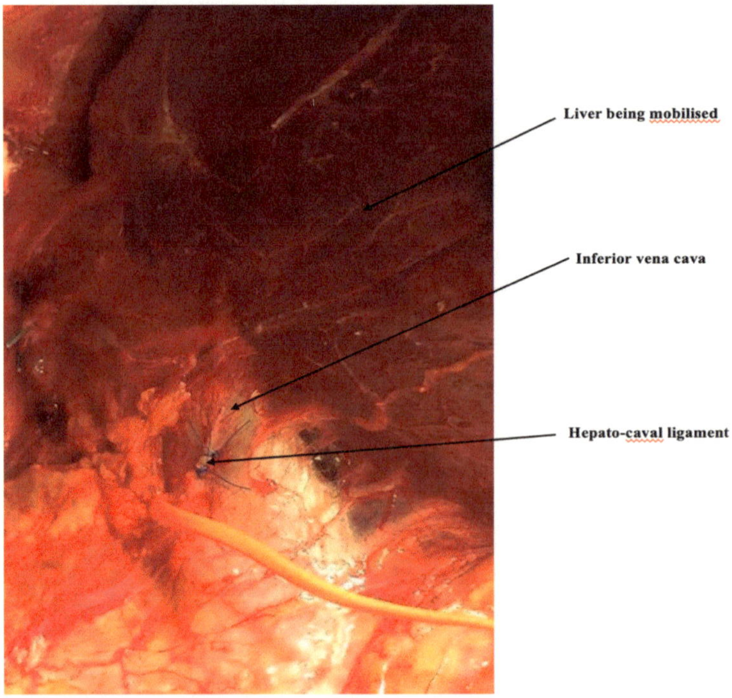

Figure 5.
Liver mobilisation.

170 patients who underwent diaphragmatic surgery and described a meticulous classification to reduce the morbidity but also achieve maximum cytoreductive effort in the upper abdomen. Soleymani majd et al. reported that in patients with diaphragmatic metastasis, 28% had disease spread to the muscle, and 20% of patients had full thickness disease involving the pleura [57–59]. Hence diaphragmatic peritonectomy alone would have left disease in the muscle and the pleura, and complete cytoreduction would not have been possible. The decision about full

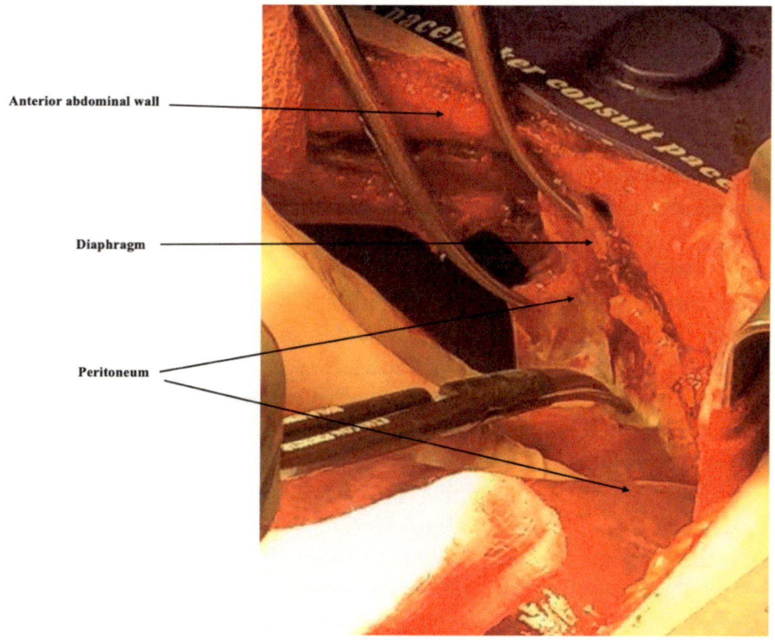

Figure 6.
Diaphragmatic peritonectomy.

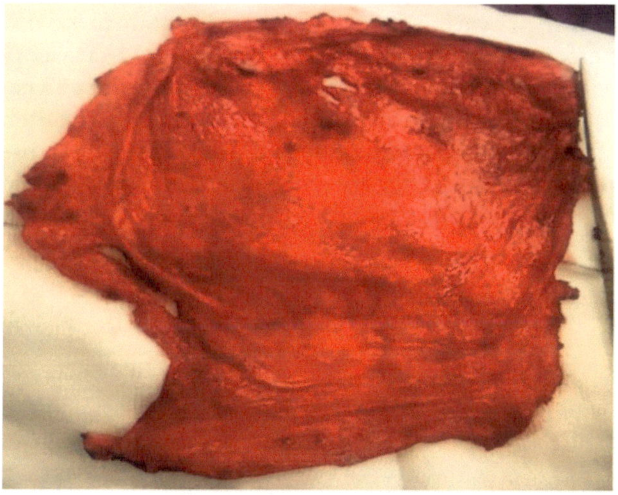

Figure 7.
Peritoneum after diaphragmatic peritonectomy (removal in one piece).

thickness diaphragmatic resection versus diaphragmatic peritonectomy requires prospective studies balancing morbidity against survival benefits [56].

The porta hepatis (PH) shall always be assessed prior to laparotomy, as encasement of the vessels is an absolute contraindication to proceed with radical debulking surgery. Inspection and palpation of the portal vein, hepatic artery, and bile duct are required, along with assessment of the hepato-coeliac lymph nodes. The pringle manoeuvre should be performed prior to liver mobilisation to maximise surgical safety.

Resection of ovarian disease at the PH was feasible in 90.3% of patients in the Tozzi et al. study [33]. No intra- or postoperative complications were associated with tumour resection at the PH, moreover the resection of PH disease was effective, significantly contributing to a 90% rate of achieving R0. Raspagliese et al. [33, 60], along with this study [33] highlight the importance of routinely exploring the PH area, if aiming for complete cytoreduction.

The excision of lymph nodes beyond abdomen and pelvis is controversial, however leaving an enlarged/bulky lymph node despite all other maximal cytoreductive efforts, may mean that no residual disease status was not achieved. Removal of the cardio-phrenic lymph nodes has to be assessed on individual circumstances and localization of the lymph nodes. In the circumstance, that an enlarged pericardiac lymph node is noted, and the gynaecological oncologist is not trained or confident in removing it, then cardiothoracic expertise would be required in order to achieve complete cytoreduction. The Lion study intraoperatively randomly assigned 647 patients with newly diagnosed advanced ovarian cancer (Stage IIB to IV) who had undergone macroscopically complete resection and had normal lymph nodes (both before and during surgery) to either undergo or not undergo lymphadenectomy. In total, 323 had lymphadenectomy whilst 324 did not. The median overall survival was 69.2 months in the non-lymphadenectomy group and 65.5 months in the lymphadenectomy group. The median progression-free survival was 25.5 months in both groups. Postoperative complications were more prevalent in the lymphadenectomy group. Therefore, the Lion study concluded that systematic pelvic and para-aortic lymphadenectomy in patients with advanced ovarian cancer, was not associated with longer overall or progression-free survival but was associated with a higher incidence of postoperative complications, when compared with those who had no lymphadenectomy [61].

Figure 8 illustrates the opening of the right pelvic side wall.

Surgical debulking in ovarian cancer (especially for advanced disease) has traditionally been performed via an open abdominal route. Laparoscopy in advanced ovarian cancer has mostly been used to explore the feasibility of a complete surgical resection [30]. However, there are a few recent studies in the literature, which report complete response to chemotherapy and no gross residual disease after a laparoscopic approach. In the past, concern about the use of laparoscopy included inadequate radicality, the risk of vaginal and/or port site metastasis secondary to

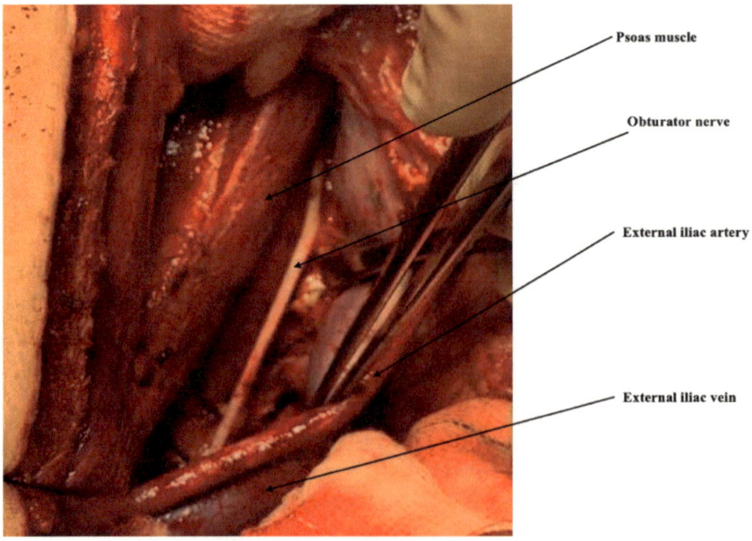

Figure 8.
Right pelvic side wall- exposure of lumbosacral and obturator fossae.

tumour contamination and the use of CO2. In the recent reports, complete resection was achieved at laparoscopy, making it a potentially feasible alternative, warranting consideration [30]. Safe laparoscopy in advanced ovarian cancer consists of thorough preoperative preparation and study of the CT scan images, matching it with the laparoscopic findings, and exploring all peritoneal surfaces. Particular care needs to be taken in avoiding tumour contamination, seeking for cleavage planes in healthy tissue and minimising tumour manipulation. Endobags should be used to extract all specimens, which should be removed intact. Tumour extraction through the vagina is ill advised, if compliance is not adequate [30].

There are a number of well-known benefits of a laparoscopic approach, including: reduced blood loss, decreased pain, earlier discontinuation of analgesia, shorter hospital stay, lower rate of complication and infection. Some researchers report that a short postoperative period is very important in the prognosis of cancer patients and affects survival [30, 62–66]. Surgery has been associated with an increased risk of metastasis and tumour recurrence. The main responsible mechanisms are tumour cell dissemination, shedding, enhanced adhesion, increased tumour growth secondary to reduced apoptosis, increased release of growth factors and angiogenesis, transient but profound suppression of cell-mediated immunity (CMI). The latter controls the minimal residual disease which is present at a cytological level in patients with ovarian cancer. The degree of surgical trauma is noted to correlate with immune depression and with tumour growth [30, 62–66]. Laparoscopy, however, causes reduced trauma and as a consequence a lower inflammatory response, an increased TH1 cytokine production, faster return to normal lymphocyte count and an absence of tumour growth factors in the serum [30, 65]. These effects contribute to a reduced recurrence rate [30, 66], as well as a faster recovery of the immune system in patients with ovarian cancer during their chemotherapy, as they are more prone to anaemia and infections [30, 66].

The data reported so far is for the use of laparoscopy in interval debulking surgery, there is no data on its use in primary debulking surgery [30].

5. Quality of Life

The Quality of Life (QoL) needs to be assessed after such a major and long surgery, which sometimes lasts up to ten hours. QoL questionnaires were sent out to the patients in the Lion study [61]. At the time of discharge, most patients had a poor quality of life, but this improved at follow up (at the end of chemotherapy).

An ultra-radical surgery with the aim of leaving no residual disease (R0) is not successful if the approach to the patient is not holistic; an assessment of whether the patient's quality of life could be improved has to be performed. This surgery should be offered to suitable patients only. Du Bois et al. demonstrated in their study that the benefit was exclusively seen in patients with complete resection (R0) indicating the importance of both the optimal selection of the patients, and of centres with expertise and a high chance of achieving R0 [26, 67, 68].

In ovarian cancer surgery, a multidisciplinary approach is required for successful cytoreductive surgery, keeping the patient at the centre of care.

Conflict of interest

The authors declare no conflict of interest.

Author details

Felicia Elena Buruiana[1*], Lamiese Ismail[2], Federico Ferrari[3] and Hooman Soleymani Majd[2]

1 PanBirmingham Gynaecological Cancer Centre, Birmingham, UK

2 Oxford University Hospitals NHS Foundation Trust, Oxford, UK

3 Department of Obstetrics and Gynecology, University of Brescia, Italy

*Address all correspondence to: f.buruiana@nhs.net

References

[1] Ovarian Cancer, Cancerresearchuk.org

[2] Reid F: Global Trends in Incidence, Mortality and Survival, The World Ovarian Cancer Coalition Atlas @World Ovarian Cancer Coalition 2018.

[3] Fotopoulou C, Hall M, Cruickshank D, Gabra H, Ganesan R, Hughes C, Kehoe S, Ledermann J, Morrison J, Naik R, Rolland P, Sundar S: British Gynaecological Cancer Society (BGCS) Epithelial Ovarian / Fallopian Tube / Primary Peritoneal Cancer Guidelines: Recommendations for Practice.

[4] Bristow R E, Tomacruz R.S., Armstrong D.K., Trimble E.L., Monts F.J.: Survival effect of maximal cytoreductive surgery for advanced ovarian carcinoma during the platinum era: a meta-analysis, J. Clin. Oncol. 20 (2002) 1248-1259.

[5] Chi D.S., Eisenhauer E.L., Zivanovic O., Sonoda Y., Abu-Rustum N.R, Levine D.A., et al.: Improved progression-free and overall survival in advanced ovarian cancer as a result of a change in surgical paradigm, Gynecol. Oncol. 114 (2009) 26-31.

[6] Eisenkop S.M, Spirtos N.M., Friedman R.L., Lin W.C., Pisani A.L: Relative influences of tumor volume before surgery and the cytoreductive outcome on survival for patients with advanced ovarian cancer: a prospective study, Gynecol. Oncol. 90 (2003) 390-396.

[7] Chi D.S., O. Zivanovic, K.L. Levinson, V. Kolev, J. Huh, J. Dottino et al:. The incidence of major complications after the performance of extensive upper abdominal surgical procedures during primary cytoreduction of advanced ovarian, tubal, and peritoneal carcinomas, Gynecol. Oncol. 119 (1) (Oct 2010) 38-42.

[8] Chang S.J., Bristow R.E., Ryu H.S.: Impact of complete cytoreduction leaving no gross residual disease associated with radical cytoreductive surgical procedures on survival in advanced ovarian cancer, Ann. Surg. Oncol. 19 (13) (Dec 2012) 4059-4067.

[9] Vergote I., Tropé C.G, Amant F., Kristensen G.B., Ehlen T., Johnson N et al.: Neoadjuvant Chemotherapy or Primary Surgery in Stage IIIC or IV Ovarian Cancer. European Organization for Research and Treatment of Cancer-Gynaecological Cancer Group; NCIC Clinical Trials Group, N. Engl. J. Med. 363 (2010) 943-953.

[10] Kommoss S., Rochon J., Harter P., Heitz F., Grabowski J.P., Ewald-Riegler N., et al.: Prognostic impact of additional extended surgical procedures in advanced-stage primary ovarian cancer, Ann. Surg. Oncol. 17 (1) (2010 Jan) 279-286.

[11] Rafii A., Stoeckle E., Jean-Laurent M., Ferron G., Morice P., Houvenaeghel G., Lecuru F. et al.: Multi-center evaluation of post-operative morbidity and mortality after optimal cytoreductive surgery for advanced ovarian cancer, PLoS One 7 (7) (2012), e39415.

[12] Soleymani Majd H et al.: Latest developments and techniques in gynaecological oncology surgery, Current opinion in Obstetrics and Gynaecology 27(4), 291-296, https://doi.org/10.1097/gco.0000000000000186.

[13] Cosin J A, Kesterson J P, Olawaiye A B: Staging of Gynaecologic Malignancies Handbook, Society of Gynecologic Oncology, 2014.

[14] Fotopoulou C et al.: Value of Neoadjuvant Chemotherapy for Newly Diagnosed Advanced Ovarian Cancer: A European Perspective, Journal of

Clinical Oncology, Vol 35, No 6 (February 20), 2017: pp 587-590.

[15] Wright AA, Bohlke K, Armstrong DK, et al: Neoadjuvant chemotherapy for newly diagnosed, advanced ovarian cancer: Society of Gynecologic Oncology and American Society of Clinical Oncology clinical practice guideline. J Clin Oncol 34: 3460-3473, 2016.

[16] Vergote I, Trope´ CG, Amant F, et al: Neoadjuvant chemotherapy or primary surgery in stage IIIC or IV ovarian cancer. N Engl J Med 363:943-953, 2010.

[17] Kehoe S, Hook J, Nankivell M, et al: Primary Chemotherapy Versus Primary Surgery for Newly Diagnosed Advanced Ovarian Cancer (CHORUS): An open-label, randomised, controlled, non-inferiority trial. Lancet 386:249-257, 2015.

[18] Bristow RE, Tomacruz RS, Armstrong DK, et al: Survival effect of maximal cytoreductive surgery for advanced ovarian carcinoma during the platinum era: A meta-analysis. J Clin Oncol 20:1248-1259, 2002.

[19] du Bois A, Reuss A, Pujade-Lauraine E, et al: Role of surgical outcome as prognostic factor in advanced epithelial ovarian cancer: A combined exploratory analysis of 3 prospectively randomized phase 3 multicenter trials: by the Arbeitsgemeinschaft Gynaekologische Onkologie Studiengruppe Ovarialkarzinom (AGOOVAR) and the Groupe d'Investigateurs Nationaux Pour les Etudes des Cancers de l'Ovaire (GINECO). Cancer 115:1234-1244, 2009.

[20] Kehoe S, Hook J, Nankivell M, Jayson GC, Kitchener H, Lopes T, Luesley D, Perren T, Bannoo S, Mascarenhas M, Dobbs S, Essapen S, Twigg J, Herod J, McCluggage G, Parmar M, Swart AM: Primary chemotherapy versus primary surgery for newly diagnosed advanced ovarian cancer (CHORUS): an open label, randomised, controlled, non-inferiority trial, Lancet. 2015 Jul 18;386(9990):249-57. doi: 10.1016/S0140-6736(14)62223-6. Epub 2015 May 19. PMID: 26002111.

[21] Reuss A et al. - TRUST: Trial of Radical Upfront Surgical Therapy in advanced ovarian cancer (ENGOT ov33/AGO-OVAR OP7), Int J Gynecol Cancer 2019; 29: 1327-1331.

[22] Barber H.R., Brunschwig A., Pelvic exenteration for locally advanced and recurrent ovarian cancer, Surgery 58 (1965) 935-937.

[23] Eisenhauer E.A., Therasse P., Bogaerts J. et al.: New response evaluation criteria in solid tumours: revised RECIST guideline (version 1.1), Eur. J. Cancer 45 (2) (2009) 228-247, http://dx.doi.org/10.1016/j.ejca.2008.10.026.

[24] Tozzi R, et al.: En-bloc resection of the pelvis (EnBRP) in patients with stage IIIC–IV ovarian cancer: A 10 steps standardised technique. Surgical and survival outcomes of primary vs interval surgery., Gynecol Oncol (2017), http://dx.doi.org/10.1016/j.ygyno.2016.12.019.

[25] Hall et al: Maximal-Effort Cytoreductive Surgery for Ovarian Cancer Patients with a High Tumor Burden: Variations in Practice and Impact on Outcome, Ann Surg Oncol (2019) 26:2943-2951.

[26] du Bois A.R., Pujade-Lauraine E., Harter P., Ray-Coquard I., Pfisterer J.: Role of surgical outcome as prognostic factor in advanced epithelial ovarian cancer: a combined exploratory analysis of 3 prospectively randomized phase 3 multicenter trials: by the arbeitsgemeinschaft gynaekologische onkologie studiengruppe ovarialkarzinom (AGO-OVAR) and the

groupe d'investigateurs nationaux pour les etudes des cancers de l"vaire (GINECO), Cancer 115 (6) (2009) 1234-1244.

[27] Querleu D, Planchamp F, Chiva L, et al.: European Society of Gynaecologic Oncology quality indicators for advanced ovarian cancer surgery. Int J Gynecol Cancer. 2016;26:1354 63.

[28] Fotopoulou C, Hall M, Cruickshank D. British Gynaecological Cancer Society (BGCS) epithelial ovarian/fallopian tube/primary peritoneal cancer guidelines: recommendations for practice. Eur J Obstet Gynecol Reprod Biol. 2017;213:123-39.

[29] Tozzi et al.: Morbidity of multiple bowel resection compared to single bowel resection after debulking surgery for ovarian cancer; European Journal of Obstetrics & Gynecology and Reproductive Biology 240 (2019) 215-219

[30] Tozzi, et al., Interval Laparoscopic En-Bloc Resection of the Pelvis (L-EnBRP) in patients with stage IIIC-IV ovarian cancer: Description of the technique and surgical outcomes, Gynecol Oncol (2016), http://dx.doi.org/10.1016/j.ygyno.2016.07.003

[31] Fotopoulou C: How to predict treatment failure in frail patients with advanced epithelial ovarian cancer: strategies to personalize surgical effort: J Gynecol Oncol. 2020 Jan;31(1): e26.

[32] Liu YL, Filippova OT, Zhou Q, Iasonos A, Chi DS, Zivanovic O, et al.: Characteristics and survival of ovarian cancer patients treated with neoadjuvant chemotherapy but not undergoing interval debulking surgery. J Gynecol Oncol 2020;31: e17.

[33] Tozzi et al.: Porta hepatis peritonectomy and hepato–celiac lymphadenectomy in patients with stage IIIC–IV ovarian cancer: Diagnostic pathway, surgical technique and outcomes, Gynecol Oncol (2016), http://dx.doi.org/10.1016/j.ygyno.2016.08.232.

[34] Tozzi et al.: Diagnostic flow-chart to identify bowel involvement in patients with stage IIIC-IV ovarian cancer: Can laparoscopy improve the accuracy of CT scan?; Gynecologic Oncology 155 (2019): 207-212.

[35] Phillips A, Sundar S, Singh K, Pounds R, Nevin J, Kehoe S, Balega J, Elattar A: The NICE classification for "Ultra-radical (extensive) surgery for advanced ovarian cancer" guidance does not meaningfully predict postoperative complications: a cohort study, BJOG, 2018, doi: 10.1111/1471-0528.15423.

[36] Tozzi, et al.: Morbidity and reversal rate of ileostomy after bowel resection during Visceral-Peritoneal Debulking (VPD) in patients with stage I..., Gynecol Oncol (2017), https://doi.org/10.1016/j.ygyno.2017.11.017.

[37] Tozzi, K. Hardern, K. Gubbala, R. Garruto Campanile, H. Soleymani Majd: En-bloc resection of the pelvis (EnBRP) in patients with stage IIIC-IV ovarian cancer: a 10 steps standardised technique. Surgical and survival outcomes of primary vs. interval surgery, Gynecol. Oncol. 144 (3) (2017) 564-570, https://doi.org/10.1016/j.ygyno. 2016.12.019.

[38] H. Soleymani Majd, F. Ferrari, S. Manek, K. Gubbala, R.G. Campanile, K. Hardern, et al.: Diaphragmatic peritonectomy vs. full thickness resection with pleurectomy during Visceral-Peritoneal Debulking (VPD) in 100 consecutive patients with stage IIIC-IV ovarian cancer: a surgical-histological analysis, Gynecol. Oncol. 140 (3) (2016) 430-435.

[39] K.K. Shih, D.S. Chi: Maximal cytoreductive effort in epithelial ovarian

cancer surgery, J. Gynecol. Oncol. 21 (2) (2010) 75-80.

[40] M. Peiretti, R.E. Bristow, I. Zapardiel, M. Gerardi, V. Zanagnolo, R. Biffi, et al.: Rectosigmoid resection at the time of primary cytoreduction for advanced ovarian cancer. A multi-center analysis of surgical and oncological outcomes, Gynecol. Oncol. 126 (2) (2012) 220-223.

[41] R.D. Clayton, A. Obermair, I.G. Hammond, Y.C. Leung, A.J. McCartney: The Western Australian experience of the use of en bloc resection of ovarian cancer with concomitant rectosigmoid colectomy, Gynecol. Oncol. 84 (1) (2002) 53-57.

[42] M.F. Sier, L. van Gelder, D.T. Ubbink, W.A. Bemelman, R.J. Oostenbroek: Factors affecting timing of closure and non-reversal of temporary ileostomies, Int. J. Color. Dis. 30 (9) (2015) 1185-1192.

[43] M. Kairaluoma, H. Rissanen, V. Kultti, J.P.Mecklin, I. Kellokumpu: Outcome of temporary stomas. A prospective study of temporary intestinal stomas constructed between 1989 and 1996, Dig. Surg. 19 (1) (2002) 45-51.

[44] A.J. Kuryba, N.A. Scott, J. Hill, J.H. van der Meulen, K.Walker: Determinants of stoma reversal in rectal cancer patients who had an anterior resection between 2009 and 2012 in the English National Health Service, Color. Dis. 18 (6) (2016) O199-205.

[45] G.G. David, J.P. Slavin, S. Willmott, D.J. Corless, A.U. Khan, C.R. Selvasekar: Loop ileostomy following anterior resection: is it really temporary? Color. Dis. 12 (5) (2010) 428 432.

[46] P. Waterland, K. Goonetilleke, D.N. Naumann, M. Sutcliff, F. Soliman: Defunctioning ileostomy reversal rates and reasons for delayed reversal: does delay impact on complications of ileostomy reversal? A study of 170 defunctioning ileostomies, J. Clin. Med. Res. 7 (9) (2015) 685-689.

[47] Tozzi et al.: Bowel resection rate but not bowel related morbidity is decreased after interval debulking surgery compared to primary surgery in patients with stage IIIC-IV ovarian cancer, j Gynecol Oncol. 2019 Mar; 30 (2): e25.

[48] F. Rondelli, P. Reboldi, A. Rulli, F. Barberini, A. Guerrisi, L. Izzo, et al.: Loop ileostomy versus loop colostomy for fecal diversion after colorectal or coloanal anastomosis: a meta-analysis, Int. J. Color. Dis. 24 (5) (2009) 479-488.

[49] G.D. Aletti, S.C. Dowdy, B.S. Gostout, M.B. Jones, C.R. Stanhope,Wilson TO, et al.: Aggressive surgical effort and improved survival in advanced-stage ovarian cancer, Obstet. Gynecol. 107 (2006) 77-85.

[50] M.A. Merideth, W.A. Cliby, G.L. Keeney, T.G. Lesnick, D.M. Nagorney, K.C. Podratz: Hepatic resection for metachronous metastases from ovarian carcinoma, Gynecol. Oncol. 89 (2003) 16-21.

[51] S.M. Eisenkop, N.M. Spirtos, W.C. Lin: Splenectomy in the context of primary cytoreductive operations for advanced epithelial ovarian cancer, Gynecol. Oncol. 100 (2006) 344-348.

[52] P.M. Magtibay, P.B. Adams, M.B. Silverman, S.S. Cha, K.C. Podratz: Splenectomy as part of cytoreductive surgery in ovarian cancer, Gynecol. Oncol. 102 (2006) 369-374.

[53] D.S. Chi, E.L. Eisenhauer, O. Zivanovic, Y. Sonoda, N.R. Abu-Rustum, D.A. Levine, et al.: Improved progression-free and overall survival in advanced ovarian cancer as a result of a change in surgical paradigm, Gynecol. Oncol. 114 (2009) 26-31.

[54] R. Salani, A. Axtell, M. Gerardi, C. Holschneider, R.E. Bristow: Limited utility of conventional criteria for predicting unresectable disease in patients with advanced stage epithelial ovarian cancer, Gynecol. Oncol. 108 (2008) 271-275.

[55] R.E. Bristow, L.R. Duska, N.C. Lambrou, E.K. Fishman,M.J. O'Neill, E.L. Trimble, et al.: A model for predicting surgical outcome in patients with advanced ovarian carcinoma using computed tomography, Cancer 89 (2000) 1532-1540.

[56] Tozzi R et al.: Classification of diaphragmatic surgery in patients with stage IIIC–IV ovarian cancer based on surgical findings and complexity, J Gynecol Oncol. 2020 Mar; 31(2): e14., https://dx.doi.org/10.3802%2Fjgo.2020.31.e14.

[57] Addley S, Yao D-S, Soleymani majd H: Primary diaphragmatic closure following diaphragmatic resection and cardiophrenic lymph node dissection during interval debulking surgery for advanced ovarian malignancy, Gynecol Oncol Reports, 36 (2021), 100744.

[58] Ciro Pinelli, Matteo Morotti, Jvan Casarin, Roberto Tozzi, Moiad Alazzam, Vasileios K Mavroeidis, Hooman Soleymani Majd: The Feasibility of Cardiophrenic Lymphnode Assessment and Removal in Patients Requiring Diaphragmatic Resection During Interval Debulking Surgery for Ovarian Cancer, J Invest Surg 2019 Dec 6;1-7. doi: 10.1080/08941939.2019.1690077.

[59] Soleymani majd H et al.: Diaphragmatic peritonectomy vs. full thickness resection with pleurectomy during Visceral-Peritoneal Debulking (VPD) in 100 consecutive patients with stage IIIC–IV ovarian cancer: A surgical-histological analysis, December 2015, Gynecologic Oncology 140(3). DOI: 10.1016/j.ygyno.2015.12.004.

[60] F. Raspagliesi, A. Ditto, F. Martinelli, E. Haeusler, D. Lorusso: Advanced ovarian cancer: omental bursa, lesser omentum, celiac, portal and triad nodes spread as cause of inaccurate evaluation of residual tumor, Gynecol. Oncol. 129 (2013) 92-96.

[61] Harter P, Sehouli J, Lorusso D, Reuss A, Vergote I et al.: A Randomized Trial of Lymphadenectomy in Patients with Advanced Ovarian Neoplasms (Lion trial), Engl J Med, 2019 Feb 28;380(9):822-832., doi: 10.1056/NEJMoa1808424.

[62] C. Evans, C. Galustian, D. Kumar, R. Hagger, D.M. Melville, M. Bodman-Smith, I. Jourdan, A.M. Gudgeon, A.G. Dalgleish: Impact of surgery on immunologic function: comparison between minimally invasive techniques and conventional laparotomy for surgical resection of colorectal tumors, Am. J. Surg. 197 (2) (2009 Feb) 238-245.

[63] M. Horowitz, E. Neeman, E. Sharon, S. Ben-Eliyahu: Exploiting the critical perioperative period to improve long-term cancer outcomes, Nat. Rev. Clin. Oncol. 12 (4) (2015 Apr) 213-226.

[64] E. Neeman, S. Ben-Eliyahu: Surgery and stress promote cancer metastasis: new outlooks on perioperative mediating mechanisms and immune involvement, Brain Behav. Immun. 30 (Suppl) (2013 Mar) S32–S40.

[65] G.J. Van der Bij, S.J. Oosterling, R.H. Beelen, S. Meijer, J.C. Coffey, M. van Egmond: The perioperative period is an underutilized window of therapeutic opportunity in patients with colorectal cancer, Ann. Surg. 249 (5) (2009 May) 727-734.

[66] G. Shakhar, S. Ben-Eliyahu: Potential prophylactic measures against postoperative immunosuppression: could they reduce recurrence rates in oncological patients? Ann. Surg. Oncol. 10 (8) (2003 Oct) 972-992 (Review).

[67] Petrillo M, Ferrandina G, Fagotti A, et al: Timing and pattern of recurrence in ovarian cancer patients with high tumor dissemination treated with primary debulking surgery versus neoadjuvant chemotherapy. Ann Surg Oncol 20: 3955-3960, 2013.

[68] du Bois A, Sehouli J, Vergotte I & co: Randomizeed Phase III study to evakuate the imoact of secondary cytoreductive surgery in recurrent ovarian cancer: Final analysis of AGO DESKTOP III/ENGOT-ov20, Journal of Clinical Oncology, Vol 38, Issue 15.

Chapter 7

Cytoreductive Procedures and HIPEC in the Treatment of Advanced Ovarian Cancer

Bogdan Moldovan, Silviu-Tiberiu Makkai-Popa, Costel Rad, Radu Pisica, Vlad Untaru and Doly Stoica

Abstract

This chapter is dedicated to cytoreductive procedures and hyperthermic intraperitoneal chemotherapy (HIPEC) in the treatment of advanced ovarian cancer. Cytoreductive procedures and HIPEC constitute nowadays an important weapon in the surgical armamentarium used to treat ovarian cancer. Our service led by Dr. Moldovan Bogdan has an experience of 235 patients that underwent a HIPEC procedure, with an average of 33,5 cases/year which places us among some of the most experienced teams worldwide. We propose a chapter describing the indications and contraindications of such procedures, the surgical approach, followed by a description of our experience, including a review of our indications, the type of chemotherapeutic agents and a case example.

Keywords: cytoreductive surgery, HIPEC, carcinomatosis, hyperthermic intraperitoneal chemotherapy, cisplatin, doxorubicin

1. Introduction

Ovarian cancer ranks as the seventh most common cancer in women worldwide, as shown by a metanalysis of 125 articles published between 1925 and 2018 [1]. This frequency also comes with a non-neglectable mortality which in the same meta-analysis is estimated at 4,4% of all the cancer cases, in 2018. The mortality index is mostly due to the fact that the diagnosis is made when the disease is already advanced with two thirds of the mortality being attributed to advanced forms of serous carcinoma. Even with the current care recommendations which involve standard cytoreductive surgery and multiple lines of chemotherapy the confounded long-term survival for all disease stages is only 20–30% and is mostly due to peritoneal carcinomatosis [1–6]. As such we find that completing the cytoreductive surgery with hyperthermic intraperitoneal chemotherapy is the best way to ensure the best possible outcomes for ovarian cancer patients. A review of the current literature shows that it improves the 5-year survival to 24–60% compared to an average life expectancy of 12 to 25 months with standard chemotherapy [4, 7].

The aim of this chapter is to bring insight into our current surgical practice of performing extensive cytoreductive surgery and hyperthermic intraperitoneal chemotherapy.

2. Historic perspective and rationale for HIPEC

Over time our view of peritoneal carcinomatosis evolved from considering it a terminal disease to considering it a form of locally advanced disease amenable to surgery which is sometimes with curative intent. The first to introduce the concept of cytoreductive surgery was Griffiths in 1975. His work shows a direct link between the radicality of the surgery and the survival of the patients [8, 9]. Five years later Spratt et al. show that hyperthermic intraperitoneal chemotherapy is feasible in peritoneal carcinomatosis [10, 11] and finally, in 1995 Sugarbaker et al. describe the technique of complete peritonectomy with an extraperitoneal approach, which in our opinion is the most suitable technique for most of the cases. He also described the combination of his technique with HIPEC [10].

If we look at the literature, we find articles clearly showing that the peritoneum in general and regions where scars exist – port sites for example are more prone to metastasis compared to solid organs and systemic chemotherapy is effective in about one third of the cases, with a complete response in only 15% of the cases [11]. Hence cytoreduction is extremely important to reduce tumor burden and HIPEC augments its efficacy by the lavage itself which, performed in a recent postoperative setting helps flush the cells resulted from manipulating bulky lesions such as is often the case. It also helps by activating heat shock proteins due to the temperature which is around 42 degrees and gives the chemotherapeutic agent a chance to act locally by putting it in direct contact with the peritoneum.

3. HIPEC indications

The established concept of cytoreduction and HIPEC in peritoneal carcinomatosis is that they are to be performed in advanced stages of the disease, however more and more articles, starting with Sugarbaker and continuing with other high-volume surgical centers propose using HIPEC as a prophylactic measure not only in ovarian cancer but also in advanced appendiceal, colonic or gastric malignancies [11–19]. Keeping this in mind, it is our opinion that in the surgical management of ovarian cancer we will soon be able to classify HIPEC procedures into prophylactic – in stages up to II B and conventional – in stages III and IV. Because of the aggressiveness of the procedure, in each and every case we operate we struggle to achieve a complete cytoreduction, otherwise known as CC0 and in order to preoperatively assess in which patients this might be achieved we use staging scores such as the Fagotti score.

Initially, the Fagotti score [20] was described as a laparoscopic means of assessing the feasibility of a HIPEC procedure, but because all surgical manipulation of the peritoneum decreases the chances to perform a radical surgery, we substitute the laparoscopic Fagotti score with an imaging score based on a good quality abdominal and pelvic contrasted, diffusion weighed magnetic resonance imaging (MRI). Besides avoiding unnecessary manipulation of the peritoneum, we consider it superior to laparoscopy because it allows us to assess the areas of the abdomen and pelvis which are difficult to evaluate surgically, especially in a patient that has had previous abdominal surgery. Similar to it is also the Bristow CT score, but in our opinion the Fagotti score based on a good quality MRI examination is better [21].

The Fagotti score contains 5 variables – omental cake, diaphragmatic carcinomatosis, mesenteric retraction, bowel/stomach infiltration and spleen/liver metastasis. If present, each variable receives 2 points. If the Fagotti score obtained on the MRI is less than 8 we go ahead and prepare the patient for HIPEC, while if the score is higher than 8 we prefer to perform a Pressurized Intraperitoneal Aerosol

Chemotherapy (PIPAC) session, continue chemotherapy and reassess the patient by the same MRI score 4–6 weeks after. We can perform 2–3 such PIPAC sessions in the hopes of achieving operability.

Besides the Fagotti score which in our opinion is the best tool for staging ovarian peritoneal carcinomatosis and the Bristow score, there are several other scores which we only mention but not describe in detail as they are not used in case of ovarian cancer carcinomatosis – the Peritoneal Cancer Index (PCI) proposed in 1996 by Sugarbaker and Jaquet [15, 16], the Gilly staging [15, 17] and the simplified PCI system proposed by Zoetmulder [18].

In conclusion to this subsection on staging scores we would like to talk about our standard preoperative workup in cases which are referred to our center as candidates for cytoreductive surgery and HIPEC. This includes an MRI of the abdomen and pelvis with contrast and diffusion weighted imaging and a chest CT.

We prefer MRI because in our experience it correlates best with what we would find on an exploratory laparoscopy allowing us to obtain a more accurate Fagotti score. The chest CT allows us to define the intrathoracic involvement and plan for an eventual diaphragmatic resection. We place bilateral chest tubes at the end of the procedure and if needed the chest drain can also be connected to the HIPEC machine in order to have cytostatic agent circulating also in the pleural cavity.

Based on the imaging findings we can define not only the patients with better chances for having a complete resection but also those where there is a contraindication for HIPEC. The contraindications can be classified in absolute and relative.

Absolute contraindications are:

- inoperable invasion of the liver hilum;
- diffuse, inoperable liver metastases;
- diffuse small bowel lesions in which resection would mean leaving less than 1 m of small bowel;
- unresectable retroperitoneal lymph node masses;
- inoperable distant metastasis.

Relative contraindications are:

- locally advanced multiple relapses, resistant to different chemotherapy regimens;
- progression under neoadjuvant therapy;
- bad performance status and comorbidities.

Pleural involvement which is common, is not a contraindication for performing HIPEC, but rather an indication to also perform hyperthermic intrathoracic chemotherapy (HITOC), eventually as staged procedures.

4. Timing of the cytoreductive and HIPEC procedures

Because of the variability of the moment when ovarian cancer is diagnosed there are several moments in the natural history of an ovarian cancer case when cytoreductive procedures and HIPEC can be performed as can be seen in the analysis performed by Helm et al. [14].

The first such moment and the one in which cytoreduction and HIPEC give the best chances of survival is when the diagnosis is made, if complete cytoreduction can be achieved [2]. In the moment of diagnosis, depending on the extent of the disease we can talk about prophylactic HIPEC or conventional HIPEC in later stages [19]. Prophylactic HIPEC in ovarian cancer refers to stages I and II in which we have a cytology sample which is positive for tumor cells, which suggests an increased risk for peritoneal relapse and a decision is made together with the patient and the oncologist to perform HIPEC with a preventive thinking in mind.

Another moment for HIPEC and cytoreduction is after neoadjuvant chemotherapy, because most ovarian cancers respond well to chemotherapy and become operable after a neoadjuvant treatment. The only disadvantage is that it might downsize the peritoneal implants, rather than really downstage the tumor and thus hide implants that otherwise would have been resected, increasing the risk for recurrence.

HIPEC can also be performed as a consolidation therapy after neoadjuvant chemotherapy, meaning that it is performed during a second look laparotomy when peritoneal biopsies reveal residual disease.

Another occasion on which these procedures might become useful in ovarian cancer is when a peritoneal relapse is diagnosed and surgery is performed usually after a new course of neoadjuvant chemotherapy which will also determine the chemotherapeutic agent to be used based on the response of the tumor.

Finally, the last situation in which we would perform HIPEC is as a last resort treatment – basically a salvage procedure.

5. Description of the technique for cytoreductive surgery

In ovarian cancer most of the authors recommend a selective peritonectomy technique and not a total peritonectomy, but in our hospital we prefer performing a total extraperitoneal (Sugarbaker) peritonectomy because we have more experience with it and we consider it more radical based on our results [22, 23]. An example of extraperitoneal peritonectomy can be seen in **Figures 1** and **2**.

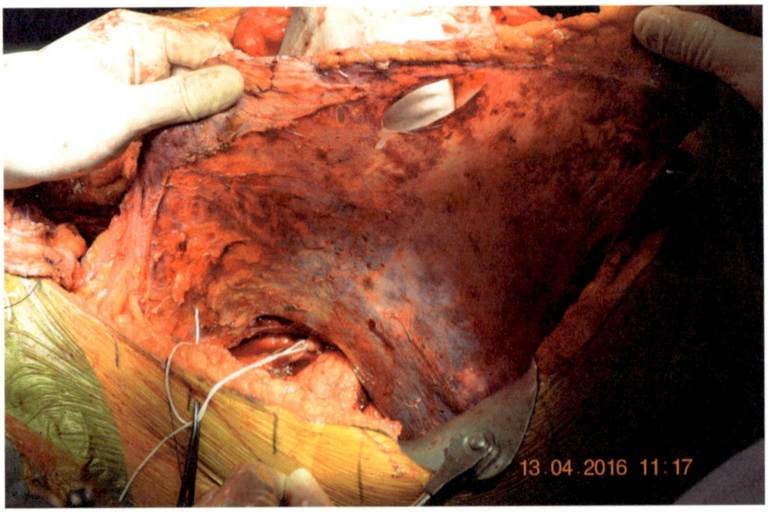

Figure 1.
Sugarbaker extraperitoneal peritonectomy.

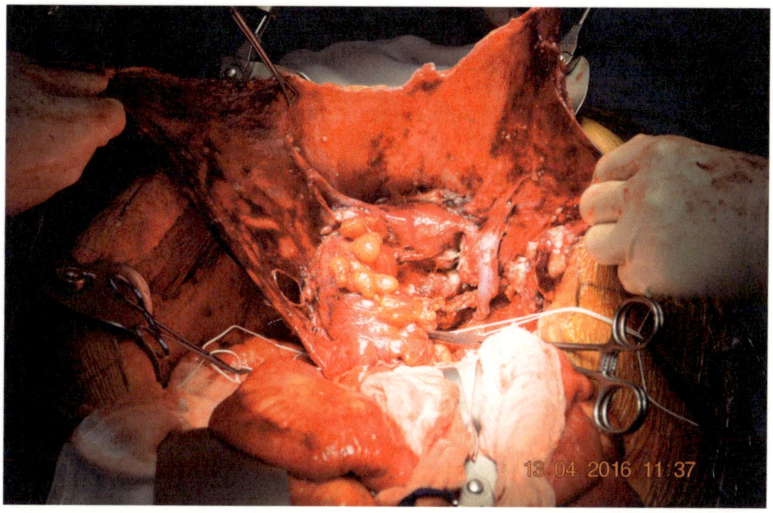

Figure 2.
Sugarbaker extraperitoneal peritonectomy view once the peritoneal cavity is opened.

We start by detaching the peritoneum completely without opening it by entering a plane located between the peritoneum and the rectus sheath. We continue in this plane laterally until reaching the peritoneum, cranially until the Glisson's capsule and inferiorly we resect the peritoneum covering the bladder with the uterus and the two adnexae, with or without the rectum. As patients usually come to us after a staging laparotomy performed elsewhere, we start by resecting the previous scars which are the most common sites of future relapses. We usually start below the umbilicus as this is the place where we can develop the correct plane at greater ease. Once the round ligament is cut at the level of the deep inguinal ring we can dissect easily laterally until reaching the retroperitoneum and exposing the iliac vessels and the ureters.

We then develop the plane cranially. Sometimes splenectomy is necessary if implants are seen on it or close to it, but it is not indicated as a rule in ovarian cancer.

Once the peritoneum is detached completely cranially and laterally, we enter the peritoneal cavity. A first resection specimen is constituted by the median scar, the umbilicus, the round ligament of the liver which is cut at the level of Rex's recess, the falciform ligament and the urachal fold down to the bladder. The remaining peritoneum will be split into four quadrants. Completing the peritonectomy of the right upper quadrant is considered the most difficult as it consists of:

- resecting the diaphragmatic peritoneum, sometimes with a piece of diaphragm;
- dissection of the Glisson's capsule, if affected, with the eventual metastases;
- cholecystectomy
- liver hilum lymph node dissection
- right colo-epiploic takedown with dissection of the posterior peritoneal sheath of the omental bursa
- resection the peritoneum of the Morison space

- selective peritonectomy of the space between the caudate lobe, the inferior vena cava and the right diaphragmatic crux

In the left upper quadrant, the peritonectomy means:

- resecting the diaphragmatic peritoneum, sometimes with a piece of diaphragm;
- left colo-epiploic takedown
- dissection of the greater curvature
- resection of the peritoneum with or without the spleen
- mobilization of the left colonic flexure, sometimes requiring a colectomy

In the lower abdomen the peritonectomy includes:

- dissection of the peritoneum covering the urinary bladder
- dissection and section of the ovarian vessels
- dissection of the ureters in order to expose and ligate the uterine vessels safely
- sectioning the vagina below the cervix
- dissection of the peritoneum of the Douglas pouch when it is normal macroscopically or with the rectum if there are visible tumor implants
- appendicectomy
- sometimes colonic resections
- pelvic and paraaortic lymphadenectomy.
- sometimes a bladder resection or vascular resections might be necessary

In the central part of the abdomen the small intestine is examined carefully on both sides. Severely affected portions of the small bowel are resected carefully, keeping in mind in mind the risk for short bowel and taking away as little bowel as possible. Mesenteric implants are either resected or Argon beam coagulated. Atypical resections of the stomach can also be performed with the use of linear staplers.

Keeping in mind that the cytoreduction is usually followed by HIPEC we are faced with some delicate decisions regarding the anastomoses we perform. For small bowel we perform a 2-layer latero-lateral continuous suture without stoma. For colorectal anastomoses we perform a mechanical anastomosis using a circular stapler and protecting the anastomosis with a colostomy which we prefer to an ileostomy. And finally, there are cases where we do not perform an anastomosis but rather an end colostomy or ileostomy. These are mostly CC1 cases, posterior pelvic exenteration cases or total colectomy cases in fragile patients, even with a CC0 resection where an anastomosis would be too risky due to the status of the patient.

6. Assessing the completeness of cytoreduction – the radicality score

It is considered the most important prognostic score, being estimated at the end of the cytoreductive stage. The penetrability of intraperitoneal chemotherapy is possible for lesions up to 2.5 mm. For most intraperitoneal neoplasms, complete CC0 cytoreduction is required, the CC1 score being considered acceptable only for peritoneal pseudomyxoma, a neoplasm with reduced aggressiveness. The radicality of resection classification is as follows: CC0 – no residual disease, CC1 – residual lesions smaller than 0,25 cm, CC2 – residual lesion between 0,25 and 2,5 cm and CC3 – residual lesions larger than 2,5 cm [18].

The impossibility of a radical surgery CC0-CC1 can determine the change of the operative strategy, either towards a palliative debulking surgery, or towards giving up any gesture of excision. In chemotherapy "naive" tumors, the maximum cytoreduction with HIPEC followed by adjuvant CT is to be considered.

7. Description of the HIPEC procedure

For reasons related to the safety of handling cytostatic substances, most HIPEC teams in Europe, including our team use the "closed abdomen" technique in which the abdomen is closed permanently or only temporarily (the skin), with 4 drains inside, coupled to extracorporeal circulation device.

In short, the Rand Performer HT device that we use in our current activity, has the following components: 1) a heater or heat exchanger; 2) a pump system, which includes one or two peristaltic pumps; 3) a tank containing the infusion solution; 4) a circuit that distributes the drugs and heated fluid to the patient's peritoneal cavity. In 1999 the Italian Biomedical Company (RanD Biotech SRL, Medolla, Italy) was the first to develop a device dedicated to HIPEC, used especially for the treatment by hyperthermic perfusion of the peritoneal cavity. The most important advantage of this device (Performer HT) is its portability and adaptability for various purposes, as it can also be used to infuse isolated anatomical regions or organs, such as the treatment of an isolated limb or the separate infusion of the liver or lung. The Performer HT device ensures a flow rate of 100–2000 ml/min and it has up to 8 temperature monitoring lines in various areas of the peritoneal cavity, which has the ability to measure temperatures between 28 °C and 46 °C. In our practice we use tubes with a diameter of 28 Fr, two for inlet (1 - subdiaphragmatic and 1 - in the pelvis) and two for the outlet (1 - subdiaphragmatic and 1 - in the pelvis). We also use two lines for monitoring the intra-abdominal temperature mounted in the pelvis and in the supramesocolic space. In terms of the perfused solution, we use 4–6 liters of warm transport solution (2/3 Ringer, 1/3 Voluven). Once an optimal infusion rate (> 800 ml/min) and an optimal intraperitoneal temperature around 42-43 °C is reached, the cytotoxic drugs are administered. We use Cisplatin (43 mg/L solution/m2) or Doxorubicin (15 mg/L solution) for carcinomatosis due to serous ovarian cancer. The duration of chemoperfusion is between 60 and 90 minutes. At the end of the procedure, the abdomen is rinsed with 3 liters of saline and the drains are left in place.

As to the choice of the chemotherapeutic drug, it takes into account the sensitivity of the tumor to platinum salts, which can be seen preoperatively by the response of the tumor to the neoadjuvant chemotherapy. Platinum-sensitive patients will follow the Cisplatin protocol, Platinum-resistant patients, the Doxorubuicin protocol.

- Cisplatin (43 mg/L solution/m2) - for Platinum CEO sensitive.
- Doxorubicin (15 mg/L solution) - for CEO resistant Platinum.

Other types of protocols using Taxol, Oxaliplatin, 5 Fluorouracil or Mitomycin C, etc. are also cited in the literature.

8. Our experience

In our experience we performed cytoreductive surgery and HIPEC on a number of 235 cases since we started performing these procedures in our hospital on the 5th of June 2013 which means an average of 33,5 cases/year. From a surgical point of view, critically speaking there were 2 stages: the initial experience 2013-December 2014, dominated by surgical caution, fear of complications, selective peritonectomy by "open" approach, after intraperitoneal exploration and the second stage, starting from January 2015, with the introduction of the Sugarbaker-Deraco extraperitoneal total peritonectomy technique, marked by increased aggression, the association of multiorgan resections often with digestive anastomoses.

Of these patients there were 188 (80%) females and 47 (20%) males. The mean age of the patients was 60,92 ± 10,64 years. The mean hospital stay was 9,23 ± 3,66 with a minimum of 4 days and a maximum of 32 days. In terms of overall survival, 182 out of 203 patients (89,65%) survived at 1 year and 15 out of 75 patients (20%) survived at 5 years. The mean operating time for these cases was 7,21 ± 0,7 hours and the mean PCI was 14,5 ± 0,3.

Because of the number of patients and the variety of the pathology we preferred to give a visual representation of the type of pathology approached (**Figure 3**), the type of chemotherapeutic agent we used (**Figure 4**) and whether or not we did a stoma and what type of stoma we did (**Figure 5**). In terms of the radicality of resection you can see in **Figure 6** the proportions of CC0, CC1 and CC2 resections.

Of particular importance in 2020, we had to reorganize our in-hospital protocols in order to ensure a COVID-free surgical department which allowed us to perform 29 cytoreductive procedures followed by HIPEC since the pandemic was declared on March 11th 2020. We were able to do this by thoroughly screening admitted patients by aligning ourselves to the guidelines emitted by the major surgical and

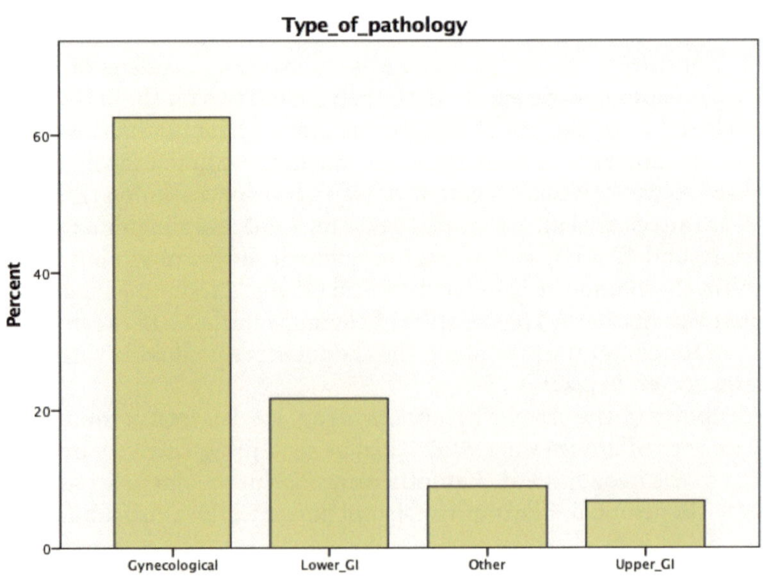

Figure 3.
Types of pathologies approached by cytoreduction and HIPEC in our experience.

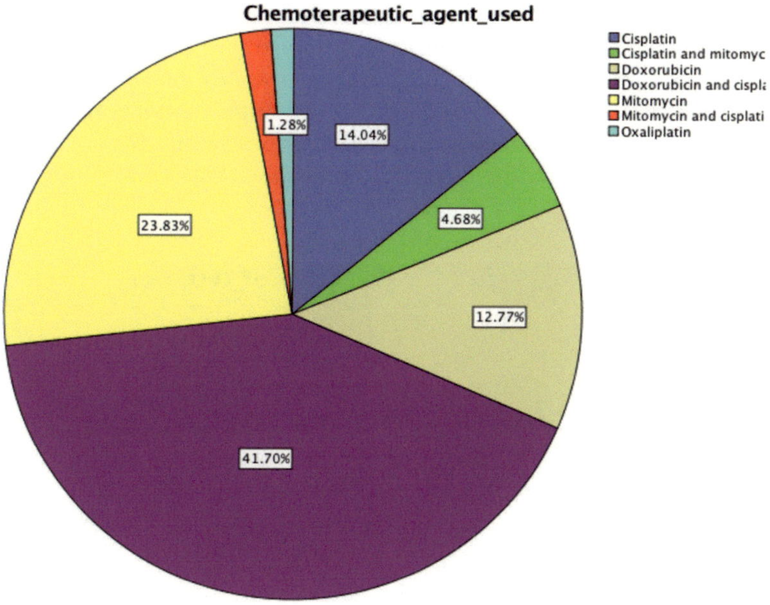

Figure 4.
Cytostatic agents used in our experience.

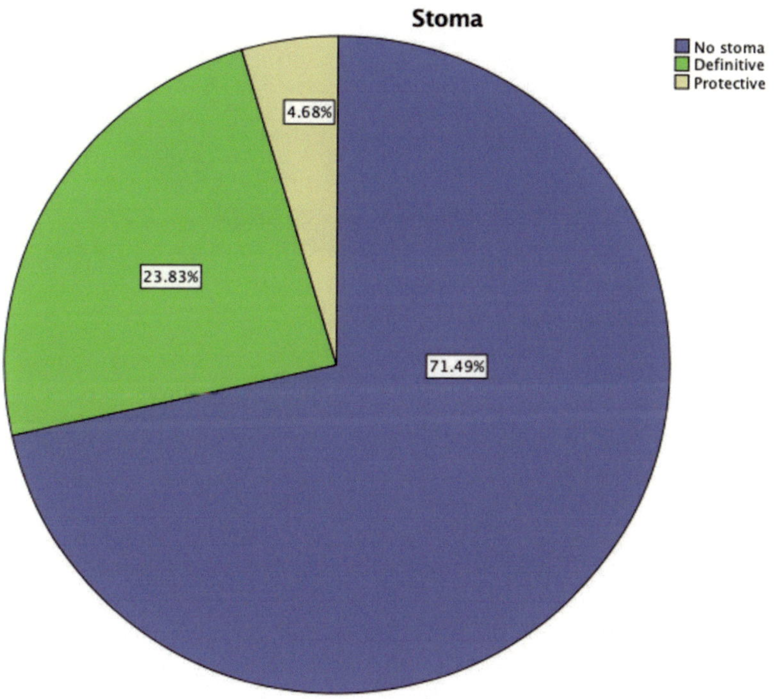

Figure 5.
Use of stomas in our experience.

oncological international societies. Initially our screening consisted in PCR tests from nasopharyngeal swab, rapid antibody test and chest CT and according to the guidelines we started only performing PCR from nasopharyngeal swab, leaving rapid antibody and antigen tests and chest CT scans only for patients in which we had a strong clinical suspicion of COVID and a negative PCR test [24].

In terms of multiorgan resections of note are cases of associations between posterior pelvic exenteration, right hemicolectomy and resection of liver metastases, resection of ureter, bladder horn and uretero-vesical reimplantation, total colectomy with extended jejuno-ileal enterectomy, entero-enteral anastomosis and right iliac terminal ileostomy, association of posterior exenteration with regulated left hepatic lobectomy and radiofrequency thermoablation of liver metastasis.

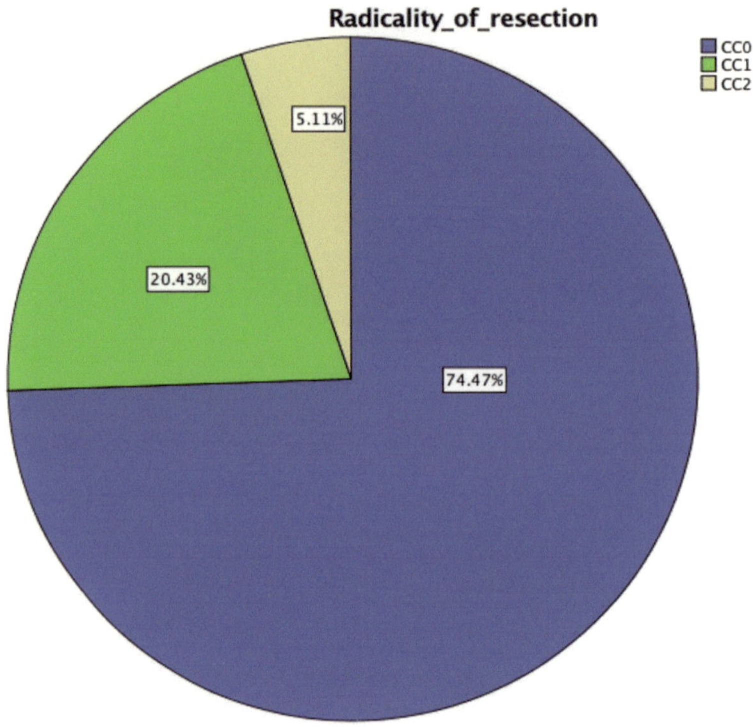

Figure 6.
Radicality of resection in our experience.

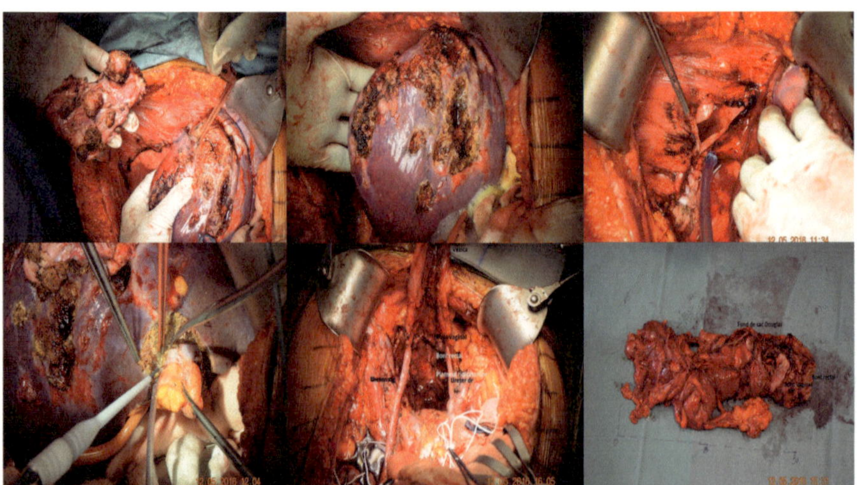

Figure 7.
Intraoperative pictures showing multiple organ resections in a patient with recurrent ovarian carcinoma.

As an example, we would like to present a case of ovarian carcinoma recurrence in a 51 years-old patient previously operated and treated by chemotherapy. The PCI was calculated to be 19 and we performed a CC0 resection with a Sugarbacker extraperitoneal approach associated with a Hartmann resection, multiple liver resections, diaphragmatic resection with phrenic reconstruction, appendicectomy, omentectomy, HIPEC - Doxorubicin 80 mg 60 minutes at 42 °C. Some intraoperative pictures can be seen in **Figure 7**. The patient is still living at 3 years after the procedure and does not show signs of recurrence, despite the fact that she was considered untreatable by other centers before coming in our service.

9. Conclusion

Cytoreductive surgery and HIPEC now offer an alternative to ovarian cancer patients that were once considered inoperable and in high-volume centers the complications are minimal. This chapter provides insight into the technique of cytoreductive surgery and HIPEC and presents our experience with these techniques.

Acknowledgements

The authors would like to thank the producers of the hyperthermic perfusion system – RanD for their excellent support in using the RanD Performer HT system which was used in this case.

Conflict of interest

The authors declare no conflict of interest.

Author details

Bogdan Moldovan[1,2]*, Silviu-Tiberiu Makkai-Popa[1], Costel Rad[1], Radu Pisica[1], Vlad Untaru[1] and Doly Stoica[1]

1 “Sf. Constantin” Hospital, Brasov, Romania

2 Academy of Science People in Romania, Romania

*Address all correspondence to: bogdan.moldovan@spitalulsfconstantin.ro

References

[1] Momenimovahed Z, Tiznobaik A, Taheri S, Salehiniya H: Ovarian cancer in the world: epidemiology and risk factors. Int J Womens Health. 2019;11:287-299. DOI: 10.2147/IJWH.S197604

[2] Deraco M, Kusamura S, Virzì S, Puccio F, Macrì A, Famulari C, Solazzo M, Bonomi S, Iusco DR, Baratti D: Cytoreductive surgery and hyperthermic intraperitoneal chemotherapy as upfront therapy for advanced epithelial ovarian cancer: multi-institutional phase-II trial. Gynecol Oncol. 2011;122:215-220

[3] Deraco M, Baratti D, Laterza B, Balestra MR, Mingrone E, Macrì A, Virzì S, Puccio F, Ravenda PS, Kusamura S: Advanced cytoreduction as surgical standard of care and hyperthermic intraperitoneal chemotherapy as promising treatment in epithelial ovarian cancer. EJSO. 2011;37:4-9

[4] Hotouras A, Desai D, Sugarbaker PH: Heated IntraPEritoneal Chemotherapy (HIPEC) for Patients With Recurrent Ovarian Cancer: A Systematic Literature Review. Int J Gynecol Cancer. 2016;26:661-670

[5] McGuire WP, Hoskin WJ, Brady MF, Kucera PR, Partridge EE, Look KY, Clarke-Pearson DL, Davidson M: Cyclophosphamide and cisplatin compared with paclitaxel an cisplatin in patients with stage III and IV ovarian cancer. N Engi J Med. 1996;334:1-6

[6] Ozols RF, Bundy BN, Greer BE, Fowler JM, Clarke-Pearson D, Burger RA, Mannel RS, DeGeest K, Hartenbach EM, Baergen R, Gynecologic Oncology Group. Phase III trial of carboplatin and paclitaxel compared with cisplatin and paclitaxel in patients with optimally resected stage III ovarian cancer: a Gynecologic Oncology Group study. J Clin Oncol. 2003;21:3194-3200

[7] Königsrainer I, Beckert S, Becker S, Zieker D, Fehm T, Grischke E-M, Lauk O, Glatzle J, Brücher B, Wallwiener D, Königsrainer A: Cytoreductive surgery and HIPEC in peritoneal recurrent ovarian cancer: experience and lessons learned. Langenbecks Arch Surg. 2011; 396:1077-1081

[8] Luyckx M, Leblanc E, Filleron Th, Morice Ph, Darai E, Classe J-M, Ferron G, Stoeckle E, Pomel Ch, Vinet B, Chereau E, Bergzoll C, Querleu D: Maximal cytoreduction in patients with FIGO stage IIIc to stage IV ovarian, fallopian and peritoneal cancer in day-to-day practice, a retrospective French multicentric study. Int.J.Gynecol.Cancer. 2012;22:1337-1343

[9] Griffiths CT: Surgical resection of tumor bulk in primary treatment of ovarian carcinoma. Natl Cancer Inst Monogr.1975;42:101-104

[10] Chua TC, Robertson G, Liauw W, Farrell R, Yan TD, Morris DL: Intraoperative HIPEC after CRS in ovarian cancer peritoneal carcinomatosis: systematic review of current results. J Cancer Res Clin Oncol. 2009;135:1637-1645.

[11] Sugarbaker PH: Colorectal cancer, prevention and management of metastatic disease. Biomed Res Int. 2014;2014:782890 DOI: 10.1155/2014/782890

[12] Spratt JS, Adcock RA, Muskovin M, Sherril W, Mc Keown J: Clinical delivery system for intraperitoneal HIPEC. Cancer Res. 1980;40:256-260

[13] Sugarbaker PH: Peritonectomy procedures. Ann Surg. 1995;221: 29-42

[14] Helm CW, Bristow RE, Kusamura S, Deraco M: Hyperthermic intraperitoneal chemotherapy with

and without cytoreductive surgery for epithelial ovarian cancer. J Surg Oncol. 2008;98:283-290

[15] Portilla AG, Kusamura S, Baratti D, Deraco M: The intraoperative staging system in the management of peritoneal surface malignancy. J Surg Oncol. 2008;98:228-231

[16] Jaquet P, Sugarbaker PH: Clinical research methodologies in diagnosis and staging of patients with PC. In: Sugarbaker PH, editor. Peritoneal carcinomatosis: principals of management. Boston: Kluwer Academic publishers 1996:359-374

[17] Gilly FN, Carry PY, Sayag AC: Regional chemotherapy (with mitomycin C) and intra-operative hyperthermia for digestive cancers with peritoneal carcinomatosis. Hepatogastroenterol. 1994;41: 124-129

[18] Witkamp AJ, de Bree E, Kaag MM, Boot H, Beijnen JH, van Slooten GW, van Coevorden F, Zoetmulder FA: Extensive cytoreductive surgery followed by intra-operative hyperthermic intraperitoneal chemotherapy with mitomycin-C in patients with peritoneal carcinomatosis of colorectal origin. Eur J Cancer. 2001;37:979-984

[19] Klaver CEL, Musters GD, Bemelman WA, Punt CJA, Verwaal VJ, Dijkgraaf MGW, Aalbers AGJ, van der Bilt JDW, Boerma D, Bremers AJA, Burger JWA, Buskens CJ, Evers P, van Ginkel RJ, van Grevenstein WMU, Hemmer PHJ, de Hingh IHJT , Lammers LA, van Leeuwen BL, Meijerink WJHJ, Nienhuijs SW, Pon J, Radema SA, van Ramshorst B, Snaebjornsson P, Tuynman JB, Te Velde EA, Wiezer MJ, de Wilt JHW, Tanis PJ: Adjuvant hyperthermic intraperitoneal chemotherapy (HIPEC) in patients with colon cancer at high risk of peritoneal carcinomatosis; the COLOPEC randomized multicentre trial. MC Cancer. 2015;15:428. DOI: 10.1186/s12885-015-1430-7

[20] Fagotti A, Ferrandina G, Fanfani F, Garganese G, Vizzielli G, Carone V, Salerno MG, Scambia G: Prospective validation of a laparoscopic predictive model for optimal cytoreduction in advanced ovarian carcinoma. Am J Obstet Gynecol. 2008;199:642.e1-6

[21] Bristow RE, Duska LR, Lambrou NC, Fishman EK, O'Neill MJ, Trimble EL, Montz FJ: A model for predicting surgical outcome in patients with advanced ovarian carcinoma using computer tomography. Cancer 2000;89:1532-1540

[22] Moldovan B, Pescaru F, Pocreata D, Capalna M: Example of multimodal oncosurgery approach used to treat peritoneal carcinomatosis in a patient with occlusive ovarian carcinoma. EJGO. 2016;2:251-254

[23] Moldovan B, Capilna M, Pocreata D, Rad CC, Pescaru F, Stan S, Ioanid N: Aspecte generale. Tehnica chirurgiei cytoreductive si HIPEC. In: Moldovan B, editor. Tratamentul carcinomului ovarian prin chirurgie citoreductiva si HIPEC. Brasov: Editura Didactica si Pedagocica, R.A. 2017 :7-42

[24] Makkai-Popa S-T, Rad C, Pisica R, Untaru V, Stoica D, Zolog A, Bosinceanu LM, Moldovan B (forthcoming): Hyperthermic intraperitoneal chemotherapy procedure for uterine sarcoma following a COVID-19 infection - case report. EJGO. 2021

Chapter 8

HIPEC for Ovarian Cancer: A Controversial Discussion

Michael Friedrich, Dominique Friedrich, Clayton Kraft, Walther Kuhn and Christoph Rogmans

Abstract

Peritoneal carcinomatosis is a sign of advanced disease of ovarian cancer. The prognosis of ovarian cancer is significantly improved after cytoreductive surgery with complete tumor debulking followed by platin based chemotherapy. If cytoreductive surgery results in a tumor free situation with remaining tumor less than 0.25 cm, HIPEC may further improve prognosis. Materials and methods: The results of the Krefeld study are presented and the literature is reviewed according to overall survival and progression free survival with or without HIPEC. In the Krefeld study, patients with ovarian cancer and peritoneal carcinomatosis underwent cytoreductive surgery. In patients with optimal tumor debulking, HIPEC was performed. The peri- and postoperative course was observed. Adverse events were recorded after the Clavien-Dindo classification. Results: 43 patients were treated with cytoreductive surgery and HIPEC. In all patients an optimal cytoreductive situation with remaining tumor less than 0.25 cm was achieved. HIPEC was performed with a cisplatin solution (50 mg/m2) at 41°C. The median age of the patients was 56 years (range: 32–74 years), the median peritoneal cancer index (PCI) was 13 (range: 4–21), the median operation time was 356 minutes (range: 192–507 minutes). The median time to postoperative systemic treatment with chemotherapy was 29 days (range 21–70). There was no postoperative surgically associated death. No adverse events were recorded in 16 (37.2%) of 43 patients, no grade III or IV adverse events were reported for 33 (76.7%) patients, and no grade IV adverse events were reported for 41 (95.3%) patients. Grade III adverse events occured in 19 (44.2%) of the 43 patients; a total of 29 grade III adverse events were reported in these 19 patients. Grade IV adverse events occured in 3 (7.0%) of the 43 patients; a total of 3 grade IV adverse events were reported. Two of them resulted in return to the operating room. This was a fistula of the distal small bowel caused by drainage and a revision of wound infection. Conclusion: In ovarian cancer multiple surgical procedures may be necessary in order to have macroscopically eradicated tumor tissue. Combined with HIPEC, this seems to have positive effects on the survival of patients with peritoneal carcinomatosis. Since we have no marked additional adverse events caused by HIPEC in our case series, HIPEC seems to be an additional treatment option of peritoneal carcinomatosis in ovarian cancer. This statement is strengthened by the literature review in that metaanalysis show significant improved OAS and PFS.

Keywords: Hyperthermic intraperitoneal intraoperative chemotherapy, HIPEC, ovarian cancer

1. Introduction

Most patients with advanced ovarian cancer will suffer from recurrence, because the five year overall survival for stage FIGO III and IV epithelial ovarian cancer is still very low with 20–30%. Thus, gynecologic oncologists are looking for better treatment strategies [1].

In most patients with advanced ovarian cancer the spread to the peritoneum is the primary site of failure. Thus, it seems reasonable to assess additional local treatment strategies apart from maximal tumor debulking. According to prior studies the intraperitoneal application of cisplatin is assiciated with a 20-fold higher concentration in the intraperitoneal space compared to that measured in plasma after intravenous administration. Furthermore it was shown that the combination of postoperative intraperitoneal and intravenous (ip/iv) chemotherapy improves survival in women with optimally resected stage III ovarian cancer compared with iv chemotherapy alone. There are many aspects like treatment-related toxicities, adhesion barriers after surgery, dysfunction of implanted i.p. catheters (Tenckhoff catheters), the absence of a standard treatment regimen, patients` preference and the inconvenience of an inpatientregimen that prevent the integration of ip/Iv chemotherapy into clinical routine [2].

2. Review and discussion

HIPEC is usually applied immediately following peritonectomy procedure with the aim of directly delivering a heated cytotoxic drug to the peritoneal surface of the abdomen. While macroscopic disease is removed by cytoreductive surgery, microscopic disease from the peritoneal surface should be eradicated by HIPEC. There are studies showing that hyperthermia enhances penetration of the cytotoxic agent and induces tumor cell death by multiple mechanisms including impaired DNA repair, inhibition of angiogenesis and induction of apoptosis. The rationale of applicatio of HIPEC is that HIPEC eradicates tumors up to a diameter of 2.5 cm. Advantages of HIPEC in comparison to postoperative ip chemotherapy are the missing adhesion barriers at the time of operation. Furthermore, the effectiveness of intraoperative intraperitoneal chemotherapy is increased by the hyperthermic application [3–9].

In our own case series analysis [10] of 43 patients treated with HIPEC (cisplatin 50 mg/m2 for 60 minutes at 42°C) for advanced or recurrent ovarian cancer there was no postoperative death. Adverse events of grade III following the Clavien Dindo classification [11] were observed in 44.2% of the patients, which suggests that HIPEC with cisplatin 50 mg/m2 after CRS in ovarian cancer is a feasable treatment option. Additionally, the time to chemotherapy (TTC) was not markedly prolonged in our setting. The main complications are caused by surgery and not by HIPEC procedure. The very low rate of insufficiences of anastomoses with only one case of a fistula of the small bowel shows the immense importance of the experience of the surgical team.

Yonemura et al. [12] described in their study with CRS and HIPEC for colorectal carcinomas one postoperative death caused by pulmonary thromboembolism. Grade IV adverse events were observed in 9.9% of cases mainly due to insufficiences of anastomosis. Grade III adverse events were reported by Kuijpers et al. [13] in 34% of the 960 patients in a simliar trial with a mortality rate of 3%, while Passot et al. [14], found an incidence of grade III and IV adverse events in 42% of 216 patients (CRS and HIPEC) with peritoneal carcinomatosis (35% ovarian cancer).

Ovarian cancer is a leading cause of cancer related death in women and is often only diagnosed at an advanced stage, then with diffuse peritoneal carcinomatosis [15–34]. Peritoneal carcinomatosis represents the advanced stage in the evolution of

EOC, which has been considered as the main cause of recurrence [23, 35, 36]. Since ovarian cancer is mainly confined to the peritoneal cavity, even after recurrence, it is an ideal target for locoregional therapy. IP chemotherapy is not a standard treatment option because of concerns of excessive toxicity [37–39]. Nevertheless IP chemotherapy is associated with improved survival of advanced EOC [6–8]. HIPEC and post-operative IP chemotherapy are differing distinctly from eachother, because HIPEC is a single treatment of intraoperative chemotherapy at the time of cytoreductive surgery. Some critical aspects of ip chemotherapy may be eliminated by this fact [21]. So far, most of the evidence for HIPEC in the treatment of advanced ovarian cancer was based on large retrospective series [15–17], a few small non-randomized prospective studies [18, 19] and a small randomized trial of low quality in regard to study design [20]. These available studies are difficult to interpret and compare due to the heterogenicity of the study groups. A clear distinction between primary and recurrent disease, extensiveness of peritonectomy surgery, various FIGO stages and types of histology is not made, although these aspects in themselves significantly influence the outcome. A systemic review of published trials [21] identified 9 comparative studies reporting an improvement in survival following CRS and HIPEC (+/− CHT) compared with CRS alone (+/− CHT). Morbidity following CRS and HIPEC was reported to be between 12% and 33% [21, 22]. The majority of complications are more likely to be due to the aggressive CRS rather than HIPEC, particularly in respect to bowel complications (anastomotic insufficiences, bowel fistula sepsis). On the other hand the addition of HIPEC is associated with renal impairment and haematological toxicity due to transient bone marrow suppression.

The results of the first RCT for HIPEC for primary ovarian cancer were published in 2018 [23]. In this study, hyperthermic intraperitoneal chemotherapy with cisplatin 100 mg/m2 was administered at 40°C over 90 min in an open technique. Sodium thiosulfate was administered by a six-hour intravenous infusion to prevent nephrotoxicity. The hazard ratio (HR) for disease recurrence or death was 0.66 (95% CI 0.50–0.87, P = 0.003), favouring the HIPEC group. The median PFS was 14.2 months in the CRS plus HIPEC group versus 10.7 months in the CRS group. At 5 years, 50% of the patients in the CRS plus HIPEC group had died versus 62% in the CRS group (HR 0.67, 95% CI 0.48–0.94, P = 0.02). The median OS was 45.7 months versus 33.9 months, showing a 11.8-month survival advantage in the CRS plus HIPEC group. There was no significant difference in grade three or four adverse events between the two groups (27% vs. 25%, P = 0.76, respectively). There was a higher rate of stoma formation in the CRS plus HIPEC group (72% vs. 43%, P = 0.04). Despite this, the overall health-related quality of life outcomes did not differ between the two groups. To date this is the best evidence that a single administration of HIPEC given at the time of cytoreductive surgery for ovarian cancer may achieve significant benefits in terms of survival without excess morbidity or loss of quality of life. However, there has been critique concerning this study, in the direction of a possible premature analysis of overall survival, the heterogeneity of results between study centres, and the results being applicable to only a small subset of patients with ovarian cancer [24]. The HIPEC arm also received an additional, high dose of cisplatin compared to the non-HIPEC arm, which in itself might explain the improved survival.

This study provided the evidence of survival benefit by HIPEC in patients with intervall debulking surgery in advanced EOC. One hast o keep in mind that the survival of the group without HIPEC was shorter than that in the Gynecologic Oncology Group–172 study perhaps because of the different inclusion criteria (intervall debuling surgery versus primary debulking surgery) [40].

In contrast to the results of Van Driehl et al., a smaller Korean RCT on HIPEC with 184 women, including only patients with stage 3 and 4 disease, did not demonstrate a significant advantage in terms of five-year survival in the HIPEC arm [25]. It is not described in how many patients the remaining tumor mass was less than 2.5 mm. In addition, women with extraperitoneal metastatic ovarian cancer were also included in the study. However, it is important for HIPEC therapy to have minimal residual tumor. Therefore, the Korean study would need to be reevaluated from these perspectives to gain valdie insights. For stage IV colorectal carcinoma, a recently published phase III RCT HIPEC trial failed to demonstrate a survival benefit over systemic chemotherapy after cytoreductive surgery [26].

Which drugs and in what dosage should be used for intraperitoneal chemotherapy is still unclear. Zivanovic et al. [27] showed in the first prospectively designed German HIPEC-ROC-I study of 12 patients with recurrence of ovarian cancer that a dose increase from 50 mg/m2 cisplatin to 100 mg/m2 is safe. Although one patient in the study experienced renal failure not requiring dialysis, a dose of 100 mg/m2 cisplatin should be used in future studies. The mean operative time was 463 minutes. In all cases, systemic chemotherapy was started within 6 weeks. We used the dosage of 50 mg/m2 cisplatin in our study, because at the beginning of the study the results of Zivanovic et al. [27] had not been published.

Nevertheless, it is not clear at which point it is appropriate to start postoperative systemic chemotherapy (TTC). The most important prognostic factor regarding OS is achieving surgical R0 resection. At the same time, Mahner et al. [28] demonstrated in a systemic review of 3,326 patients from three AGO-OVAR trials [3, 5, 7] that delayed initiation of therapy of more than 19 days in R0 resected patients was associated with significantly decreased overall survival. In contrast, patients with macroscopic residual tumor did not benefit from an earlier start of chemotherapy. Hofstetter et al. [29] support these findings. An analysis of the European multicenter OVCAD trial in which the median start of chemotherapy was 28 days (range 4 to 158 days) demonstrated that patients with macroscopic R1 resection had significantly worse overall survival, when chemotherapy was started after 28 days or later. In contrast, Feng et al. [30] demonstrated in 625 patients with advanced ovarian cancer that an interval of up to 6 weeks between cytoreductive surgery and start of chemotherapy did not negatively affect overall survival. The median TTC in our study was 29 days (range 21–70 days). The late start of therapy with a TTC of 70 days was due to a fistula at the ileum that required multiple surgeries.

As already mentioned, surgical R0 resection is the most important prognostic factor associated with significantly improved overall survival. When evaluating the studies described above, this must be taken into account. In Hofstetter et al. [29], 63.4% of the patients had R0 resection, whereas in Feng et al. [30], this was 33.4%. In our study, R0 resection was achieved in 93% of cases, and only 7% of cases had R1 resection.

Wu et al. [41] demonstrate in their metaanalysis, that HIPEC can significantly improve the OS and PFS of EOC. But so far HIPEC is not accepted as a standard treatment in clinical routine [21] because of the heterogeneity of the inclusion criteria and the study methods.

Wu et al. [41] demonstrate in their metaanalysis, that HIPEC significantly improves the OS and PFS of EOC. But so far HIPEC is not accepted as a standard treatment in clinical routine [21] because of the heterogeneity of the inclusion criteria and the study methods. Subgroup analysis, which considered study design, adjusted for heterogeneity. Nevertheless, there are only two RCTs on HIPEC in ovarian cancer. The different lengths of follow-up made it necessary to perform further analyses regarding to OS and PFS.

Even in this analysis there is the suggestion that HIPEC could significantly improve survival. Consistent with previous studies [23, 42] Wu et al. [41] also found that the administration of HIPEC is safe, with limited and less morbidity and mortality compared with no HIPEC group in the majority of included studies. In primary EOC patients, Wu et al. demonstrated that HIPEC improved OS, PFS and each year survival rate. In addition, these results are consistent with previous meta-analysis of HIPEC [21] suggesting that the incorporation of HIPEC may result in better prognosis of primary EOC [40]. Most previous evidence of a beneficial effect from HIPEC in primary EOC has been limited to single-group trials or retrospective cohorts [43–48]. Until recently, van Driel et al. [23] reported the first RCT about primary EOC and HIPEC with the evidence of HIPEC's survival benefit in advanced EOC after NAC.

Lei et al. [49] perfomed a cohort study from January 2010 to May 2017 at 5 high-volume institutions in China to compare survival outcomes between PCS with HIPEC vs. PCS alone for patients with stage III epithelial ovarian cancer. A total of 584 patients with stage III primary epithelial ovarian cancer were treated with either PCS alone or PCS with HIPEC. The median follow-up period was 42.2 (33.3–51.0) months.

In addition, a distinction was made how the resection grade of tumor mass affected the 3-year overall survival rate and median survival time. In patients with R0 resection with additional HIPEC, median survival was 53.9 months (95% CI, 46.6–63.7) and 3-year overall survival was 65.9% (95% CI, 60.1%–71.2%). Patients with residual tumor who underwent HIPEC therapy had a median survival of 29.2 months (95% CI, 22.3–45.5) and a 3-year overall survival rate of 44.3% (95% CI, 34.6%–53.4%). In patients with complete tumor mass reduction who received PCS only, median survival was 42.3 months (95% CI, 31.1–59.3), and 3-year overall survival was 55.4% (95% CI, 44.7%–64.8%). Incomplete tumor mass resection without HIPEC, exhibits the worst outcome with a median survival of 19.9 months (95% CI, 11.6–39.1) and a 3-year overall survival rate of 36.7% (95% CI, 23.4%–50.1%). This leads to the conclusion that PCS with HIPEC results in significantly better overall survival, especially with R0 resection of tumor mass.

In contrast, several studies in the past lead to opposing results. This could be due to heterogeneous study designs, different treatment regimens, and different inclusion criteria of patients. Mendivil et al. [50] performed a comparative study in primary advanced EOC, highlighting survival rates of patients with and without HIPEC treatment. Here, a significant PFS advantage was evident in the HIPEC group, although overall survival was not prolonged. The reason could be the different recruitment period of the cohorts. The control group was recruited much earlier (2008–2014) and thus had a longer median follow-up time in contrast to the HIPEC group, which was collected in 2012–2015. This could be the reason for the similar median OS of both groups. Wu et al. [45] also failed to show a significant PFS benefit in their study regarding HIPEC therapy. Interestingly, the rate of complete tumor reduction was only 14.58% in the control group and 8.33% in the HIPEC group. As shown above, this could have a strong impact on the data analysis.

Additional trials are still needed to determine the optimal time for HIPEC administration and whether HIPEC is also effective after primary cytoreductive surgery in aprospective randomized trial.

For recurrent ovarian cancer, Wu et al. showed that HIPEC therapy significantly increased OS and PFS. These results are in accordance with similar meta-analysis of Huo et al. on HIPEC [21]. Cascales-Campos et al. confirmed the results regarding significant differences in 2-, 4-, and 5-year PFS with and without HIPEC therapy [42]. It is well known that the standard treatment of relapsed EOC is systemic chemotherapy. The median OS is less than 30 months [21]. Nevertheless, there is evidence that even in relapsed EOS, prognosis can be improved by CRS, provided that the tumor can be completely resected [51, 52]. Bristow et al. showed that patients who underwent CRS had OS ranging from 41 to 60 months. The PFI was

30.3 months [51, 52]. Again, the complete tumor mass reduction was crucial for median overall survival (R0 45.2 vs. R1 19.7, HR¼3.71, $p < 0.001$) [53]. These data demonstrates that overall survival in relapsed EOS can be significantly increased by CRS. Implementation of CRS in the therapy of relapsed EOC would improve overall survival. This may be a reason, which could have led to insignificant difference for 1- and 2-year PFS for therapy with and without HIPEC. Baiocchi et al. [54] showed that overall survival cannot be improved by combining CRS and HIPEC in relapsed platinum-sensitive EOC. Further studies are needed for recurrent EOC, especially considering tumor resectability.

But this result might be based on a selection bias with regard to the different extent of disease or surgery status. It has to be taken under consideration, if the result might be based on a selection bias with regard to the different extent of disease or surgery status. Spiliotis et al. [20] demonstrated in their randomized trial of 120 relapsed EOC patients that the combination of CRS and HIPEC was superior to CRS only. Surprisingly, overall survival rates were the same in the HIPEC cohorts regardless of the presence or absence of platinum resistance. This was not the case in the CRS group. The reason for this could be sensitization of tumor cells by hyperthermia. It is conceivable that molecular mechanisms, such as heat shock proteins or epigenetic changes, could be triggered to sensitize the tumor cells [55, 56]. Again, complete tumor reduction is shown to prolong median overall survival. A limitation could be the randomization process and primary endpoints of the study are not clearly defined [23, 57]. In conclusion, further RCS on relapsed EOC need to be performed as the study situation is very heterogeneous regarding PFS, median follow-up and first-line postoperative treatment [19].

There are some limitations existing in the meta-analysis by Wu et al. First, the inclusion criteria and HIPEC drug regimens for EOC are varying with regard to the extent of disease status and CRS, to the standardization of IPEC protocols. Second, no standard quantitative measurement of the morbidity related to HIPEC was established. Third, the potential publication bias of included studies was unavoidable due to insufficient RCTs data so far.

It is expected that additional RCS will be performed in the future to elucidate the value of HIPEC in primary and recurrent EOC. In previous studies, the common thread was the performance of HIPEC following CRS. Platinum and/or paclitaxel were usually chosen as therapeutic agents. Only one study evaluated the combination of cisplatin and doxirubicin.

3. Conclusion

Taken together, Wu et al. support with their meta-analysis that HIPEC therapy has a positive impact, both in primary and recurrent EOC on patients' OS and PFS. Nevertheless, no improvement in 1- and 2-year PFS was achieved in recurrent EOC. Therefore, especially for relapsed disease, it is essential to design clearly structured studies that support the value of HIPEC in the treatment of EOC.

Conflict of interest

The authors declare no conflicts of interest.

Author details

Michael Friedrich[1*], Dominique Friedrich[1], Clayton Kraft[2], Walther Kuhn[3] and Christoph Rogmans[4]

1 Klinik für Frauenheilkunde und Geburtshilfe, Helios Klinikum, Krefeld, Germany

2 Klinik für Orthopädie und Unfallchirurgie, Helios Klinikum, Krefeld, Germany

3 Klinik für Frauenheilkunde und Geburtshilfe, DonauIsar Klinikum Deggendorf, Deggendorf, Germany

4 Klinik für Frauenheilkunde und Gebursthilfe, Universitätsklinikum Schleswig-Holstein, Campus Kiel, Germany

*Address all correspondence to: michael.friedrich@helios-gesundheit.de

References

[1] RKI https://www.krebsdaten.de/Krebs/DE/Content/Krebsarten/Ovarialkrebs/ovarialkrebs_node.html

[2] Jaaback K, Johnson N, Lawrie TA. Intraperitoneal chemotherapy for the initial management of primary epithelial ovarian cancer. In: The Cochrane database of systematic reviews 2016; 1, CD005340. DOI: 10.1002/14651858.CD005340.pub4.

[3] Farrell R. Review article: Is peritonectomy and hyperthermic intraperitoneal chemotherapy a new standard of treatment for advanced epithelial ovarian cancer? Aust N Z J Obstet Gynaecol 2019;1-6.

[4] Ohno S, Siddik ZH, Kido Y, et al. Thermal enhancement of drug uptake and DNA adducts as a possible mechanism for the effect of sequencing hyperthermia on cisplatin-induced toxicity in L1210 cells. Cancer Chemother Pharmacol 1994; 34: 302-306.

[5] Van de Vaart PJ, van der Vange N, Zoetmulder FA. Intraperitoneal cisplatin with regional hyperthermia in advanced ovarian cancer: pharmacokinetics and cisplatin-DANN adduct formation in patients and ovarian cancer cell lines. Eur J Cancer 1998; 34: 148-154.

[6] Los G, Mutsaers PHA, van der Vijgh WJF, Mc Vie JG. Direct diffusion of cis-diamminedichloroplatinum (II) in intraperitoneal rat tumours after intraperitoneal chemotherapy: a comparison with systemic chemotherapy. Cancer Res 1989; 49: 3380-3384.

[7] Spratt JS, Adcock RA, Muskovin M, et al. Clinical delivery system for intraperitoneal hyperthermic chemotherapy. Cancer Res 1980; 40: 256-260.

[8] Blinman P, Gainford C, Donoghoe M, et al. Feasibility, acceptability, and preferences for intraperitoneal chemotherapy with paclitaxel and cisplatin after optimal debulking surgery for ovarian and related cancers: an ANZGOG study. J Gynecol Oncol 2013; 24: 359-366.

[9] Sugarbaker PH. Peritonectomy Procedures. Annals of Surgery 1995; 221 (1): 29-42. DOI: 10.1097/00000658-199501000-00004.

[10] Friedrich M, Zinn W, Kolnsberg L, et al. Hyperthermic Intraperitoneal Chemotherapy (HIPEC) for Ovarian Cancer: Evaluation of Side Effects in a Single Institution Cohort. Anticancer Res 2020; 40: 545-550.

[11] Dindo D, Demartines N, Clavien PA. Classification of Surgical Complications. In: Annals of Surgery 2004; 240 (2): 205-213. DOI: 10.1097/01.sla.0000133083.54934.ae.

[12] Yonemura Y, Canbay E, Ishibashi H. Prognostic factors of peritoneal metastases from colorectal cancer following cytoreductive surgery and perioperative chemotherapy. Scientific World Journal 2013; 978394. DOI: 10.1155/2013/978394.

[13] Kuijpers AMJ, Mirck B, Aalbers AGJ, Nienhuijs SW, de Hingh IJHT, Wiezer MJ, et al. Cytoreduction and HIPEC in the Netherlands: nationwide long-term outcome following the Dutch protocol. Ann. Surg. Oncol. 2013; 20 (13): 4224-4230. DOI: 10.1245/s10434-013-3145-9.

[14] Passot G, Bakrin N, Roux AS, Vaudoyer D, Gilly FN, Glehen O, Cotte E. Quality of life after cytoreductive surgery plus hyperthermic intraperitoneal chemotherapy: a prospective study of 216 patients. Eur J Surg Oncol 2014; 40 (5): 529-535. DOI: 10.1016/j.ejso.2013.11.019.

[15] Bakrin N, Bereder JM, Decullier E, et al. Peritoneal carcinomatosis treated with

cytoreductive surgery and hyperthermic intraperitoneal chemotherapy (HIPEC) for advanced ovarian carcinoma: a French multicentre retrospective cohort study of 566 patients. Eur J Surg Oncol 2013; 39: 1435-1443.

[16] Di Gorgio A, De Iaco P, De Simone M, et al. Cytoreduction (peritonectomy procedures) combined with hyperthermic intraperitoneal chemotherapy (HIPEC) in advanced ovarian cancer: retrospective Italian multicentre observational study of 511 cases. Ann Surg Oncol 2016; 24: 914-922.

[17] Munoz-Casares FC, Medina-Fernandez FJ, Arjona-Sanchez A, et al. Peritonectomy procedures and HIPEC in the treatment of peritoneal carcinomatosis from ovarian cancer: long term outcomes and perspectives from a high-volume center. Eur J Surg Oncol 2016; 42: 224-233.

[18] Coccolini F, Campanati L, Catena F, et al. Hyperthermic intraperitoneal chemotherapy with cisplatin and paclitaxel in advanced ovarian cancer: a multicentre prospective observational study. J Gynecol Oncol 2015; 26: 54-61.

[19] Deraco M, Kusamura S, Virzi S, et al. Cytoreductive surgery and hyperthermic intraperitoneal chempotherapy as upfront therapy for advanced epithelial ovarian cancer: multi-institutional phase-II trial. Gynecol Oncol 2011; 122: 215-220.

[20] Spiliotis J, Halkia E, Lianos E, et al. Cytoreductive surgery and HIPEC in recurrent epithelial ovarian cancer: a prospective randomised phase III study. Ann Surg Oncol 2015; 22: 1570-1575.

[21] Huo YR, Richards A, Liauw W, Morris DL. Hyperthermic intraperitoneal chemotherapy (HIPEC) and cytoreductive surgery (CRS) in ovarian cancer: a systematic review and meta-analysis. Eur J Surg Oncol 2015; 41: 1578-1589.

[22] Hotouras A, Desai D, Bhan C, et al. Heated intraperitoneal chemotherapy (HIPEC) for patients with recurrent ovarian cancer: a systematic literature review. Int J Gynecol Cancer 2016; 26: 661-670.

[23] Van Driehl WJ; Koole SN; Sikorska K, et al. Hyperthermic intraperitoneal chemitherapy in ovarian cancer. N Engl J Med 2018; 378: 230 – 240.

[24] Fotopoulou C, Sehouli J, Mahner S, et al. Editorial, Hipec: hope or hype in the fight against advanced ovarian cancer? Ann Oncol 2018; 29: 1610-1613.

[25] Lim MC, Chang SJ, Heong JY, et al. Randomised trial of hyperthermic intraperitoneal chemotherapy (HIPEC) in women with advanced peritoneal, ovarian and tubal cancer. J Clin Oncol 2017; 35(15_suppl): 5520-5520.

[26] Quenet F, Elias D, Roca L, et al. A UNICANCER phase III trial of hyperthermic intraperitoneal chemotherapy (HIPEC) for colorectal carcinomatosis (PC): PRODIGE 7. J Clin Oncol 2018; 36: (18_suppl): LBA3503-LBA3503.

[27] Zivanovic O, Abramian A, Kullmann M, et al. HIPEC ROC I: A phase I study of cisplatin administered as hyperthermic intraoperative intraperitoneal chemoperfusion followed by postoperative intravenous platinum-based chemotherapy in patients with platinum-sensitive recurrent epithelial ovarian cancer. Int. J. Cancer 2015; 136 (3): 699-708. DOI: 10.1002/ijc.29011.

[28] Mahner S, Eulenburg C, Staehle A, Wegscheider K, Reuss A, Pujade-Lauraine E, et al. Prognostic impact of the time interval between surgery and chemotherapy in advanced ovarian cancer: analysis of prospective randomised phase III trials. Eur. J. Cancer 2013; 49 (1): 142-149. DOI: 10.1016/j.ejca.2012.07.023.

[29] Hofstetter G, Concin N, Braicu I, Chekerov R, Sehouli J, Cadron I, et al. The time interval from surgery to start of chemotherapy significantly impacts prognosis in patients with advanced serous ovarian carcinoma - analysis of patient data in the prospective OVCAD study. Gynecologic oncology 2013; 131 (1): 15-20. DOI: 10.1016/j.ygyno.2013.07.086.

[30] Feng Z, Wen H, Bi R, Yang W, Wu X. Prognostic impact of the time interval from primary surgery to intravenous chemotherapy in high grade serous ovarian cancer. Gynecologic oncology 2016; 141 (3): 466-470. DOI: 10.1016/j.ygyno.2016.04.016.

[31] Bristow RE, Cliby WA, Powell MA, Al-Hammadi N, Chen L, Philip Miller J, et al. Ovarian cancer in the United States: contemporary patterns of care associated with improved survival. Gynecologic oncology 2015; 136 (1): 11-17. DOI: 10.1016/j.ygyno.2014.10.023.

[32] Bristow RE, Tomacruz RS, Armstrong DK, Trimble EL, Montz FJ. Survival effect of maximal cytoreductive surgery for advanced ovarian carcinoma during the platinum era: a meta-analysis. J. Clin. Oncol. 2002; 20 (5): 1248-1259.

[33] Harter P, Beutel B, Alesina PF, Lorenz D, Boergers A, Heitz F, et al. Prognostic and predictive value of the Arbeitsgemeinschaft Gynaekologische Onkologie (AGO) score in surgery for recurrent ovarian cancer. Gynecol. Oncol. 2014; 132 (3): 537-541. DOI: 10.1016/j.ygyno.2014.01.027.

[34] Wimberger P, Lehmann N, Kimmig R, Burges A, Meier W, Du Bois A. Prognostic factors for complete debulking in advanced ovarian cancer and its impact on survival. An exploratory analysis of a prospectively randomized phase III study of the Arbeitsgemeinschaft Gynaekologische Onkologie Ovarian Cancer Study Group (AGO-OVAR). Gynecol. Oncol. 2007; 106 (1): 69-74. DOI: 10.1016/j.ygyno.2007.02.026.

[35] Munoz-Casares FC, Rufian S, Rubio MJ, et al. The role of hyperthermic intraoperative intraperitoneal chemotherapy (HIPEC) in the treatment of peritoneal carcinomatosis in recurrent ovarian cancer. Clin Transl Oncol. 2009;11:753-759.

[36] Spiliotis J, Halkia E, de Bree E. Treatment of peritoneal surface malignancies with hyperthermic intraperitoneal chemotherapy current perspectives. Curr Oncol. 2016;23:e266-275.

[37] Wright AA, Cronin A, Milne DE, et al. Use and effectiveness of intraperitoneal chemotherapy for treatment of ovarian cancer. JCO. 2015;33:2841-2847.

[38] Tewari D, Java JJ, Salani R, et al. Long-term survival advantage and prognostic factors associated with intraperitoneal chemotherapy treatment in advanced ovarian cancer: a gynecologic oncology group study. JCO. 2015;33:1460-1466.

[39] Cascales PA, Gil J, Galindo PJ, et al. Heterogeneity in patients and methods. A problem for hyperthermic intraoperative intraperitoneal chemotherapy (HIPEC) in ovarian carcinoma. Eur J Obstet Gynecol Reprod Biol. 2011;158:361-362.

[40] Armstrong DK, Bundy B, Wenzel L, et al. Intraperitoneal cisplatin and paclitaxel in ovarian cancer. N Engl J Med. 2006;354:34-43.

[41] Wu Q, Wu Q, Xu J. Efficacy of hyperthermic intraperitoneal chemotherapy in patients with epithelial ovarian cancer: a meta-analysis. International Journal of Hyperthermia 2019; 36:1, 562-572.

[42] Cascales-Campos PA, Gil J, Feliciangeli E, et al. The role of

hyperthermic intraperitoneal chemotherapy using paclitaxel in platinum- sensitive recurrent epithelial ovarian cancer patients with microscopic residual disease after cytoreduction. Ann Surg Oncol. 2015;22:987-993.

[43] van Driel WJ, Lok CA, Verwaal V, et al. The role of hyperthermic intraperitoneal intraoperative chemotherapy in ovarian cancer. Curr Treat Options Oncol. 2015;16:14.

[44] Cowan RA, O'Cearbhaill RE, Zivanovic O, et al. Current status and future prospects of hyperthermic intraoperative intraperitoneal chemotherapy (HIPEC) clinical trials in ovarian cancer. Int J Hyperthermia. 2017;33:548-553.

[45] Wu Y, Chen L, Zhao Y, et al. Efficacy and safety of hyperthermic intraoperative intraperitoneal chemotherapy with Paclitaxel and Cisplatin in the treatment of ovarian cancer. Anti-Tumor Pharmacy. 2016;6:291-295.

[46] Cascales-Campos PA, Gil J, Gil E, et al. Treatment of microscopic disease with hyperthermic intraoperative intraperitoneal chemotherapy after complete cytoreduction improves disease-free survival in patients with stage IIIC/IV ovarian cancer. Ann Surg Oncol. 2014;21:2383-2389.

[47] Kim JH, Lee JM, Ryu KS, et al. Consolidation hyperthermic intraperitoneal chemotherapy using paclitaxel in patients with epithelial ovarian cancer. J Surg Oncol. 2010;101:149-155.

[48] Ryu KS, Kim JH, Ko HS, et al. Effects of intraperitoneal hyperthermic chemotherapy in ovarian cancer. Gynecol Oncol. 2004;94: 325-332.

[49] Lei Z, Wang Y, Wang J, et al. Evaluation of Cytoreductive Surgery With or Without Hyperthermic Intraperitoneal Chemotherapy for Stage III Epithelial Ovarian Cancer. *JAMA Network Open.* 2020;3(8):e2013940. doi:10.1001/jamanetworkopen.2020.13940

[50] Mendivil AA, Rettenmaier MA, Abaid LN, et al. Consolidation hyperthermic intraperitoneal chemotherapy for the treatment of advanced stage ovarian carcinoma: a 3 year experience. Cancer Chemother Pharmacol. 2017;80:405-410.

[51] Bristow RE, Puri I, Chi DS. Cytoreductive surgery for recurrent ovarian cancer: a meta-analysis. Gynecol Oncol. 2009;112:265-274.

[52] Munkarah AR, Coleman RL. Critical evaluation of secondary cytoreduction in recurrent ovarian cancer. Gynecol Oncol. 2004;95: 273-280.

[53] Harter P, Du Bois A, Hahmann M, et al. Surgery in recurrent ovarian cancer: the Arbeitsgemeinschaft Gynaekologische Onkologie (AGO) DESKTOP OVAR trial. Ann Surg Oncol. 2006;13: 1702-1710.

[54] Baiocchi G, Ferreira FO, Mantoan H, et al. Hyperthermic intraperitoneal chemotherapy after secondary cytoreduction in epithelial ovarian cancer: a single-center comparative analysis. Ann Surg Oncol. 2016;23:1294-1301.

[55] Didelot C, Lanneau D, Brunet M, et al. Anti-cancer therapeutic approaches based on intracellular and extracellular heat shock proteins. CMC. 2007;14:2839-2847.

[56] Hegyi G, Szigeti GP, Szasz A. Hyperthermia versus oncothermia: cellular effects in complementary cancer therapy. Evid Based Complement Alternat Med. 2013;2013:672873.

[57] Harter P, Reuss A, Sehouli J, et al. Brief report about the role of hyperthermic intraperitoneal chemotherapy in a prospective randomized phase 3 study in recurrent ovarian cancer from Spiliotis et al. Int J Gynecol Cancer. 2017;27:246-247.

Section 3

Novel Ovarian Cancer Therapeutics

Chapter 9

Targeting Leader Cells in Ovarian Cancer as an Effective Therapeutic Option

Nazanin Karimnia, Gwo-Yaw Ho, Andrew N. Stephens and Maree Bilandzic

Abstract

Majority of ovarian cancers are diagnosed at advanced stages with intra-peritoneal spread as the most common mode of disease metastasis. The formation of cancer spheroids is essential for the collective migration process, where shed tumour cells from the primary tumour form aggregates rather than disseminating as individual cells and seed within the peritoneal cavity. These cancer spheroids consist of leader cells (LC) and follower cells (FC), with the LC subset as key drivers of cellular movement and invasion. LCs have stem cell-like properties and are highly chemo-resistant with a specific survival addiction to several cell signalling pathways, such as the PI3K/AKT/mTOR pathway. We explore in this book chapter, the evidence supporting the role of LC in OC metastasis and the suppression of LC as an attractive therapeutic option for the treatment of advanced OC.

Keywords: Ovarian cancer, Leader Cells, KRT14, PI3K/AKT/mTOR, Collective migration

1. Introduction

1.1 The majority of ovarian cancers disseminate passively within the intraperitoneal space via ascitic fluid

The majority of ovarian cancers (OC), up to 70%, are diagnosed at advanced stages (stage III-IV) with intra-peritoneal spread as the most common mode of metastasis [1]. OC dissemination is often accompanied by the formation of ascitic fluid within the peritoneal cavity [2–4]. Under normal conditions, a small amount of fluid is secreted by the peritoneal capillaries into the cavity to lubricate the movement of abdominal organs which is normally re-absorbed by the lymphatic channels as a result of intrathoracic pressure [5]. However, in the presence of malignant cells, fluid can accumulate in large volumes in the peritoneum and facilitate passive cancer cell dissemination [6]. Whilst haematogenous spread may account for some ovarian tumour metastasis [7], it is largely the passive peritoneal dissemination of spheroids that results in ovarian cancer spread [8].

Prior to detachment from the primary tumour, OC cells are believed to exhibit a unique gene expression profile. This includes co-expression of both epithelial and mesenchymal markers and the acquisition of an epithelial-mesenchymal transition

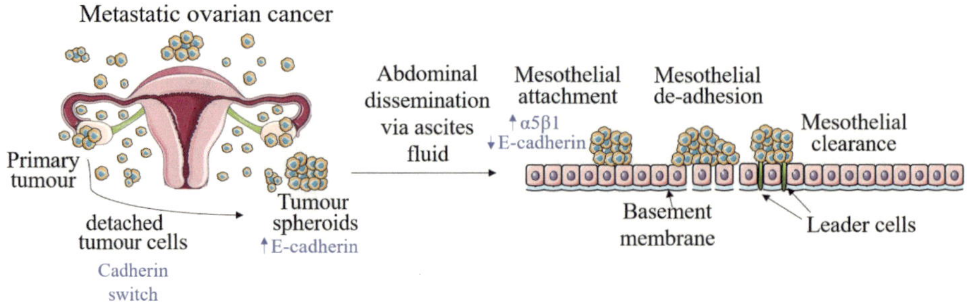

Figure 1.
Ovarian cancer passive mode of metastasis. Ovarian cancer cells from the primary tumour are exfoliated into the peritoneal cavity. Exfoliated cancer cells aggregate to form compact multicellular spheroids and disseminate within the peritoneal cavity, where single cells are subject to anoikis. Spheroids further attach to and invade the perineal lining by displacing the mesothelial cell layer in a process mediated by ovarian cancer leader cells.

(EMT)-like phenotype [9, 10]. The detached OC cells are then shed into the peritoneal cavity and simultaneously, E-cadherin expression is replaced by P-cadherin and N-cadherin, an event known as the global cadherin switch [11]. A fluctuation in E-cadherin levels is once again observed when detached cells form multicellular spheroids and E-cadherin levels are elevated [12], collectively demonstrating OC phenotypic plasticity is crucial for each step of the metastatic process [13].

1.2 OC spheroids play a key role in intra-peritoneal spread of malignant cells

Detached tumour cells from the primary tumour aggregate as spheroids in the ascites to overcome anoikis [2]. We believe that these cancer cell spheroids "floating" in the ascites are a key component in OC passive dissemination and play a pivotal role in both invasion and metastasis [6]. Furthermore, OC spheroids exhibit remarkable chemoresistance and progenitor-like properties [14, 15].

The mesothelial monolayer covering all of the abdominal organs is the initial point of contact for the disseminating spheroids during the metastatic process [16]. This layer lies on top of basement membrane, which is composed of collagen I, IV, laminin and fibronectin and contains a milieu of macrophages and fibroblasts populating the extracellular matrix (ECM) space [17–19]. It was observed that transcriptional reprogramming occurred within the floating spheroids which transformed tumour cells from a proliferative to an invasive phenotype to facilitate invasion through the mesothelium via the ECM [6]. Studies have shown that α5β1-integrin expression by spheroids binds fibronectin expressed by mesothelial cells and is critical for spheroid adhesion to the mesothelial lining [20–24]. However, multiple preclinical studies targeting individual integrin complexes failed to prevent the adhesion of spheroids to the peritoneum, hence the role of non-integrin-based adhesion molecules, such as CD44 and L1CAM, may be crucial to the spheroid adhesion process [25]. The attachment of OC spheroids to the peritoneum initiates the process of infiltration and invasion. The process of passive dissemination is illustrated in **Figure 1**.

2. Collective migration and leader cells

2.1 Collective migration occurs during epithelial cancer metastasis

During embryonic development, tissue homeostasis and also cancer invasion, cells migrate as multicellular clusters with a directed and coordinated movement – this process is called collective migration [26]. Collective migration is characteristic of metastatic tumours in transit, particularly cancers with epithelial origin [27, 28] including pancreatic cancer [29], colon cancer [30], sebaceous cancer [31], melanoma [32], breast cancer [33–35], lung cancer [36] and OC [37, 38]. There are three key features that define the collective phenomenon; (i) the preservation of the physical connections and cell–cell junctions to orchestrate collective movement; (ii) the shared cytoskeletal dynamics within the cell clusters, allowing groups of cells to proceed as a single unit and maintain multicellular polarity; and (iii) the interactions with other cells and ECM along the migration path [26, 39, 40]. Interestingly, not all cells within the collective invading cell cluster are invasion competent [26] and it is now understood that the complex cohesive movement of collective invasion is orchestrated by a subset of cells called "leader cells" (LCs) [37, 41–44].

2.2 Cancer leader cells are the key drivers in cancer cell migration

The LCs have been well characterised in the context of collective migration in normal physiological events such as wound healing [41], nephric ducts growth [45], angiogenesis [46], and mammary branching [47]. More recently, cancer LCs have been identified in bladder [48–50], breast [34, 35, 51], prostate [50], pancreatic [52], small cell lung cancer (SCLC) [53], and now in metastatic OC [37]. These cells have a distinct front-rear polarity and membrane protrusions to sense environmental cues in order to direct the invading cluster [28, 54]. Studies have shown that within a collectively migrating cancer cluster the cancer LCs will be situated at the invasive front, followed by follower cells (FCs) in a packed morphology [28, 54, 55]. It has been shown that the removal of the LCs from an invading cluster of kidney epithelial cells results in the loss of orientation and speed in movement of the FCs - this highlighted the importance of LCs in the organisation of collective movement [44]. However, the dynamic interaction between the LCs and FCs is required to ensure the success of collective movement. Therefore, the FCs play a critical role in LCs polarisation, gradient sensing, and chemotaxis [54, 56, 57], and thus in return actively influence LC function.

2.3 Leader cells exhibit remarkable ability to alter their surrounding tissue micro-environment, which is crucial in their role as cell migration drivers

Within the collective migration process, LCs are able to lose or rearrange their baso-apical polarity during cellular elongation, while maintaining attachment to FCs by retaining molecular plasticity through the expression of epithelial markers such as *CDH1,* which encodes for E-cadherin [34, 55, 58]. LCs can mediate cytoskeletal organisation by displaying front-to-rear polarisation [28, 59]. Activation of phosphoinositide 3-kinase (PI3K) [60], GTPase proteins, cell division cycle 42 (Cdc42) and Ras-related C3 botulinum toxin substrate (Rac) [54] at the front of the spheroid induces actin polymerisation and integrin-based interactions with ECM components [61], while the expression of matrix metalloproteinases (MMPs) by LCs generates a track within the ECM and the basement membrane allowing for cell invasion into these spaces [62].

In the absence of a known LC marker, earlier studies have focused on the physical positioning of LCs within a collectively invading cluster to investigate the LCs profile. Carey et al., shed light on heterogeneous tumour subpopulations within 3D spheroids and showed different invasion and ECM remodelling capacities with LCs driving malignant protrusions [63]. Later, Yamaguchi et al., used the same approach and showed that by removing the LCs from a collectively invading cluster of epithelial kidney cells, the follower population movement lost direction [44].

This study further showed that LCs express high level of proteins involved in cell migration and polarisation, such as Rac, integrin β1 and PI3K [44]. Konen and colleagues established a novel image-guided manipulation technique to isolate the LCs from collectively invading lung cancer spheroids [64]. The spatiotemporal genomic and cellular analysis (SaGA) technique involved labelling cells within the spheroid with a green-to-red photoconvertible fluorescent protein. Invasive cells at the front were tagged with a laser beam which converted the fluorescence to red allowing the isolation of the invasive LCs by fluorescent activated cell sorting (FACS) [64, 65]. Using SaGA, transcriptomic analysis of lung cancer LCs identified 788 differentially expressed genes comparing LCs and FCs. Among them, genes involved in VEGF signalling, focal adhesion and RNA polymerase II transcription were significantly over-expressed in the LCs population [64]. The authors further demonstrated that although LC function was not dependent on VEGF signalling, it was necessary to drive the collective movement of FCs [64]. In SCLC, a distinctive mutation profile between LCs and FCs showed that mutations in the actin related protein-3 (*ARP3*) gene enhanced LCs function [53]. Further, introducing this mutation into the non-invasive follower population promoted invasion and collective movement [53].

2.4 Cancer LCs have stem cell-like phenotype

Cancer LCs play a critical role in early-stage invasion and tumour micrometastatic seeding [34, 35, 42, 66, 67]. Multiple studies investigating cancer micrometastasis in patient-derived-xenograft (PDX) models further characterised cancer LCs at a single cell level. A study by Lawson et al. analysing breast cancer PDX micrometastases by single cell sequencing demonstrated a distinct basal/stem-cell signature in early-stage metastatic cells [68]. This study demonstrated a distinctive molecular signature for low and high- burden metastatic tumours with elevated stem cell signatures and dormancy in low burden tumours and high proliferation and differentiation signatures in high-burden tumours [68]. Another study with the same approach for the analysis of breast cancer micrometastasis identified 330 differentially expressed genes. Among the genes significantly upregulated in the micrometastatic lesions were those encoding heat shock proteins HSPB1, HSPA8 and HSPE1 as well as cytokeratins KRT14, KRT16, KRT7 and KRT17 [69]. HSPB1 is involved in protein folding, apoptosis evasion and actin remodelling [70, 71], whereas KRT14 is a marker of invasion driving LCs in breast and ovarian cancer [34, 37]. This study also showed that mitochondrial oxidative phosphorylation (OXPHOS) was significantly up-regulated in metastatic cell seedings, suggesting a potential alternative metabolic pathway is utilised by the LCs to fuel the metastatic process [72–74].

2.5 KRT14 is a reliable dynamic cancer LC marker

KRT14 is a member of the intermediate filaments (IFs) and is generally expressed within the basal layer of epithelium to provide structural support [75]. In cancer cells, the direction of collective migration cell cluster movement and formation of protrusive structures are mediated via the interplay between the keratin IFs and cadherin [76]. Elevated expression of KRT14 has been identified in invasive LCs of breast [34], ovarian [37], bladder [49], and salivary adenoid cystic carcinoma (SACC) [77]. *In vitro* studies on KRT14 expressing LCs in OC demonstrated that spheroids generated from KRT14 depleted cells failed to maintain stable attachment with the mesothelial layer and to generate invasive protrusions [37]. RNA-sequencing revealed that the $KRT14^+$ breast cancer LCs show a significantly higher level of DSG3, encoding a major desmosomal protein, as well as gene expression signatures associated with cell and matrix adhesion [34]. Desmosomes play a critical role in maintaining cell–cell adhesion throughout the collective movement via intracellular connection of keratin filaments in neighbouring cells [78, 79]. However, the exact mechanisms of KRT14 involvement in driving collective invasion remains unknown. It was hypothesised that keratin IFs may regulate focal adhesions via intertwined interactions with the AKT and integrin/focal adhesion kinase (FAK) pathways [80–83]. More specifically, KRT14 has been shown to stabilise hemidesmosomes by regulating the levels of integrin β4 on the surface of keratinocytes [80]. Furthermore, KRT14 can mediate the phosphorylation of desmosomal cell junctions via PKCα, which is important in regulating epithelial cell adhesion [81, 82]. These results suggest that the KRT14 expression in LCs can be a determining factor to maintain the integrity of the collective movement via cell–cell and cell-matrix adhesion [54, 83].

Study		**Model**	**LC-specific signatures**
Yamaguchi et al. [43]	LCs isolated from invasive strands of a spheroid embedded in collagen matrix using a micromanipulator	Kidney epithelial cells	Rac Integrin β1 PI3K
Lawson et al. [66]	FACS-based isolation of single metastatic cells followed by Fluidigm dynamic array experiments identified signatures of micrometastases.	Breast cancer PDX model	Differentiation Proliferation Dormancy exit
Cheung et al. [33]	RNA-sequencing identified 239 DEGs comparing KRT14$^+$ LCs and KRT14$^-$ FCs	Breast cancer cells/ PDX model	ECM proteins Immune system regulators Cell–cell and cell-matrix adhesion Regulators of the metastatic niche
Konen et al. [62]	SAGA identification of 788 DEGs in the LCs isolated from a collectively invading spheroid model	Lung cancer	VEGF signalling Focal adhesion molecules RNA polymerase II transcription
Sonzogni et al. [50]	RNA sequencing and secretome analysis of KRT14$^+$ LCs and KRT14$^-$ FCs	Breast cancer	Pro-metastatic genes Matrix adhesion
Zoeller et al. [52]	SAGA identification of genomic and transcriptomic signatures for LCs via parallel mutation and RNA-seq analysis	NSCLC	collective movement Actin filament proteins Mitochondrial enzymes
Davis et al. [67]	Single-cell RNA sequencing of micrometastases compared to the primary tumour.	Breast cancer / PDX model	Heat shock proteins Cytokeratins OXPHOS Mitochondrial electron transport Mitochondrial ribosomal genes

Table 1.
Summary of studies investigating LCs profile.

2.6 KRT14 positive cells are linked to LC with distinct gene expression profile

Transcriptome analysis of the KRT14 expressing LCs in breast cancer by RNA sequencing identified 239 differentially expressed signatures between the $KRT14^+$ LCs and the $KRT14^-$ FC population. Gene ontology (GO) analyses, revealed that the expression of genes encoding ECM proteins, intermediate filaments, cytoskeleton organisation, and cell adhesion were significantly elevated in LCs compared to the FC population [34]. Interestingly, this study demonstrated that the LC subset is not a fixed lineage, however, the mechanisms regulating the interconversion of LCs and FCs remains unclear [34]. Recent studies suggest that the behaviour of breast cancer LCs can be mediated by CD44 expression levels where a high level of expression induces a shift towards an invasive LC phenotype [84]. Sonzogni et al. showed that KRT14 expressing LCs have a significantly higher expression of genes involved in metastasis progression including metallothionein-2 (*Mt2*), glycoprotein non-metastatic B (*Gpnmb*), and adhesion molecule Amigo2, and secrete significantly higher levels of the collagen VI subunit A (*Col6a1*) [51]. In bladder cancer, stem-like $KRT14^+$ cells gave rise to differentiated cells and were shown to be necessary for epithelial layer establishment following tissue damage [49]. A summary of studies and pathways involved in LC function is provided in **Table 1**.

2.7 LCs are implicated in OC metastasis and invasion

We have recently identified the OC LCs [37]. A study using spheroid-mesothelium co-culture model was utilised to identify molecules that were specifically expressed at the early stages of invasion via matrix-assisted laser desorption/ionisation (MALDI) tissue imaging. Among the identified proteins, KRT14 was shown to mark the invading cells universally across the different subtypes of EOC, while KRT14 expression was absent from the normal ovarian and fallopian tube tissue [37]. This study confirmed that cells lacking KRT14 proliferate at the same rate as the WT cells, however, demonstrate significantly impaired migration and matrix-adhesion [37]. These results suggest the explicit role of LCs in invasion and metastasis in OC.

3. Novel OC therapeutic approach by targeting the collectively migrating cell population

3.1 Collectively migrating cell clusters may be targeted to reduce cancer spread

Current cancer therapies are mainly evaluated by cytotoxicity and their effect on tumour shrinkage; however, bulk tumour regression is not the only factor in effective cancer therapies [85]. In OC, the majority of patients are diagnosed with metastatic disease which is associated with a significantly poorer prognosis, hence strategies to interrupt metastasis through the disruption of cell motility, collective movement, directed cell migration and invasion have gained interest [86]. Targeting the cytoskeletal stability through actin is one such approach that has shown inhibitory effects on invadopodia formation and outgrowth in lung [87, 88], melanoma [88] and prostate [89] cancers. Unfortunately, these drugs are usually associated with significant toxicities due to the lack of discriminative drug effects between the malignant and healthy cells [88, 89]. Targeting other processes involved in actin polymerisation such as Rho GTPases and RhoA/Rho-associated kinase (ROCK) signalling pathway is potentially beneficial since the cytoskeletal dynamics play an important role during invasion and metastasis of a collectively invading cluster [90, 91]. However, cancer cells generally are able to establish alternative mechanisms to bypass these targets leading to early drug resistance [92].

3.2 Targeting LCs within the collectively migrating cluster may be a better therapeutic option for the treatment of OC

As highlighted earlier, the molecular features of LCs are cancer-specific and this represents a challenge for developing clinically relevant therapies against LCs. Despite this, multiple targets have emerged from LCs studies (listed in **Table 1**: Summary of studies investigating LCs profile). These include targeting the LC stimulatory pathways such as the PI3K/mTOR pathway (with tyrosine kinase inhibitors and Ivermectin), metabolic/energy pathways (statins, cardiac glycosides and metformin) and inflammatory pathways (non-steroidal anti-inflammatory drugs).

3.3 Disrupting the PI3K/AKT/mTOR pathway is an attractive therapeutic strategy to inhibit LCs

There is an enrichment of LCs observed in late-stage OC associated with the up-regulation of the PI3K/AKT/mTOR pathway [37, 93]. Yamaguchi et al.'s study revealed the up-regulation of PI3K in kidney epithelial LCs [44] implicating this pathway as a potential target for LC inhibition. The PI3K/AKT/mTOR signalling pathway mediates major cellular events such as growth, motility, metabolism, and survival [94].

PI3Ks are a group of membrane-associated kinases that form heterodimeric structures comprised of regulatory and catalytic subunits classified based on their structure, regulation and substrates [95]. Class I PI3Ks are hugely implicated in cancer and are comprised of a p85 regulatory and a p110 catalytic subunit [96]. The catalytic subunit in class IA has three variants including p110α, p110β, and p110δ encoded by *PIK3CA*, *PIK3CB* and *PIK3CD* respectively, whilst the catalytic subunit of the only class IB PI3K, p110γ, is produced from *PIK3CG* gene [96]. Class IA PI3Ks are activated via ligand binding to receptor tyrosine kinases (RTKs), while activation IB PI3Ks is mediated by G-protein-coupled receptors (GCPRs) [97]. Upon ligand binding, activated PI3Ks catalyse phosphorylation of phosphatidylinositol (PtdIns) [4, 5] P2 (PIP2) to produce PtdIns [3–5] P3 (PIP3), an event that is inhibited by the tumour suppressor Phosphatase and tensin homologue (PTEN) in normal cells [94]. Following PIP2 to PIP3 conversion, proteins with a PH domain are recruited to the plasma membrane to activate downstream signalling proteins such as AKT, triggering multiple downstream pathways regulating survival, growth and invasion [94, 98]. AKT, also known as protein kinase B (PKB) is the main effector of PI3K and other than direct activation by PI3K, can be activated indirectly by mTOR and phosphoinositide-dependent kinase-1 (PDK1) that phosphorylate AKT at Ser 473 and Tyr 308 residues, respectively [99–101]. A schematic overview of the PI3K/AKT/mTOR pathway is demonstrated in (**Figure 2**).

3.4 Dual PI3K/mTOR kinase inhibitors may be required to effectively suppress OC leader cells

Activation of PI3K/AKT/mTOR pathway is frequently observed in oncogenic events contributing to tumour development, metastasis and therapy resistance [98] and irregularities in the PI3K/AKT/mTOR pathway corresponds with a poor prognosis in OC patients [99, 102, 103]. Activating mutations and genomic amplification of *PIK3CA* [104] and AKT and mTOR are more prevalent in women with

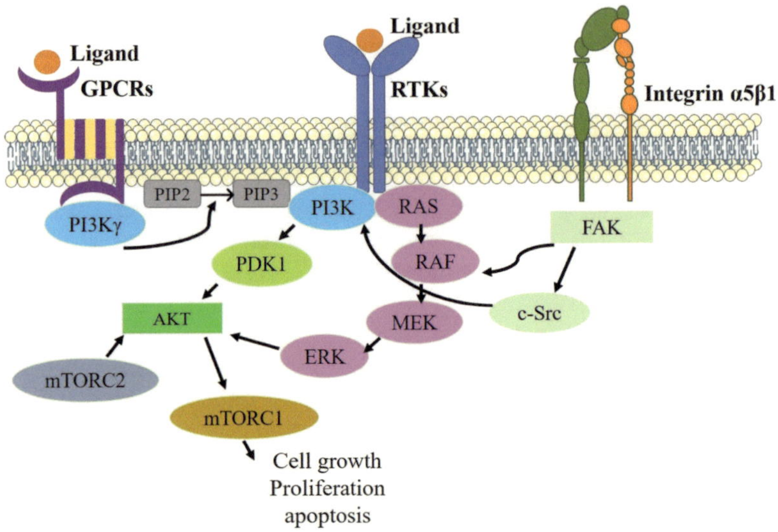

Figure 2.
Overview of the PI3K/AKT/mTOR pathway. Class IA PI3Ks are activated via ligand binding of receptor tyrosine kinases (RTKs), while class IB PI3Ks depend on G protein-coupled receptor (GPCRs) activation. Activated PI3K facilitates the conversion of PIP2 to PIP3 and in turn induces AKT phosphorylation. Activated AKT mediates the phosphorylation mTOR and a signalling cascade that drives cellular proliferation and cell death. In concert, the RAS/RAF/MEK/ERK pathway is activated by RTKs, acting as an escape mechanism for PI3K inhibition. The focal adhesion kinase (FAK) pathway also feeds into the PI3K pathway through c-Src activated by integrin-based adhesion molecules including integrin α5β1.

clear cell ovarian carcinoma and associated with drug resistance phenotype [101]. Importantly, pharmaceutical inhibition of the PI3K/AKT/mTOR pathway was shown to increase *in vitro* sensitivity of OC cell lines to multiple chemotherapy agents [105, 106]. Moreover, PI3K inhibition via LY294002 disrupted the directional movement of kidney LCs [44], further highlighting the importance of the PI3K pathway for LC function. Inhibition of PI3K/AKT/mTOR pathway can be achieved via pan or isoform specific PI3K inhibitors, AKT inhibitors or dual pan PI3K/mTOR inhibitors [107–109]. However, PI3K/AKT/mTOR inhibition as a therapeutic option can be challenging due to the potential toxicities compounded by the activation of compensatory pathways and enhanced insulin production upon inhibition of PI3K [94, 98, 100, 101, 104, 110]. Currently, the PI3K inhibitor idelalisib and the mTOR inhibitor everolimus have gained FDA approval for the treatment of lymphoma [111] and renal cancer [112], respectively. Unfortunately, the clinical use of single agent inhibitors has shown minimal efficacy and high toxicities in treatment of OC [113–115].

The PI3K/AKT/mTOR pathway is interconnected with other signalling pathways including focal adhesion kinases [116] and RAS/RAF/MEK/ERK [117]. There are multiple canonical and non-canonical crosslinked pathways that could bypass single protein inhibition resulting in therapeutic failure. Therefore, targeting the pathway cascade at multiple levels via dual PI3K/mTOR inhibitors, might circumvent the negative feedback loops that occur with single target inhibitors [118]. Pre-clinical data from the PI3K/mTOR dual inhibitors omipalisib (GSK2126458), CMG002 and BEZ235 have indicated effective inhibition of ovarian cancer tumour growth and progression *in vitro* and *in vivo* [93, 106, 119, 120]. Currently, there are no ongoing clinical trials investigating the efficacy of dual inhibitors in OC patients mainly due to toxicity and off target effects of the dual inhibitors in clinical setting [121].

3.5 Anti-helminth, Ivermectin, may be effective in sensitising OC LCs to chemotherapy by disrupting the AKT/mTOR pathway

Ivermectin belongs to a family of drugs widely used to treat parasites and pest insects [122]. The anti-cancer property of ivermectin can be related to the inhibition of the Pgp pumps and MDR protein expression [123], inhibition of AKT/mTOR pathway [124], and targeting the yes-associated protein 1 (YAP1) [125], all of which are involved in the OC tumorigenesis [100, 126–128]. *In vivo,* ivermectin treatment of a xenograft mouse model of EOC showed a significant reduction in tumour growth and a reversal in tumour growth without severe toxicity effects when the drug was combined with cisplatin [129]. Currently there is a phase II clinical trial in recruitment to study the long-term effect of ivermectin treatment (NCT02366884).

3.6 The mevalonate pathway in LC can be potentially targeted with HMG-CoA inhibitors

Statins are among the most commonly prescribed medications to reduce cholesterol and inflammation through blocking 3-hydroxy-3-methyl-glutaryl-CoA (HMG-CoA) reductase [130]. Inhibiting the mevalonate pathway can have a protective effect against cancer progression and reduce LC activity [131, 132]. Furthermore, the mevalonate pathway has been shown to be significantly activated in *TP53* mutated cells [133]. Therapeutic effects of statins in OC are further supported by the *in vitro* studies showing anti-metastatic and anti-tumorigenic effects through the inhibition of MAPK and mTOR pathways [134]. Lovastatin significantly reduced the development of serous tubal intraepithelial carcinomas, the purported precursor ovarian cancer lesions, in mice through the inhibition of the mevalonate pathway and dysregulation of the Rho signalling pathway [135]. Currently, a phase III clinical study for evaluating the safety, tolerability and effects on tumour progression of Atorvastatin is at the recruitment stage for ovarian and pancreatic cancer patients (NCT 02201381).

3.7 Cardiac glycosides, such as digoxin, may be able to suppress LC population

Cardiac glycosidases (CGs) are a family of drugs used for the treatment of congestive heart failure and cardiac arrhythmia by regulating cardiac muscle contraction through the inhibition of the NA^{+}-K^{+}-ATPase pump [136]. The first anti-proliferative effects of CGs were reported more than five decades ago in HeLa cells [137] and since then, multiple studies have highlighted the anti-neoplastic effects of CGs by inducing cancer cell apoptosis [138], activating autophagic cell death through the Ras-dependent extracellular signal-regulated kinase (ERK1/2) pathway [139], inhibiting hypoxia-inducible factor-1 alpha (HIF-1α) protein synthesis [140] and inhibiting FA/BRCA pathway activation [141]. CGs have been shown to have a higher cytotoxicity effect when combined with chemotherapy in prostate, breast, non-small cell lung, colorectal, and pancreatic cell lines as well as advanced stage melanoma patients compared to single agents [141–144]. However, so far epidemiological studies have yielded inconsistent results. For example, while digoxin was found to inhibit tumour growth *in vitro* and was associated with a 25% lower prostate cancer risk [145], systematic review and meta-analyses indicated an increased prostate cancer risk in digoxin users [146]. Nevertheless, the number of clinical trials specifically designed for cancer patients being treated with CGs is very limited and most of these conflicting results come from re-analysing data present in the medical databases with limited numbers of patients. So far, there are no clinical trials designed to investigate the relationship between CGs and OC. Despite this, there is a recent study retrospectively analysing the Surveillance, Epidemiology, and End Results (SEER) program, the national cancer institute (NCI), and Medicare healthcare claim record data to assess whether digoxin use enhances chemotherapeutic responses in OC treatment [147]. The study suggested that digoxin use during chemotherapy did not have any survival benefits in patients with EOC, however, the research was limited by small sample size. Furthermore, 46% of the patients had a prior history of heart disease complicating the interpretation of subject fatality rates. More importantly, only 7% of the studied population were treated with digoxin during chemotherapy which may describe the opposing results with other cancer types. Since cardiac glycosidases regulate ion transport via the NA^+/K^+-ATPase, they interact with a wide variety of the intracellular signalling pathways, including those driving cellular proliferation and apoptosis [148], therefore, future clinical trials specifically designed for OC patients is highly expected. Our laboratory drug screening pipeline used to identify therapies against LCs has identified digoxin as a potent LC inhibitor, demonstrating synergistic effects when sublethal concentrations of digoxin were combined with platinum-based chemotherapies (result not published).

3.8 Metformin is a potential LC targeting agent by suppressing the AMPK pathway

Metformin is an anti-diabetic drug reducing blood glucose and insulin levels through activation of adenosine monophosphate-activated protein kinase (AMPK) to inhibit gluconeogenesis in the liver [149]. In cancer cells, AMPK activation results in mTOR pathway inhibition and therefore inhibition of cell proliferation [150]. So far, several epidemiological studies focusing on ovarian cancer patients with type 2 diabetes who were taking metformin at the time of diagnosis showed that these patients had a significantly improved 5-year survival rate compared to those who did not take metformin [151, 152]. Currently, there are multiple clinical trials submitted in the national institute of health (NIH) clinical trial database focusing on non-diabetic ovarian cancer patients being treated with a combination of metformin and first line chemotherapy. The results from one of the completed phase II studies (NCT01579812) showed that the tumours in women treated with metformin had a significantly fewer $ALDH1^+$ cells representing OC stem cells [153], therefore, supporting the use of this drug in the next phase of clinical trials. Furthermore, investigations in our lab evaluated the effect of sitagliptin, a drug used for the treatment of type 2 diabetes, in a murine model of ovarian cancer showing that sitagliptin enhanced the immune response via T cell recruitment to the tumour and inhibited several pro-tumorigenic cytokines, therefore reducing tumour burden and improving survival [154].

3.9 Non-steroidal anti-inflammatory drugs are potent cytotoxic LC inhibitors

Non-steroidal anti-inflammatory drugs (NSAIDs), such as aspirin, diclofenac and celecoxib are mainly prescribed to reduce pain, fever and inflammation [155]. Inflammation has a key role in cancer development and progression, therefore, NSAIDs have been shown to exhibit protective roles against this disease [156]. This effect is mediated through the inhibition of cyclooxygenase-1 and 2 (COX-1,2) enzymes inhibiting prostaglandin (PG) synthesis [157]. While constitutive expression of COX-1 regulates tissue homeostasis through PG synthesis, COX-2 is not expressed in normal epithelial tissues and is only induced during inflammation.

In addition, this marker is found to be overexpressed in epithelial tumours [158]. COX-2 inhibition eventually leads to the induction of apoptosis and the inhibition of tumour invasion [159]. The action of NSAIDs has been further linked to PI3K signalling pathway [160, 161] and the inhibition of $NF_{K}B$ that leads to dysregulation of the genes involved in cancer progression and apoptosis [162]. The benefit of NSAIDs in cancer prevention and treatment remains controversial and tumour type dependant [156]. Re-assessing case–control and cohort studies from 1950 to 2011, that reported associations between aspirin uptake and cancer, showed that cancer prevention becomes significant only when the aspirin usage proceeds 5 years [162] and in this case, the overall benefit from the long-term use of NSAIDs was compromised by side-effects, such as gastrointestinal bleeding [163–165]. *In vitro* investigation of a panel of NSAIDs in ovarian cancer, showed significant apoptosis induction and reduced tumour growth in four cell lines treated with diclofenac [166]. Moreover, *in vivo* evaluation of diclofenac in mice implanted with ovarian cancer cells, showed significantly smaller tumours formed in diclofenac-treated animals compared to the control group [166, 167]. In line with this data, the drug screening platform established in our laboratory also identified diclofenac as a potent cytotoxic LC inhibitor. However, despite the growing body of evidence regarding the anti-neoplastic effects of diclofenac in OC, currently there are no clinical trials evaluating the effectiveness of this drug in patients. A phase II clinical trial to examine the effect of celecoxib treatment in combination with carboplatin in recurrent resistant ovarian cancer patients has shown promising results with a 28% RR and PFS [168], however this study did not provide any evidence of COX-2 inhibition in patients after treatment. Likewise, a phase II investigation of celecoxib plus carboplatin and docetaxel as a first-line treatment for ovarian cancer failed to demonstrate COX-2 inhibition with 82% of patients expressing COX-2 and no improvement in PFS or OS observed [169]. Furthermore, two systematic analyses on the effect of NSAID use and OC risk on big cohorts of patients failed to show such an association [170, 171]. However, both studies have indeed critical limitations with regards to the cancer subtypes, type of NSAIDs used, drug doses and the duration of treatments.

4. Conclusion

Despite the introduction of several novel therapeutics that include targeting DNA repair pathways with Poly (ADP-ribose) polymerase (PARP) inhibitors (PARPi), and vascular endothelial growth factor (VEGF) pathways with bevacizumab, the overall survival outcome for women with platinum-resistant OC remains poor. Unfortunately, women with advanced metastatic OC will eventually succumb to their disease due to the emergence of drug resistance. Understanding the mechanisms of OC migration and metastasis is crucial for the development of an effective therapeutic approach. Targeting the OC LC population serves as an attractive strategy given LCs are instrumental in orchestrating OC spread within the intra-peritoneal cavity. LCs are often highly chemo-resistant due to their stem cell-like nature and their survival post cytotoxic chemotherapy treatment may lead to therapy resistance and tumour recurrence. Multiple potential targets have been identified based on the understanding of LC biology, some of which may be targeted by re-proposing established drugs, such as dual PI3K/mTOR inhibitors, anti-helminths, statins, NSAIDs and metformin. Suppressing and eliminating LCs may be an effective therapeutic option for management of this lethal disease and is worth further exploration.

Acknowledgements

This work is supported by an Ovarian Cancer Research Foundation research grant to MB (GA-2019-20) and by the Victorian Government's Operational Infrastructure Support Program. AS and MB are supported by fellowships from the Ovarian Cancer Research Foundation (OCRF.com.au). NK is supported by the Dr Sue Fowler PhD Scholarship.

Author details

Nazanin Karimnia[1,2], Gwo-Yaw Ho[3,4], Andrew N. Stephens[1,2] and Maree Bilandzic[1,2*]

1 Hudson Institute of Medical Research, Clayton, VIC, Australia

2 Department of Molecular and Translational Sciences, Monash University, Clayton, VIC, Australia

3 School of Clinical Sciences, Monash University, Clayton, VIC, Australia

4 Monash Health, Clayton, VIC, Australia

*Address all correspondence to: maree.bilandzic@hudson.org.au

References

[1] Torre, L.A., *et al.* Ovarian cancer statistics, 2018. CA Cancer J Clin **68**, 284-296 (2018).

[2] Ahmed, N. & Stenvers, K.L. Getting to know ovarian cancer ascites: opportunities for targeted therapy-based translational research. Frontiers in oncology **3**, 256 (2013).

[3] Garrison, N.R., Kaelin, D.L., Heuser, S.L. & Galloway, H.R. Malignant Ascites: Clinical and Experimental Observations. Annals of Surgery **203**, 644-651 (1986).

[4] Adam, R.A. & Adam, Y.G. Malignant ascites: past, present, and future. Journal of the American College of Surgeons **198**, 999-1011 (2004).

[5] Feldman, G.B. & Knapp, R.C. Lymphatic drainage of the peritoneal cavity and its significance in ovarian cancer. American journal of obstetrics and gynecology **119**, 991 (1974).

[6] Yeung, T.-L., *et al.* Cellular and molecular processes in ovarian cancer metastasis. A Review in the Theme: Cell and Molecular Processes in Cancer Metastasis. American journal of physiology. Cell physiology **309**, C444 (2015).

[7] Pradeep, S., *et al.* Hematogenous Metastasis of Ovarian Cancer: Rethinking Mode of Spread. Cancer Cell **26**(2014).

[8] Carmignani, C., Sugarbaker, T., Bromley, C. & Sugarbaker, P. Intraperitoneal cancer dissemination: Mechanisms of the patterns of spread. Cancer and Metastasis Reviews **22**, 465-472 (2003).

[9] Ahmed, N., Thompson, E.W. & Quinn, M.A. Epithelial-mesenchymal interconversions in normal ovarian surface epithelium and ovarian carcinomas: an exception to the norm. Journal of cellular physiology **213**, 581 (2007).

[10] Kalluri, R. & Weinberg, R.A. The basics of epithelial-mesenchymal transition. The Journal of clinical investigation **119**, 1420-1428 (2009).

[11] Patel Ila, S., Madan, P., Getsios, S., Bertrand Monique, A. & MacCalman Colin, D. Cadherin switching in ovarian cancer progression. International Journal of Cancer **106**, 172-177 (2003).

[12] Wintzell, M., Hjerpe, E., Åvall Lundqvist, E. & Shoshan, M. Protein markers of cancer-associated fibroblasts and tumor-initiating cells reveal subpopulations in freshly isolated ovarian cancer ascites. BMC Cancer **12**, 359 (2012).

[13] Mitra, A.K. Ovarian Cancer Metastasis: A Unique Mechanism of Dissemination, Tumor Metastasis in *Tumor Metastasis* (InTechOpen, 2016).

[14] Ahmed, N., Abubaker, K., Findlay, J. & Quinn, M. Cancerous ovarian stem cells: Obscure targets for therapy but relevant to chemoresistance. Journal of Cellular Biochemistry **114**, 21-34 (2013).

[15] Bapat, S.A., Mali, A.M., Koppikar, C.B. & Kurrey, N.K. Stem and progenitor-like cells contribute to the aggressive behavior of human epithelial ovarian cancer. Cancer research **65**, 3025 (2005).

[16] Kenny Hilary, A., Krausz, T., Yamada Seiko, D. & Lengyel, E. Use of a novel 3D culture model to elucidate the role of mesothelial cells, fibroblasts and extra-cellular matrices on adhesion and invasion of ovarian cancer cells to the omentum. International Journal of Cancer **121**, 1463-1472 (2007).

[17] Kenny, H.A., Krausz, T., Yamada, S.D. & Lengyel, E. Use of a novel 3D

culture model to elucidate the role of mesothelial cells, fibroblasts and extra-cellular matrices on adhesion and invasion of ovarian cancer cells to the omentum. International Journal of Cancer **121**, 1463-1472 (2007).

[18] Kenny, H.A., Kaur, S., Coussens, L.M. & Lengyel, E. The initial steps of ovarian cancer cell metastasis are mediated by MMP-2 cleavage of vitronectin and fibronectin. The Journal of clinical investigation **118**, 1367-1379 (2008).

[19] Witz, C.A., *et al.* Composition of the Extracellular Matrix of the Peritoneum. Journal of the Society for Gynecologic Investigation **8**, 299-304 (2001).

[20] Shield, K., *et al.* Alpha2beta1 integrin affects metastatic potential of ovarian carcinoma spheroids by supporting disaggregation and proteolysis. Journal of carcinogenesis **6**, 11 (2007).

[21] Iwanicki, M.P., *et al.* Ovarian cancer spheroids use myosin-generated force to clear the mesothelium. Cancer discovery **1**, 144 (2011).

[22] Casey, R.C., *et al.* Beta 1-integrins regulate the formation and adhesion of ovarian carcinoma multicellular spheroids. Am J Pathol **159**, 2071-2080 (2001).

[23] Burleson, K.M., Boente, M.P., Pambuccian, S.E. & Skubitz, A.P. Disaggregation and invasion of ovarian carcinoma ascites spheroids. J Transl Med **4**, 6 (2006).

[24] Burleson, K.M., *et al.* Ovarian carcinoma ascites spheroids adhere to extracellular matrix components and mesothelial cell monolayers. Gynecol Oncol **93**, 170-181 (2004).

[25] van Baal, J.O.A.M., *et al.* Development of Peritoneal Carcinomatosis in Epithelial Ovarian Cancer: A Review. *The journal of histochemistry and cytochemistry: official journal of the Histochemistry* Society **66**, 67-83 (2018).

[26] Peter, F. & Darren, G. Collective cell migration in morphogenesis, regeneration and cancer. Nature Reviews Molecular Cell Biology **10**, 445 (2009).

[27] Wang, X., Enomoto, A., Asai, N., Kato, T. & Takahashi, M. Collective invasion of cancer: Perspectives from pathology and development. Pathology international **66**, 183-192 (2016).

[28] Friedl, P., Locker, J., Sahai, E. & Segall, J.E. Classifying collective cancer cell invasion. Nature cell biology **14**, 777 (2012).

[29] Beerling, E., Oosterom, I., Voest, E., Lolkema, M. & van Rheenen, J. Intravital characterization of tumor cell migration in pancreatic cancer. Intravital **5**, e1261773-e1261773 (2016).

[30] Sonoshita, M., *et al.* Promotion of colorectal cancer invasion and metastasis through activation of NOTCH-DAB1-ABL-RHOGEF protein TRIO. Cancer Discov **5**, 198-211 (2015).

[31] Hesse, K., *et al.* Characterisation of Prognosis and Invasion of Cutaneous Squamous Cell Carcinoma by Podoplanin and E-Cadherin Expression. Dermatology **232**, 558-565 (2016).

[32] Hegerfeldt, Y., Tusch, M., Brocker, E.B. & Friedl, P. Collective cell movement in primary melanoma explants: plasticity of cell-cell interaction, beta1-integrin function, and migration strategies. Cancer research **62**, 2125-2130 (2002).

[33] Ewald, A.J., *et al.* Mammary collective cell migration involves transient loss of epithelial features and individual cell migration within the

epithelium. J Cell Sci **125**, 2638-2654 (2012).

[34] Cheung, K.J., *et al.* Polyclonal breast cancer metastases arise from collective dissemination of keratin 14-expressing tumor cell clusters. Proceedings of the National Academy of Sciences of the United States of America **113**, E854 (2016).

[35] Cheung, K.J., Gabrielson, E., Werb, Z. & Ewald, A.J. Collective invasion in breast cancer requires a conserved basal epithelial program. Cell **155**, 1639 (2013).

[36] Haney, S., Konen, J., Marcus, A.I. & Bazhenov, M. The complex ecosystem in non small cell lung cancer invasion. PLoS computational biology **14**, e1006131-e1006131 (2018).

[37] Bilandzic, M., *et al.* Keratin-14 (KRT14) Positive Leader Cells Mediate Mesothelial Clearance and Invasion by Ovarian Cancer Cells. Cancers (Basel) **11**(2019).

[38] Moffitt, L., Karimnia, N., Stephens, A. & Bilandzic, M. Therapeutic Targeting of Collective Invasion in Ovarian Cancer. Int J Mol Sci **20**(2019).

[39] Montell, D. Morphogenetic Cell Movements: Diversity from Modular Mechanical Properties. Vol. 322 1502-1505 (The American Association for the Advancement of Science, Washington, 2008).

[40] Carlos, C.-F., *et al.* Contact inhibition of locomotion in vivo controls neural crest directional migration. Nature **456**, 957 (2008).

[41] Khalil, A.A. & Friedl, P. Determinants of leader cells in collective cell migration. Integrative biology: quantitative biosciences from nano to macro **2**, 568-574 (2010).

[42] Cheung, K.J. & Ewald, A.J. Invasive leader cells: metastatic oncotarget. Oncotarget **5**, 1390 (2014).

[43] Chapnick, D.A. & Liu, X. Leader cell positioning drives wound-directed collective migration in TGFbeta-stimulated epithelial sheets. Molecular biology of the cell **25**, 1586-1593 (2014).

[44] Yamaguchi, N., Mizutani, T., Kawabata, K. & Haga, H. Leader cells regulate collective cell migration via Rac activation in the downstream signaling of integrin β1 and PI3K. Scientific Reports **5**, 7656 (2015).

[45] Attia, L., Schneider, J., Yelin, R. & Schultheiss, T.M. Collective cell migration of the nephric duct requires FGF signaling. Developmental dynamics: an official publication of the American Association of Anatomists **244**, 157-167 (2015).

[46] Gerhardt, H., *et al.* VEGF guides angiogenic sprouting utilizing endothelial tip cell filopodia. J Cell Biol **161**, 1163-1177 (2003).

[47] Shamir, E.R. & Ewald, A.J. Adhesion in mammary development: novel roles for E-cadherin in individual and collective cell migration. Current topics in developmental biology **112**, 353-382 (2015).

[48] Volkmer, J.-P., *et al.* Three differentiation states risk-stratify bladder cancer into distinct subtypes. Proceedings of the National Academy of Sciences of the United States of America **109**, 2078 (2012).

[49] Papafotiou, G., *et al.* KRT14 marks a subpopulation of bladder basal cells with pivotal role in regeneration and tumorigenesis. Nature Communications **7**(2016).

[50] Hu, W.-Y., *et al.* Isolation and functional interrogation of adult human prostate epithelial stem cells at single cell resolution. Stem Cell Research **23**, 1-12 (2017).

[51] Sonzogni, O., *et al.* Reporters to mark and eliminate basal or luminal

epithelial cells in culture and in vivo. PLoS biology **16**, e2004049 (2018).

[52] Beerling, E., Oosterom, I., Voest, E., Lolkema, M. & van Rheenen, J. Intravital characterization of tumor cell migration in pancreatic cancer. IntraVital **5**, e1261773 (2016).

[53] Zoeller, E.L., *et al.* Genetic heterogeneity within collective invasion packs drives leader and follower cell phenotypes. *Journal of Cell Science* **132**, jcs231514 (2019).

[54] Mayor, R. & Etienne-Manneville, S. The front and rear of collective cell migration. Nature Reviews. Molecular Cell Biology **17**, 97-109 (2016).

[55] Lebreton, G. & Casanova, J. Specification of leading and trailing cell features during collective migration in the Drosophila trachea. Journal of cell science **127**, 465 (2014).

[56] Theveneau, E. & Linker, C. Leaders in collective migration: are front cells really endowed with a particular set of skills? F1000Research **6**, 1899 (2017).

[57] Venhuizen, J.-H. & Zegers, M.M. Making Heads or Tails of It: Cell–Cell Adhesion in Cellular and Supracellular Polarity in Collective Migration. Cold Spring Harbor Perspectives in Biology **9**(2017).

[58] Friedl, P. & Wolf, K. Plasticity of cell migration: a multiscale tuning model. Vol. 188 11 (Rockefeller University Press, New York, 2010).

[59] Caswell, P.T. & Zech, T. Actin-Based Cell Protrusion in a 3D Matrix. Trends Cell Biol **28**, 823-834 (2018).

[60] Campa, C.C., Ciraolo, E., Ghigo, A., Germena, G. & Hirsch, E. Crossroads of PI3K and Rac pathways. Small GTPases **6**, 71-80 (2015).

[61] Pollard, T.D. & Cooper, J.A. Actin, a central player in cell shape and movement. Science **326**, 1208-1212 (2009).

[62] Gialeli, C., Theocharis, A.D. & Karamanos, N.K. Roles of matrix metalloproteinases in cancer progression and their pharmacological targeting. The FEBS Journal **278**, 16-27 (2011).

[63] Carey, S., Starchenko, A., McGregor, A. & Reinhart-King, C. Leading malignant cells initiate collective epithelial cell invasion in a three-dimensional heterotypic tumor spheroid model. Official Journal of the Metastasis Research Society **30**, 615-630 (2013).

[64] Konen, J., *et al.* Image-guided genomics of phenotypically heterogeneous populations reveals vascular signalling during symbiotic collective cancer invasion. Nature Communications **8**, 15078 (2017).

[65] Hou, Y., Konen, J., Brat, D.J., Marcus, A.I. & Cooper, L.A.D. TASI: A software tool for spatial-temporal quantification of tumor spheroid dynamics. Scientific reports **8**, 7248-7248 (2018).

[66] Cheung, K.J. & Ewald, A.J. A collective route to metastasis: Seeding by tumor cell clusters. Science (New York, N.Y.) **352**, 167 (2016).

[67] Cheung, K.J. & Ewald, A.J. Illuminating breast cancer invasion: diverse roles for cell–cell interactions. Current Opinion in Cell Biology **30**, 99-111 (2014).

[68] Lawson, D.A., *et al.* Single-cell analysis reveals a stem-cell program in human metastatic breast cancer cells. Nature **526**, 131-135 (2015).

[69] Davis, R.T., *et al.* Transcriptional diversity and bioenergetic shift in human breast cancer metastasis revealed by single-cell RNA sequencing. Nature Cell Biology **22**, 310-320 (2020).

[70] Chatterjee, S. & Burns, T.F. Targeting Heat Shock Proteins in Cancer: A Promising Therapeutic Approach. Int J Mol Sci **18**(2017).

[71] Hoter, A. & Naim, H.Y. Heat Shock Proteins and Ovarian Cancer: Important Roles and Therapeutic Opportunities. Cancers **11**, 1389 (2019).

[72] Porporato, P.E., *et al.* A mitochondrial switch promotes tumor metastasis. Cell reports **8**, 754-766 (2014).

[73] Zielonka, J. & Kalyanaraman, B. "ROS-generating mitochondrial DNA mutations can regulate tumor cell metastasis"--a critical commentary. Free radical biology & medicine **45**, 1217-1219 (2008).

[74] Dai, X., *et al.* Breast cancer intrinsic subtype classification, clinical use and future trends. *American journal of cancer research* **5**, 2929-2943 (2015).

[75] Karantza, V. Keratins in health and cancer: more than mere epithelial cell markers. Oncogene **30**, 127-138 (2011).

[76] Weber, Gregory f., Bjerke, Maureen a. & Desimone, Douglas w. A Mechanoresponsive Cadherin-Keratin Complex Directs Polarized Protrusive Behavior and Collective Cell Migration. Developmental cell **22**, 104-115 (2012).

[77] Xiao-Lei, G., *et al.* Cytokeratin-14 contributes to collective invasion of salivary adenoid cystic carcinoma. PLoS One **12**, e0171341 (2017).

[78] Collins, C. & Nelson, W.J. Running with neighbors: coordinating cell migration and cell-cell adhesion. Curr Opin Cell Biol **36**, 62-70 (2015).

[79] Friedl, P. & Mayor, R. Tuning Collective Cell Migration by Cell-Cell Junction Regulation. Cold Spring Harb Perspect Biol **9**(2017).

[80] Seltmann, K., Cheng, F., Wiche, G., Eriksson, J.E. & Magin, T.M. Keratins Stabilize Hemidesmosomes through Regulation of β4-Integrin Turnover. Journal of Investigative Dermatology **135**, 1609-1620 (2015).

[81] Kröger, C., *et al.* Keratins control intercellular adhesion involving PKC-α–mediated desmoplakin phosphorylation. Journal of Cell Biology **201**, 681-692 (2013).

[82] Loschke, F., Homberg, M. & Magin, T.M. Keratin isotypes control desmosome stability and dynamics through PKCα. Journal of Investigative Dermatology **136**, 202-213 (2016).

[83] Haeger, A., Krause, M., Wolf, K. & Friedl, P. Cell jamming: Collective invasion of mesenchymal tumor cells imposed by tissue confinement. Biochimica et Biophysica Acta (BBA) - General Subjects **1840**, 2386-2395 (2014).

[84] Yang, C., *et al.* Inducible formation of leader cells driven by CD44 switching gives rise to collective invasion and metastases in luminal breast carcinomas. Oncogene **38**, 7113-7132 (2019).

[85] Hanin, L. Paradoxical Effects of Tumor Shrinkage on Long-Term Survival of Cancer Patients. Frontiers in Applied Mathematics and Statistics **6**(2020).

[86] Gandalovicova, A., *et al.* Migrastatics-Anti-metastatic and Anti-invasion Drugs: Promises and Challenges. Trends in cancer **3**, 391-406 (2017).

[87] Trendowski, M. Exploiting the cytoskeletal filaments of neoplastic cells to potentiate a novel therapeutic approach. Biochimica et Biophysica Acta (BBA) - Reviews on Cancer **1846**, 599-616 (2014).

[88] Bousquet, P.F., *et al.* Effects of cytochalasin B in culture and in vivo on murine Madison 109 lung carcinoma and on B16 melanoma. Cancer Res **50**, 1431-1439 (1990).

[89] Senderowicz, A.M., *et al.* Jasplakinolide's inhibition of the growth of prostate carcinoma cells in vitro with disruption of the actin cytoskeleton. Journal of the National Cancer Institute **87**, 46-51 (1995).

[90] Sadok, A. & Marshall, C.J. Rho GTPases: masters of cell migration. Small GTPases **5**, e29710 (2014).

[91] Matsubara, M. & Bissell, M.J. Inhibitors of Rho kinase (ROCK) signaling revert the malignant phenotype of breast cancer cells in 3D context. Oncotarget **7**(2016).

[92] Gillis, N.K. & McLeod, H.L. The pharmacogenomics of drug resistance to protein kinase inhibitors. Drug Resistance Updates **28**, 28-42 (2016).

[93] Xiao, Y., *et al.* The PI3K/mTOR dual inhibitor GSK458 potently impedes ovarian cancer tumorigenesis and metastasis. Cellular oncology (Dordrecht) **43**, 669-680 (2020).

[94] Ersahin, T., Tuncbag, N. & Cetin-Atalay, R. The PI3K/AKT/mTOR interactive pathway. Molecular bioSystems **11**, 1946-1954 (2015).

[95] Leevers, S.J., Vanhaesebroeck, B. & Waterfield, M.D. Signalling through phosphoinositide 3-kinases: the lipids take centre stage. Curr Opin Cell Biol **11**, 219-225 (1999).

[96] Engelman, J.A., Luo, J. & Cantley, L.C. The evolution of phosphatidylinositol 3-kinases as regulators of growth and metabolism. Nature Reviews Genetics **7**, 606-619 (2006).

[97] Cui, W., Cai, Y. & Zhou, X. Advances in subunits of PI3K class I in cancer. Pathology **46**, 169-176 (2014).

[98] Martini, M., De Santis, M.C., Braccini, L., Gulluni, F. & Hirsch, E. PI3K/AKT signaling pathway and cancer: an updated review. Annals of medicine **46**, 372-383 (2014).

[99] Gasparri, M.L., *et al.* PI3K/AKT/mTOR Pathway in Ovarian Cancer Treatment: Are We on the Right Track? Geburtshilfe und Frauenheilkunde **77**, 1095-1103 (2017).

[100] Dobbin, Z.C. & Landen, C.N. The importance of the PI3K/AKT/MTOR pathway in the progression of ovarian cancer. International journal of molecular sciences **14**, 8213-8227 (2013).

[101] Mabuchi, S., Kuroda, H., Takahashi, R. & Sasano, T. The PI3K/AKT/mTOR pathway as a therapeutic target in ovarian cancer. Gynecol Oncol **137**, 173-179 (2015).

[102] Cai, J., *et al.* The role of the PTEN/PI3K/Akt pathway on prognosis in epithelial ovarian cancer: a meta-analysis. The oncologist **19**, 528 (2014).

[103] Huang, J., *et al.* Frequent genetic abnormalities of the PI3K/AKT pathway in primary ovarian cancer predict patient outcome. Genes, chromosomes & cancer **50**, 606-618 (2011).

[104] Ediriweera, M.K., Tennekoon, K.H. & Samarakoon, S.R. Role of the PI3K/AKT/mTOR signaling pathway in ovarian cancer: Biological and therapeutic significance. in *Seminars in cancer biology*, Vol. 59 147-160 (Elsevier, 2019).

[105] Westfall, S.D. & Skinner, M.K. Inhibition of phosphatidylinositol 3-kinase sensitizes ovarian cancer cells to carboplatin and allows adjunct chemotherapy treatment. Molecular Cancer Therapeutics **4**, 1764 (2005).

[106] Choi, H.J., *et al.* A novel PI3K/mTOR dual inhibitor, CMG002,

overcomes the chemoresistance in ovarian cancer. Gynecol Oncol **153**, 135-148 (2019).

[107] Yang, J., *et al.* Targeting PI3K in cancer: mechanisms and advances in clinical trials. Molecular Cancer **18**, 26 (2019).

[108] Janku, F. Phosphoinositide 3-kinase (PI3K) pathway inhibitors in solid tumors: From laboratory to patients. Cancer treatment reviews **59**, 93-101 (2017).

[109] Janku, F., Yap, T.A. & Meric-Bernstam, F. Targeting the PI3K pathway in cancer: are we making headway? Nature reviews Clinical oncology **15**, 273 (2018).

[110] Ghoneum, A. & Said, N. PI3K-AKT-mTOR and NFκB Pathways in Ovarian Cancer: Implications for Targeted Therapeutics. Cancers **11**, 949 (2019).

[111] Miller, B.W., *et al.* FDA approval: idelalisib monotherapy for the treatment of patients with follicular lymphoma and small lymphocytic lymphoma. Clinical cancer research: an official journal of the American Association for Cancer Research **21**, 1525-1529 (2015).

[112] Buti, S., Leonetti, A., Dallatomasina, A. & Bersanelli, M. Everolimus in the management of metastatic renal cell carcinoma: an evidence-based review of its place in therapy. Core Evid **11**, 23-36 (2016).

[113] Taylor, S.E., Chu, T., Elvin, J.A., Edwards, R.P. & Zorn, K.K. Phase II study of everolimus and bevacizumab in recurrent ovarian, peritoneal, and fallopian tube cancer. Gynecologic Oncology **156**, 32-37 (2020).

[114] Behbakht, K., *et al.* Phase II trial of the mTOR inhibitor, temsirolimus and evaluation of circulating tumor cells and tumor biomarkers in persistent and recurrent epithelial ovarian and primary peritoneal malignancies: a Gynecologic Oncology Group study. Gynecol Oncol **123**, 19-26 (2011).

[115] Emons, G., *et al.* Temsirolimus in women with platinum-refractory/resistant ovarian cancer or advanced/recurrent endometrial carcinoma. A phase II study of the AGO-study group (AGO-GYN8). Gynecol Oncol **140**, 450-456 (2016).

[116] Thamilselvan, V., Craig, D.H. & Basson, M.D. FAK association with multiple signal proteins mediates pressure-induced colon cancer cell adhesion via a Src-dependent PI3K/Akt pathway. The FASEB Journal **21**, 1730-1741 (2007).

[117] Asati, V., Mahapatra, D.K. & Bharti, S.K. PI3K/Akt/mTOR and Ras/Raf/MEK/ERK signaling pathways inhibitors as anticancer agents: Structural and pharmacological perspectives. European Journal of Medicinal Chemistry **109**, 314-341 (2016).

[118] Dienstmann, R., Rodon, J., Serra, V. & Tabernero, J. Picking the point of inhibition: a comparative review of PI3K/AKT/mTOR pathway inhibitors. Mol Cancer Ther **13**, 1021-1031 (2014).

[119] Narov, K., *et al.* The dual PI3K/mTOR inhibitor GSK2126458 is effective for treating solid renal tumours in Tsc2(+/-) mice through suppression of cell proliferation and induction of apoptosis. Oncotarget **8**, 58504-58512 (2017).

[120] Jebahi, A., *et al.* PI3K/mTOR dual inhibitor NVP-BEZ235 decreases Mcl-1 expression and sensitizes ovarian carcinoma cells to Bcl-xL-targeting strategies, provided that Bim expression is induced. Cancer Lett **348**, 38-49 (2014).

[121] Wu, Y.-H., Huang, Y.-F., Chen, C.-C., Huang, C.-Y. & Chou, C.-Y. Comparing PI3K/Akt Inhibitors Used in Ovarian Cancer Treatment. Front Pharmacol **11**, 206-206 (2020).

[122] Bai, S.H. & Ogbourne, S. Eco-toxicological effects of the avermectin family with a focus on abamectin and ivermectin. Chemosphere **154**, 204-214 (2016).

[123] Didier, A. & Loor, F. The abamectin derivative ivermectin is a potent P-glycoprotein inhibitor. Anti-cancer drugs **7**, 745-751 (1996).

[124] Liu, Y., Fang, S., Sun, Q. & Liu, B. Anthelmintic drug ivermectin inhibits angiogenesis, growth and survival of glioblastoma through inducing mitochondrial dysfunction and oxidative stress. Biochem Biophys Res Commun **480**, 415-421 (2016).

[125] Nambara, S., *et al.* Antitumor effects of the antiparasitic agent ivermectin via inhibition of Yes-associated protein 1 expression in gastric cancer. Oncotarget **8**, 107666-107677 (2017).

[126] Seiden, M.V., *et al.* A phase II study of the MDR inhibitor biricodar (INCEL, VX-710) and paclitaxel in women with advanced ovarian cancer refractory to paclitaxel therapy. Gynecol Oncol **86**, 302-310 (2002).

[127] Kelly, R.J., *et al.* A pharmacodynamic study of docetaxel in combination with the P-glycoprotein antagonist tariquidar (XR9576) in patients with lung, ovarian, and cervical cancer. Clinical cancer research: an official journal of the American Association for Cancer Research **17**, 569-580 (2011).

[128] Xia, Y., *et al.* YAP promotes ovarian cancer cell tumorigenesis and is indicative of a poor prognosis for ovarian cancer patients. PLoS One **9**, e91770 (2014).

[129] Zhang, X., *et al.* Ivermectin Augments the In Vitro and In Vivo Efficacy of Cisplatin in Epithelial Ovarian Cancer by Suppressing Akt/mTOR Signaling. The American Journal of the Medical Sciences **359**, 123-129 (2020).

[130] Antonopoulos, A.S., Margaritis, M., Lee, R., Channon, K. & Antoniades, C. Statins as anti-inflammatory agents in atherogenesis: molecular mechanisms and lessons from the recent clinical trials. Curr Pharm Des **18**, 1519-1530 (2012).

[131] Stryjkowska-Góra, A., Karczmarek-Borowska, B., Góra, T. & Krawczak, K. Statins and cancers. Contemporary Oncology **19**, 167 (2015).

[132] Wong, W.W., Dimitroulakos, J., Minden, M. & Penn, L. HMG-CoA reductase inhibitors and the malignant cell: the statin family of drugs as triggers of tumor-specific apoptosis. Leukemia **16**, 508-519 (2002).

[133] Freed-Pastor, W.A., *et al.* Mutant p53 disrupts mammary tissue architecture via the mevalonate pathway. Cell **148**, 244-258 (2012).

[134] Stine, J.E., *et al.* The HMG-CoA reductase inhibitor, simvastatin, exhibits anti-metastatic and anti-tumorigenic effects in ovarian cancer. Oncotarget **7**, 946-960 (2016).

[135] Kobayashi, Y., *et al.* Mevalonate Pathway Antagonist Suppresses Formation of Serous Tubal Intraepithelial Carcinoma and Ovarian Carcinoma in Mouse Models. Clinical cancer research: an official journal of the American Association for Cancer Research **21**, 4652-4662 (2015).

[136] Fozzard, H.A. & Sheets, M.F. Cellular mechanism of action of cardiac glycosides. *Journal of the American College of Cardiology* **5**, 10a-15a (1985).

[137] Shiratori, O. Growth inhibitory effect of cardiac glycosides and aglycones on neoplastic cells: in vitro and in vivo studies. Gan **58**, 521-528 (1967).

[138] Orrenius, S., Zhivotovsky, B. & Nicotera, P. Regulation of cell death: the calcium-apoptosis link. Nat Rev Mol Cell Biol **4**, 552-565 (2003).

[139] Wang, Y., *et al.* Src mediates extracellular signal-regulated kinase 1/2 activation and autophagic cell death induced by cardiac glycosides in human non-small cell lung cancer cell lines. Molecular Carcinogenesis **54**, E26-E34 (2015).

[140] Zhang, H., *et al.* Digoxin and other cardiac glycosides inhibit HIF-1alpha synthesis and block tumor growth. Proc Natl Acad Sci U S A **105**, 19579-19586 (2008).

[141] Jun, D.W., *et al.* Ouabain, a cardiac glycoside, inhibits the Fanconi anemia/BRCA pathway activated by DNA interstrand cross-linking agents. PloS one **8**, e75905-e75905 (2013).

[142] Apostolou, P., *et al.* Anvirzel™ in combination with cisplatin in breast, colon, lung, prostate, melanoma and pancreatic cancer cell lines. BMC Pharmacology and Toxicology **14**, 18 (2013).

[143] Felth, J., *et al.* Cytotoxic Effects of Cardiac Glycosides in Colon Cancer Cells, Alone and in Combination with Standard Chemotherapeutic Drugs. *Journal of Natural Products* **72**, 1969-1974 (2009).

[144] Khan, M., *et al.* A phase II trial of biochemotherapy with cisplatin, vinblastine, dacarbazine, interleukin-2, interferon, and digoxin in melanoma matients. Journal of Clinical Oncology **25**, 8573-8573 (2007).

[145] Platz, E.A., *et al.* A novel two-stage, transdisciplinary study identifies digoxin as a possible drug for prostate cancer treatment. Cancer discovery **1**, 68-77 (2011).

[146] Osman, M.H., *et al.* Cardiac glycosides use and the risk and mortality of cancer; systematic review and meta-analysis of observational studies. PLoS One **12**, e0178611 (2017).

[147] Vogel, T.J., Jeon, C., Karlan, B. & Walsh, C. Digoxin therapy is not associated with improved survival in epithelial ovarian cancer: A SEER-Medicare database analysis. Gynecol Oncol **140**, 285-288 (2016).

[148] Menger, L., *et al.* Cardiac Glycosides Exert Anticancer Effects by Inducing Immunogenic Cell Death. *Science translational medicine* **4**, 143ra199 (2012).

[149] Rena, G., Hardie, D.G. & Pearson, E.R. The mechanisms of action of metformin. Diabetologia **60**, 1577-1585 (2017).

[150] Ben Sahra, I., Le Marchand-Brustel, Y., Tanti, J.F. & Bost, F. Metformin in cancer therapy: a new perspective for an old antidiabetic drug? Mol Cancer Ther **9**, 1092-1099 (2010).

[151] Romero, I.L., *et al.* Relationship of type II diabetes and metformin use to ovarian cancer progression, survival, and chemosensitivity. Obstetrics and gynecology **119**, 61-67 (2012).

[152] Kumar, S., *et al.* Metformin intake is associated with better survival in ovarian cancer: a case-control study. Cancer **119**, 555-562 (2013).

[153] Buckanovich, R.J., *et al.* A phase II clinical trial of metformin as a cancer stem cell targeting agent in stage IIc/III/IV ovarian, fallopian tube, and primary peritoneal cancer. Journal of Clinical Oncology **35**, 5556-5556 (2017).

[154] Wilson, A.L., *et al.* DPP4 Inhibitor Sitagliptin Enhances Lymphocyte Recruitment and Prolongs Survival in a Syngeneic Ovarian Cancer Mouse Model. *Cancers (Basel)* **13**(2021).

[155] Singh, N., *et al.* Inflammation and cancer. Ann Afr Med **18**, 121-126 (2019).

[156] Wong, R.S.Y. Role of Nonsteroidal Anti-Inflammatory Drugs (NSAIDs) in Cancer Prevention and Cancer Promotion. Advances in Pharmacological Sciences **2019**, 3418975 (2019).

[157] Patrono, C., García Rodríguez, L.A., Landolfi, R. & Baigent, C. Low-dose aspirin for the prevention of atherothrombosis. New England Journal of Medicine **353**, 2373-2383 (2005).

[158] Fischer, S.M., Hawk, E.T. & Lubet, R.A. Coxibs and other nonsteroidal anti-inflammatory drugs in animal models of cancer chemoprevention. *Cancer prevention research (Philadelphia, Pa.)* **4**, 1728-1735 (2011).

[159] Xu, X.C. COX-2 inhibitors in cancer treatment and prevention, a recent development. Anti-cancer drugs **13**, 127-137 (2002).

[160] Henry, W.S., *et al.* Aspirin Suppresses Growth in PI3K-Mutant Breast Cancer by Activating AMPK and Inhibiting mTORC1 Signaling. Cancer Res **77**, 790-801 (2017).

[161] Chen, Z., *et al.* Aspirin has a better effect on PIK3CA mutant colorectal cancer cells by PI3K/Akt/Raptor pathway. *Molecular medicine (Cambridge, Mass.)* **26**, 14 (2020).

[162] Thorat, M.A. & Cuzick, J. Role of aspirin in cancer prevention. Current oncology reports **15**, 533-540 (2013).

[163] Berger, J.S., Lala, A., Krantz, M.J., Baker, G.S. & Hiatt, W.R. Aspirin for the prevention of cardiovascular events in patients without clinical cardiovascular disease: a meta-analysis of randomized trials. *American heart journal* **162**, 115-124. e112 (2011).

[164] Thiagarajan, P. & Jankowski, J.A. Aspirin and NSAIDs; benefits and harms for the gut. Best Practice & Research Clinical Gastroenterology **26**, 197-206 (2012).

[165] He, J., Whelton, P.K., Vu, B. & Klag, M.J. Aspirin and risk of hemorrhagic stroke: a meta-analysis of randomized controlled trials. Jama **280**, 1930-1935 (1998).

[166] Zerbini, L.F., *et al.* A novel pathway involving melanoma differentiation associated gene-7/interleukin-24 mediates nonsteroidal anti-inflammatory drug-induced apoptosis and growth arrest of cancer cells. Cancer Res **66**, 11922-11931 (2006).

[167] Valle, B.L., *et al.* Non-steroidal anti-inflammatory drugs decrease E2F1 expression and inhibit cell growth in ovarian cancer cells. PloS one **8**, e61836-e61836 (2013).

[168] Legge, F., *et al.* Phase II study of the combination carboplatin plus celecoxib in heavily pre-treated recurrent ovarian cancer patients. BMC cancer **11**, 214-214 (2011).

[169] Reyners, A.K.L., *et al.* A randomized phase II study investigating the addition of the specific COX-2 inhibitor celecoxib to docetaxel plus carboplatin as first-line chemotherapy for stage IC to IV epithelial ovarian cancer, Fallopian tube or primary peritoneal carcinomas: the DoCaCel study. *Ann Oncol* **23**, 2896-2902 (2012).

[170] Merritt, M.A., Green, A.C., Nagle, C.M. & Webb, P.M. Talcum powder,

chronic pelvic inflammation and NSAIDs in relation to risk of epithelial ovarian cancer. Int J Cancer **122**, 170-176 (2008).

[171] Murphy, M.A., *et al.* Non-steroidal anti-inflammatory drug use and ovarian cancer risk: findings from the NIH-AARP Diet and Health Study and systematic review. Cancer Causes Control **23**, 1839-1852 (2012).

Chapter 10

The Roles of Nanoparticle in the Treatment and Diagnosis of Ovarian Cancer

Mohammed E. Mansur

Abstract

Ovarian cancer is the most common type of cancer worldwide among women, and it is usually diagnosed at an advanced stage. The initial treatment for ovarian cancer is surgical debulking, but this is only effective in the treatment of early stage disease. Surgery alone is insufficient for treatment of advanced disease and systemic therapies, in particular chemotherapies, are indicated. The main aim of this book chapter is to review the role of nano-therapy in treatment of advance ovarian cancer, in comparison to the use of traditional chemotherapies. Nano-therapies are thought to have advantages in terms of improving drug stability in the human body, chemotherapy toxicity profile, and drug delivery to the target cells thus enhancing drug penetration into the cancer cells. This book chapter also covers the development of nano-therapy and also the type of potential cargos. In summary, the types of nanocarrier, and their roles ovarian cancer diagnosis and treatment will be discussed.

Keywords: ovarian cancer, nanocarrier, Doxil, TPGS, PEG

1. Introduction

Although ovarian cancer represents only 5% of all cancer cases among women, it is ranked fifth for cancer deaths among women [1]. It is the most common among gynecological cancers and ranks third after uterine and cervical cancer, as it represents the highest, worst warning, and highest mortality rates [2]. Ovarian cancer, in particularly high grade serous subtype, is often regarded as systemic disease. I think you need to re-do this statement as up to 75% of OC is diagnosed at an advanced stage – stage III and IV. It is expected that in the next twenty years, the death rate of this type of cancer will increase significantly, the reason for the high death rate is that the disease grows secretly and without symptoms, the appearance of symptoms is delayed, and the lack of appropriate examination that detects the disease at certain stages, and this is why it is called the silent killer [3, 4].

Until recently, methods of prevention and early detection of ovarian cancer did not achieve satisfactory results, partly due to its heterogeneous nature [5]. In the past, ovarian cancer prevention methods were characterized by modifying risk factors and creating protective factors. Unfortunately, these modifications did not significantly reduce the incidence of the disease [6]. The initial treatment of ovarian- either with upfront cytoreductive surgery or chemotherapy (neoadjuvant) followed by interval debulking surgery, Almost the main reason behind recurring ovarian cancer Is due to the aggressive nature of the disease and unfortunately all metastatic ovarian cancer will develop resistance to conventional systemic therapies, and it is known that cancer cells develop resistance especially through certain mechanisms such as reduced absorption, increasing elimination, inactivation/detoxification of drugs, and accelerating DNA repair [7, 8].

Currently, many new approaches have been developed to improve delivery of drug to the target cancer cells, including the use of nanotechnology, and may be one of the solution to overcome the obstacles in treating advance ovarian cancer, nanotechnology was found to have extensively investigated for molecular imaging, drug delivery, treatment and tumor targeting [9, 10]. In addition, this type of nano-based drug can overcome the systemic toxicity towards normal cells as well as the toxicological effects of conventional chemotherapy, In addition, it is possible through this technique to control the systemic toxicity of normal cells and reduce the toxicity of chemotherapy agents. Thus the new method can be followed by using multiple chemotherapeutic drugs with a suitable nanocarrier as a solution for the future of cancer treatment. Of course, this can be done by passive targeting and active targeting where both methods are used to ensure a certain and specific targeting of cancer cells [11, 12].

2. Nanotechnology application

Nanotechnology can be defined as a practical application that results in a process or product based on the single or multi-component nanoscale, which is a fairly recent field, nanoscale components having at least one dimension in the size range of 1–100 nm. This technology is referred to in the field of biology, nanobiotechnology and in the medical field of nanomedicine, and the main principle of nanotechnology is to increase the effectiveness of the techniques used in the diagnosis and treatment of cancer.

Due to the lack of early diagnosis and the vague and multiple methods in clinical procedures for detecting ovarian cancer, there are many attempts that would modify the course in this area, which is the use of nanotechnology and its platforms.

2.1 Nanocarriers

They are the same nanomaterials used in treatment and diagnosis, Nanocarriers are a multifunctional compound that can be loaded with several types of molecules through physical absorption and chemical conjugations reactions including drugs, imaging agents, targeting moieties such as ligands or antibodies, and polyethylene glycol. There are several types, including liposomes, micelles, and dendrimers (**Figure 1**) [13].

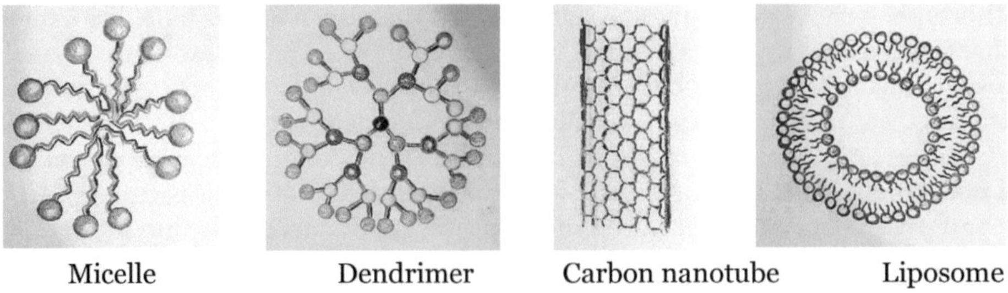

Figure 1.
Examples of some nanocarriers employed in therapy and diagnosis.

Nanocarriers can be used as an alternative to conventional chemotherapy for drug delivery because they have many advantages, including the delivery of poorly soluble drugs, as they surround them within the hydrophobic interfaces or act as carriers for them in the blood, reduce the systemic toxicity of chemical treatments, regulate the stability of drugs by prolonging their existence In the blood circulation and protecting it from disruption and reducing the renal clearance, reducing drug resistance by targeting cancer cells, where nanocarriers are taken up by the method of endocytosis [14, 15].

2.1.1 Liposomes

Liposomes have multiple properties as they are characterized by the presence of two parts, an inner hydrophilic part and an outer hydrophobic part, and of course in the form of a lipid bilayer, and it is also possible to modify the polar heads of these particles. This arrangement makes it easy to include various hydrophilic and hydrophobic drugs in the liposomes as well as to load various drugs.

They are delivery compounds that serve greatly in enhancing the efficiency of pharmaceutical components, as these compounds can hide from the immune system, simulate biological membranes, increase the chance of a drug remaining for a longer period until it reaches its destination, serve to help solubilize highly lipophilic drug molecules or, modulate the pharmacokinetics and biodistribution of the API—thereby helping to minimize side effects and enhance the product safety profile [16, 17].

2.1.2 Dendrimers

Dendrimers are radially symmetric molecules with a well-known structure that are homogeneous and monodisperse structure by tree-like arms or branches, they are hyperbranched macromolecules with a carefully tailored architecture, the end-groups, which can be functionalized, thus modifying their physicochemical or biological properties. Dendrimers have gained a broad range of applications in supramolecular chemistry, particularly in host-guest reactions and self-assembly processes. They are highly defined artificial macromolecules, which are characterized by a combination of a high number of functional groups and a compact molecular structure [18].

2.1.3 Micelles

This type of nanocomposite has gained very great importance as it has been well studied in the diagnosis and treatment of tumors. These interesting nanostructures comprise of spherically shaped, self-assembled amphiphilic block co-polymers made up of a hydrophobic core and a hydrophilic corona in an aqueous medium, with a diameter between 10 and 100 nm. The core of the micelle can accommodate hydrophobic drugs [19].

Polymeric micelles are gaining popularity as drug delivery systems because they not only provide increased solubility, but they also may enhance the stability of their drug cargo, in addition to providing in vivo pharmacokinetic advantages compared with the free drug [20].

2.1.4 Carbon nanotube

After discovering this nanotransmitter, it has enjoyed very great interest in the medical fields due to its unique structure and properties in terms of It has a large surface area, large aspect ratio, nanoscale size stability and multiple chemical functions and they are especially important as carriers for transporting drugs and biomolecules. In this regard, this type has been used due to the functional properties it possesses as an important transporter for the delivery of anti-cancer drugs and many proteins and genes. Likewise, to directly kill cancer cells, it was used as a carrier for photothermal therapy (PTT) and photodynamic therapy (PDT) [21, 22].

3. Diagnosis and imaging

In recent times, there have been many improvements and major developments in the field of diagnosis and imaging with the help of nanotechnology, where it has been used the technologies of biosensors and point of care systems as well as the updated and improved imaging technologies as well as the integration of bioinformatics together with multiplexed assays. At present, there are many nanoparticle platforms and microelectromechanical systems to strengthen and improve diagnostic processes, largely as a means of diagnosing biomarkers and of course by enhancing the contrast agents used in imaging [23]. And the real mechanics of the imaging agent used to improve visualization and accumulation within the target cells in many imaging mechanisms on its subtype. There are different imaging methods that use imaging agents such as Optical Imaging, X-ray Imaging, positron emission tomography (PET), Magnetic resonance imaging (MRI) [24].

3.1 Targeted imaging agents

Targeted contrast agents are placed in a specific type of tissue or cellular receptors, including certain types, such as target agents designated for imaging fibrin, which are molecules associated with fibrin, which are molecules associated with fibrin, and other molecules to track stem cells from super magnetic iron oxide, and there are others for imaging angiogenesis, which are of the multimodal type of carbon fluorinated, liposomes are used to target the sclerotic components, and to visualize transplant rejection, microscopic bubbles were used in MRI and ultrasound [25].

3.2 Activatable imaging agents

There are many nanoparticles that are actually designed to have better performance and are imaging agents called operable molecular probes that can produce a signal or some kind of change that can be recorded or detected, for example, when enzymatic activity or a specific response to important chemical reactions, Two imaging technologies are combined into a single activatable lifetime imaging agent. This is applied by combining the high specificity of luminescence lifetime imaging with the high signal-to-background ratio of activatable fluorescence imaging [26].

3.3 Nano-liposomal imaging agents

Liposomes can encapsulate biomolecules that are hydrophilic and increase their internalization and solubility through the lipid bilayers of the cells, Among the drawbacks that can occur in the case of imaging by means of high elimination agents and low systemic retention degrees, and because the rapid removal process from the bloodstream or the body reduces the period and efficiency of imaging, so it is necessary to add a molecule that increases the efficiency of imaging, and this is done by encapsulating the imaging agent with a liposome, can leverage the enhanced permeability and retention (EPR) effect seen in tumors [27, 28].

4. Fluorescent images and guided surgery

To increase the sensitivity, efficiency and strength of the imaging techniques used with surgery and increase their clinical efficiency, there is an actual need to develop new material, Therefore, many fluorescent nanoparticles essential for Image-supported surgeries were developed, tested and designed and tested in preclinical surgery there are some examples of that:

1. CF800 liposomes: This type is used to encapsulate iohexol contrast agent and is commercially available with clinically approved indocyanine green at ratio of 1000: 1 (iohexol to indocyanine green).

2. magnetic iron oxide nanoparticles: A HER - 2 particle that can be combined with optical magnetic resonance imaging. It is a targeting ligands. I learned a rare near-infrared dye called NIR-830 while magnetic iron oxide nanoparticles provide MRI contrast.

3. Porphyrin-lipoprotein mimicking nanoparticle: This type is based on the formation of a nanoscale in which several techniques are combined, photodynamic therapy, fluorescence imaging, positron emission tomography, where the size of the nanoparticle is 20 nanometers.

4. Fluorescent gold nanoparticles: This type is based on CT and fluorescent imaging platform an iodine based contrast agent is combined with aptamer with nucleolin specific targeting functions.

5. conjugated dendrimers: In this type activatable cell penetrating peptides are used Dendrimeric encapsulation and marker with gadolinium and Cy5 and sensitive in vivo to MMP-9 and MMP-2.

5. Nanoparticle therapeutics (anti-cancer)

Usually, nanoparticle treatments consist of therapeutic lines such as small-molecule drugs as well as peptides, nucleic acids, proteins, and other components or compounds that combine with them to form nanoparticles. As we previously knew that nanoparticles have a direct, targeted and improved anti-cancer effect compared to conventional treatments. This is owing to more specific targeting to tumor tissues via improved pharmacokinetics and pharmacodynamics, and active intracellular delivery. These properties depend on the size and surface properties (including the presence of targeting ligands) of the nanoparticles (**Figure 2**) [29].

5.1 Nanoparticle size

Naturally, the size of the anti-cancer nanoparticles should be between 10 and 100 nm. This measurement is based on the rates of glomerular sieving of the capillary wall of the kidneys. Research has indicated on size estimates where the

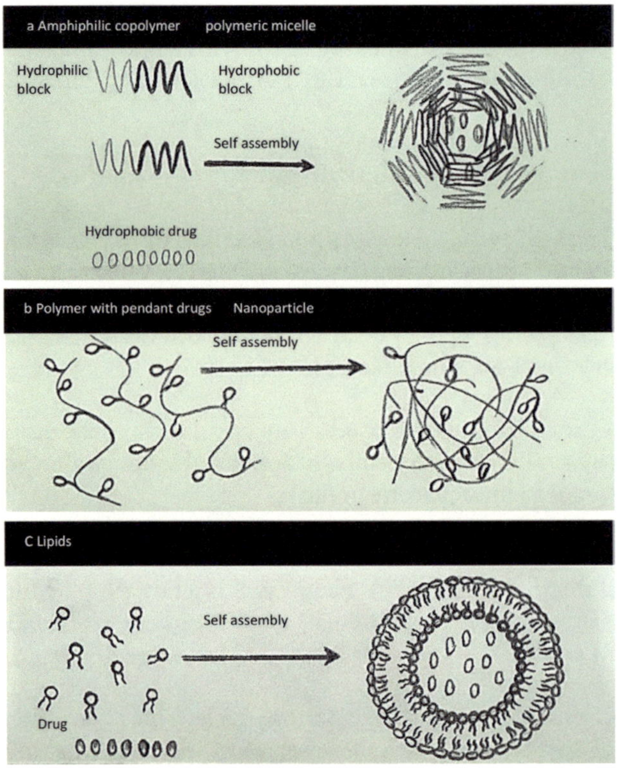

Figure 2.
Basic nanoparticles used in clinical trials. (a) Nanoparticles composed of therapeutic components. (b) the nanoparticles that are formed from polymer/drug. (c) Nanoparticles that are a liposome component.

minimum is 10 nanometers as a threshold for renal excretion and where it is known that vessels in tumor cases are subject to leak Macromolecules in a certain way, so the nanoparticles should not be able to circulate for a long time in the bloodstream and have a chance to reach the bloodstream through the vessels of the tumor tissue and enter the tumor tissue where the size of the nanoparticles is greater than 6–12 nm, which is the diameter of the sieve in the blood vessels of normal tissues and It is prevented from entering and not damaging the normal tissue, and it is known that the diameter of the sieve in the tumor blood vessels ranges from 40 to 200 nm (**Figure 3**) [30].

5.2 Nanoparticle surface

Nanoparticles have a very large surface area compared to the size of the nanoparticle and compared to normal particles, and this space provides a high degree of interaction with the molecule and its environment, and of course it is possible to almost determine the final fate of the nanoparticle inside the body through determining the strength of the interaction between the nanoparticle and its surroundings, and it depends largely on a mixture of size. And surface properties. Nanoparticles that are sterically stabilized polymers on their surface and have surface charges that are either slightly negative or slightly positive tend to have minimal self–self and self–non-self-interactions, Nanoparticles often have unexpected visible properties because they are small enough to confine their electrons and produce quantum effects. This provides a tremendous driving force for diffusion, especially at elevated temperatures [31, 32].

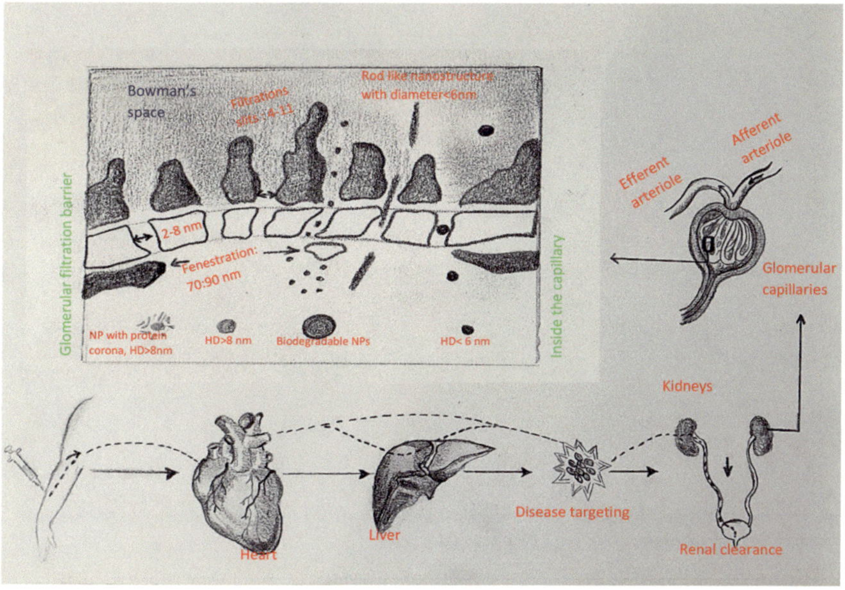

Figure 3.
The idea of special targeting of cancer cells to the nanoparticles that can be filtered through the kidney. As the nanoparticles target cancerous diseases, the residue that is not targeted is removed.

5.3 Nano-chemical therapeutics

The rare properties of nanoparticles have been exploited to present the science of chemical therapeutics in a unique way and as we previously knew that nanoparticles and the reason for their special composition can exploit the vascular infusion and absorption mechanisms associated with tumor cells to enter and implement a specific therapeutic effect where the particles accumulate in the tumor tissue, taking advantage of the enhanced permeability and retention effect, of course, when comparing the usual systemic chemotherapy by systemic administration with the science of chemotherapy coated with nanoparticles, where it can deliver the desired dose to the tissue environment of the tumor. In almost the same way, special bonds to cancer cells are added to nanoparticles to arrive in a uniform and targeted way to reduce the toxicity of systemic chemotherapy, we will mention the most common therapeutics [33].

A present example is a (PEGylated liposomal doxorubicin) formulation that has been.

U.S. Food and Drug Administration (FDA) approved for use in recurrent and platinum-resistant cancers (**Figure 4**) [34].

We previously knew that the liposomes remain less time in the circulatory system, and this affects the drug levels that reach the tumor tissue, and this can be bypassed by reducing the size of the carrier, but this may affect the levels of the drug and its required quantity, so to get rid of problems, the carrier is coated with polymers such as polyethylene glycol (PEG). As this system works to mask the immune system and increase circulation time [35]. The proposed mechanism of action and accumulation of DOXIL is as follows:

The liposomes coated with doxoribicin remain in circulation for 2–3 weeks after the injection process until the end of their estimated effective life, these particles enter the tumor tissue and settle in it through defects and gaps in the tumor vessels and then settle near the blood vessel, The extravasated liposomes release the drug

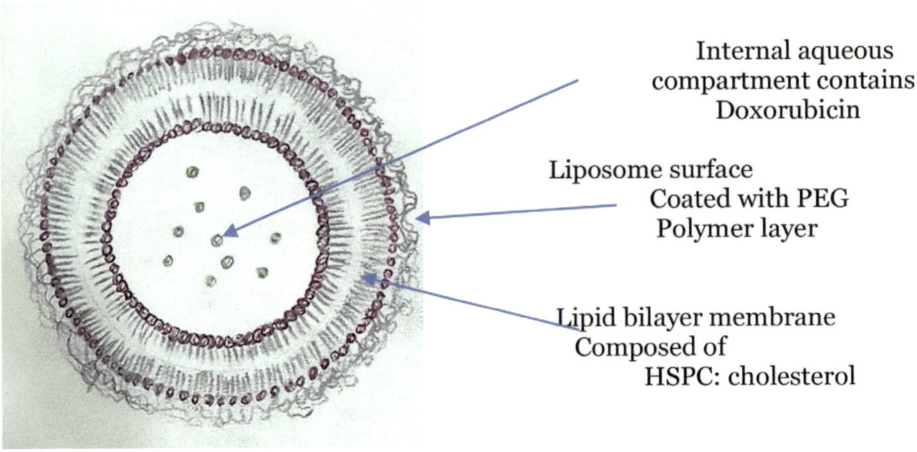

Figure 4.
This shape represents a Doxil liposome where doxorubicin is confined and encapsulated in the internal compartment where drug molecules are tightly packed.

components, and drug molecules enter deeply into the tumor tissue, where they reach and kill cancer cells. It is noted that this mechanism does not need a physical encounter and contact between the liposome and the cell, where the drug can reach and penetrate the barriers that intercept the particles [36].

There is another example of a nano-drug transporter (micelle) these structures typically contain a more hydrophobic component that helps solubilize/encapsulate therapeutic compounds, while a hydrophilic component provides stability of the assembly in aqueous environments and offers conjugation sites for eventual targeting ligands. This type of nanostructure has been widely used recently, an example being the D-α-tocopheryl polyethylene glycol (PEG) 1000 succinate (TPGS) (**Figure 5**) [37].

It is an amphiphilic water-soluble derivative of natural source vitamin E and PEG, that has been widely employed as a micelle-former biomaterial. Also, it has been reported that TPGS can inhibit the efflux pump that mediates multidrug

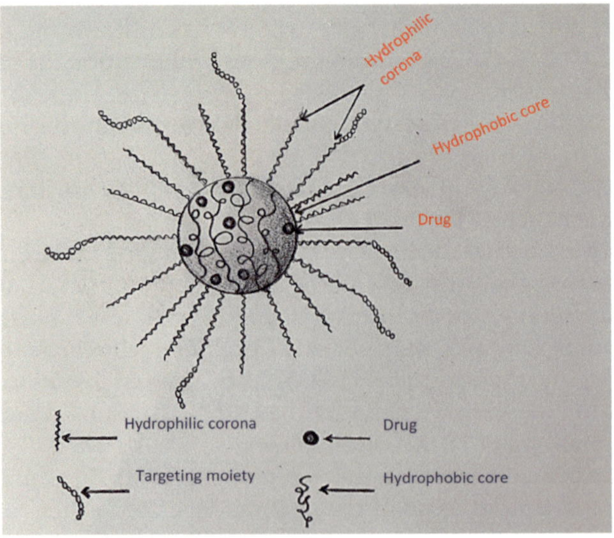

Figure 5.
A typical structure of polymeric micelle representing the drug encapsulated and targeting moiety attached.

resistance in tumor cells, known as P-glycoprotein (P-gp), In this context, TPGS has been employed for DOX encapsulation within polymeric micelles, Single polymers are the most acceptable type in recent times because they increase the solubility and stability of hydrophobic drugs, increase cellular absorption capacity, and to increase the susceptibility, two micelles were combined to obtain mixed micelles to increase strength. as enhanced thermodynamic and kinetic stabilities, higher drug loading (DL) capacity, more accurate size control and easier ways to modify their surface with different moieties [38, 39].

6. Conclusion

From the foregoing that nanoparticles are more efficient in the diagnosis and treatment of ovarian cancer as a basic alternative to chemotherapy and a highly efficient pre and postoperative adjuvant due to their great ability to reach the target tissue and high efficiency to stay in vivo for acceptable periods.

Author details

Mohammed E. Mansur
University of Kufa, Najaf, Iraq

*Address all correspondence to: mohammed.alghurabi@uokufa.edu.iq

References

[1] Engelberth S, Hempel N, Bergkvist M. Development of Nanoscale Approaches for Ovarian Cancer Therapeutics and Diagnostics. Critical. Reviews™ in Oncogenesis. 2014;19(3-4):281-315. DOI: 10.1615/CritRevOncog.2014011455.

[2] Z Momenimovahed Z, Tiznobaik A, Taheri S, Salehiniya H. Ovarian cancer in the world: epidemiology and risk factors. Int J Womens Health. 2019;11: 287-299. DOI:10.2147/IJWH.S197604.

[3] Coburn S, Bray F, Sherman M, Trabert B. International patterns and trends in ovarian cancer incidence, overall and by histologic subtype. Int J Cancer. 2017;140(11):2451-2460. doi:10.1002/ijc.30676.

[4] Yoneda A, Lendorf ME, Couchman JR, Multhaupt HA. Breast and ovarian cancers: a survey and possible roles for the cell surface heparan sulfate proteoglycans. J Histochem Cytochem. 2012;60(1):9-21. doi:10.1369/0022155411428469.

[5] Budiana N, Angelina M, Gede T, Pemayun A. Ovarian cancer: Pathogenesis and current recommendations for prophylactic surgery. J Turk Ger Gynecol Assoc. 2019; 20(1): 47-54. doi: 10.4274/jtgga.galenos.2018.2018.0119.

[6] Kwon JS. Ovarian cancer risk reduction through opportunistic salpingectomy. J Gynecol Oncol. 2015;26:83-86. doi: 10.3802/jgo.2015.26.2.83.

[7] Hasciceka C, Gun O. Nano drug delivery systems for ovarian cancer therapy. Integr Cancer Sci Therap. 2017;4(2):1-4. doi: 10.15761/ICST.1000235.

[8] Florea AM, Busselberg D. Cisplatin as an anti-tumor drug: cellular mechanisms of activity, drug resistance and induced side effects. Cancers (Basel).2011; 3: 1351-1371. doi: 10.3390/cancers3011351.

[9] Tomasina J, Lheureux S, Gauduchon P, Rault S, Malzert-Fréon A. Nanocarriers for the targeted treatment of ovarian cancers. Biomaterials.2013;34: 1073-1101. doi: 10.1016/j.biomaterials.2012.10.055.

[10] Steichen SD, Caldorera-Moore M, Peppas NA. A review of current nanoparticle and targeting moieties for the delivery of cancer therapeutics. Eur J Pharm Sci.2013;48: 416-427. doi: 10.1016/j.ejps.2012.12.006.

[11] Gupta S, Pathak Y, Gupta M, Vyas S. Nanoscale drug delivery strategies for therapy of ovarian cancer: conventional vs targeted. Artificial Cells, Nanomedicine, and Biotechnology. 2019;47(1):4066-4088.doi.org/10.1080/21691401.2019.1677680.

[12] Kim PS, Djazayeri S, Zeineldin R. Novel nanotechnology approaches to diagnosis and therapy of ovarian cancer. Gynecol Oncol. 2011;120(3):393-403. dOI: 10.1016/j.ygyno.2010.11.029.

[13] Longmire M, Choyke PL, Kobayashi H. Clearance properties of nano-sized particles and molecules as imaging agents: considerations and caveats. Nanomed. 2008;3:703-17.

[14] Chen AM, Zhang M, Wei D, Stueber D, Taratula O, Minko T. Co-delivery of doxorubicin and Bcl-2 siRNA by mesoporous silica nanoparticles enhances the efficacy of chemotherapy in multidrug-resistant cancer cells. Small 2009;5:2673-2677.

[15] Kraft JC, Freeling JP, Wang Z, Ho RJY. Emerging Research and Clinical Development Trends of Liposome and Lipid Nanoparticle Drug Delivery

Systems. Journal of pharmaceutical sciences. 2014;103(1):29-52. doi:10.1002/jps.23773.

[16] Gao W, Hu C-MJ, Fang RH, Zhang L. Liposome-like Nanostructures for Drug Delivery. Journal of materials chemistry B, Materials for biology and medicine. 2013;1(48):10.1039/C3TB21238F. doi:10.1039/C3TB21238F.

[17] Abbasi E, Aval S, Akbarzadeh A, Milani M, Nasrabadi H, Joo S, Hanifehpour Y, Koshki K, Asl R. Dendrimers: synthesis, applications, and properties. Nanoscale Research Letters. 2014;9(1):247. doi: 10.1186/1556-276X-9-247.

[18] Majumder N, Das N, Das S. Polymeric micelles for anticancer drug delivery. Ther. Deliv.2020;11(10), 613-635. doi.org/10.4155/tde-2020-0008.

[19] Doppalapudi S, Jain A, Domb AJ, Khan W. Biodegradable polymers for targeted delivery of anti-cancer drugs. Expert Opin. Drug Deliv.2016;13(6),891-909.

[20] Son K, Hong J, Lee J. Carbon nanotubes as cancer therapeutic carriers and mediators. International Journal of Nanomedicine.2016;11 5163-5185

[21] Elhissi AM, Ahmed W, Hassan IU, Dhanak VR, D'Emanuele A. Carbon nanotubes in cancer therapy and drug delivery. J Drug Deliv. 2012;2012:837327.

[22] Engelberth S, Hempel N, Bergkvist M. Development of Nanoscale Approaches for Ovarian Cancer Therapeutics and Diagnostics. Critical Reviews in Oncogenesis.2014;19(3-4):281-315. https://www.ncbi.nlm.nih.gov/pmc/articles/PMC4183979/.

[23] Hindy S. Evaluating the accumulation of dualmodal indocyanine green-containing liposomes in pre-clinical models for visualizing human lung cancer. A thesis for the degree of Master of Health Science, Clinical Engineering Institute of Biomaterials and Biomedical Engineering University of Toronto.2018. https://tspace.library.utoronto.ca/bitstream/1807/89629/3/Hindy_Salma_201806_MHSc_thesis.pdf

[24] Thomas E, Menon J, Owen J, Koukelli I, Wallington S, Gray M, Mannaris C, Kersemans V, Allen D, Kinchesh P, Smart S, Carlisle R, Katherine A. Vallis Ultrasound-mediated cavitation enhances the delivery of an EGFR-targeting liposomal formulation designed for chemo-radionuclide therapy. Theranostics. 2019; 9(19): 5595-5609. doi: 10.7150/thno.34669.

[25] Ta H, Arndt N, Wu Y, Lim H, Landeen S, Zhang R, Kamato D, Little P, Whittaker A, Xu Z. Activatable Magnetic Resonance Nanosensor as a Potential Imaging Agent for Detecting and Discriminating Thrombosis.2018;31(10):15103-15115. DOI: 10.1039/C8NR05095C.

[26] Lamichhane N, Udayakumar T, D'Souza W, Simone C, Raghavan S, Jerimy Polf J, Mahmood J. Liposomes: Clinical Applications and Potential for Image-Guided Drug Delivery.2018;23(288)1-17. doi:10.3390/molecules23020288

[27] Lorenzo G, Ricci G, Severini G, Romano F, Biffi S. Imaging and therapy of ovarian cancer: clinicalapplication of nanoparticles and future perspectives. Theranostics. 2018; 8(16): 4279-4294. doi: 10.7150/thno.26345.

[28] Davis E, Chen Z, Shin M. Nanoparticle therapeutics: an emerging treatment modality for cancer. Nature Reviews Drug Discovery.2008;7(9), 771-782. doi:10.1038/nrd2614.

[29] Zein R, Sharrouf W, Selting K. Physical Properties of Nanoparticles That Result in Improved Cancer

Targeting. Journal of Oncology.2020. Article ID 5194780 https://doi.org/10.1155/2020/5194780.

[30] Liu J, Yu M, Zhou C, Zheng J. Renal clearable inorganic nanoparticles:a new frontier of bionanotechnology. Materials Today.2013;16(12): 477-486. http://dx.doi.org/10.1016/j.mattod.2013.11.003.

[31] Gatoo M, Sufia Naseem S, Arfat M, Dar A, Qasim K, Zubair S. Physicochemical Properties of Nanomaterials: Implication in Associated Toxic Manifestations. BioMed Research International. Volume 2014, Article ID 498420, 8, pages. http://dx.doi.org/10.1155/2014/498420

[32] Amgoth C, Phan C, Banavoth M, Rompivalasa S, Tang G, Polymer Properties: Functionalization and Surface Modified Nanoparticles.2019; DOI: 10.5772/intechopen.84424.

[33] Patra J, Das G, Fraceto L, Campos E, Torres M, Torres L, Torres L, Grillo R, Sharma S, Habtemariam S, Shin H. Nano based drug delivery systems:recent developments and future prospects. Nanobiotechnol.2018;16(71):1-33. https://doi.org/10.1186/s12951-018-0392-8.

[34] Gabizon A. Pegylated Liposomal Doxorubicin:Metamorphosis of an Old Drug into a New Form of Chemotherapy.2001;Cancer Investigation, 19(4), 424-436.

[35] Pandey H, Rani R, Agarwal V. Liposome and Their Applications in Cancer Therapy.2016; BRAZILIAN ARCHIVES OF BIOLOGY AND TECHNOLOGY. Vol. 59: e16150477. http://dx.doi.org/10.1590/1678-4324-2016150477.

[36] Green A, Rose P. Pegylated liposomal doxorubicin in ovarian cancer. 2006; International Journal of Nanomedicine.1(3) 229-239.

[37] Gothwal A, Khan L, Gupta U. Polymeric Micelles: Recent Advancements in the Delivery of Anticancer Drugs. Pharmaceutical Research 33:18-39. DOI 10.1007/s11095-015-1784-1.

[38] Ahmad Z, Shah A, Siddiqa M, Kraatz H. Polymeric micelles as drug delivery vehicles.2014; 4:17028-17038 DOI: 10.1039/c3ra47370h.

[39] Muthu M, Kulkarni S, Liu Y, Feng S. Development of docetaxel-loaded vitamin E TPGS micelles: formulation optimization, effects on brain cancer cells and biodistribution in rats.2012; Nanomedicine. 7(3), 353-364. DOI: 10.2217/nnm.11.111 · Source: PubMed.

Chapter 11

Nano Technology and Gas Plasma as Novel Therapeutic Strategies for Ovarian Cancer Oncotherapy

Milad Rasouli, Nadia Fallah and Kostya (Ken) Ostrikov

Abstract

Ovarian cancer (OC) is associated with a high rate of resistance to most chemotherapy drugs and thus novel therapies are crucial to overcoming these obstacles. The technological advances in nanotechnology make it possible to adapt these approaches for the treatment of chemo-resistant OC. In parallel, it is also evident that this emerging technology plays crucial roles in other medical areas including wound healing, treatment of viral infection and applications in dentistry. With the advancement of nanotechnology, nano dependent therapies are attractive viable alternatives to conventional therapies for various diseases, especially cancers. Nanoparticles (NPs) are a suitable platform for cytotoxic agent delivery and aiding early diagnosis of disease, which can lead to improving outcomes for these patients. Gas plasma oncotherapy is an innovative modality and shows huge potentials in cancer treatment and may emerge as the fifth cancer treatment modality together with surgery, radiotherapy, chemotherapy, targeted therapy and immunotherapy. The combination of nanoparticle and gas plasma therapy could lead to the discovery of an alternative effective treatment approach in these resistant tumors leading to improvement of OC prognosis. Here, we highlighted the two novel modalities with known multiple biological targets and underlying mechanisms appropriate for their application in OC treatment. This chapter explores the utility of combination or multimodal of novel nanotherapeutic agents in the treatment of OC.

Keywords: ovarian cancer (OC), gas plasma, nanoparticles, chemoresistance, reactive oxygen and nitrogen species (RONS), physical effects (UV, EM)

1. Introduction

Emerging clinical evidence indicates OC is a disease associated with poor survival and high mortality and the current situation of OC oncotherapy has created a major problem for the health system [1, 2]. Due to the limited therapeutic results of conventional modalities, the majority of efforts in OC treatment studies focus on new therapeutic strategy achievement. The new perspectives for OC management should not have been unwanted side effects such as drug resistance and toxicity [3, 4]. Nanotechnology and gas plasma offering a promising alternative to conventional OC therapies [5–7].

Nanotechnology uses nanomaterial for a wide range of various purposes including biomedicine, energy, electronics, environment, food, and textile. Nanoparticles (NPs) have been engineered from various materials with unique properties as drug

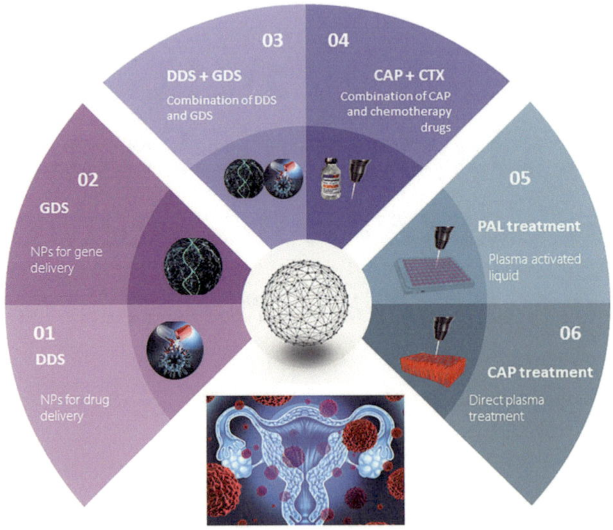

Figure 1.
Schematic illustrating of all reviewed treatment modalities for OC oncotherapy. DDS (drug delivery system), GDS (gene delivery system), CAP (cold atmospheric plasma), PAL (plasma activated liquid), CTX (chemotherapy).

vehicles to treat a peculiar disease [8–10]. Cancer nanomedicine creates a suitable strategy for modern oncotherapy and has attracted a lot of attention in recent years. The therapeutic nature of nanoparticles, drug delivery, and gene delivery are important foundations for increased attention to this new field [10–12].

The gas plasma that generates through conducting noble gas to the paired electrode at room temperature offers a new category of oncotherapy strategy in a short time [13]. Gas plasma oncotherapy will become an option for cancer treatment shortly, given its fast-development and multifunctional nature. This technology has provided the link between multidisciplinary scientific areas including physics, chemistry, biology, and medicine to address problems and offers an effective route for various oncotherapy challenges [14–16]. Multiple physical and chemical agents including charged particles, electric fields, ultraviolet (UV) radiation, and reactive oxygen and nitrogen species (RONS) involved in the efficacy of gas plasma [15].

NPs and gas plasma have risen as a promising therapeutic option for the treatment of ovarian malignant. These technologies exhibit comparable selectivity against tumor cells and provide a more efficacious and safe option for OC oncotherapy. The literature has been shown that NPs and gas plasma remarkably enhance the delivery of anticancer drugs and improve the efficacy of treatment and minimize the adverse effects of chemotherapeutic agents in healthy cells [16, 17].

This chapter presents the antitumor effect of gas plasma in combination with nanoparticle-based technology, as a new and most promising multimodal cancer therapy (**Figure 1**). Here, we provide a comprehensive and prospective review of the application of novel plasma and nanotechnology for the combination or multimodal OC oncotherapy.

2. Ovarian cancer: conventional treatment and resistance to chemotherapy

OC is one of the most common gynecological malignancies throughout the world and the fifth leading cause of cancer-related deaths among women in the

United States [18]. According to the American Cancer Society statistics, it was estimated that there would be 22,530 women who will receive a new diagnosis of OC and about 13,980 women will die from the disease in 2019. Carboplatin and platinum-based chemotherapy were used as the first choice to treat this type of cancer. Findings indicate who patients respond well to the initial treatment regime acquired drug resistance of the tumor after a time duration [19].

The main mechanisms of carboplatin resistance include reducing drug accumulation by altering the uptake/flow index, inactivating cisplatin by increasing the level of intracellular thiols such as glutathione, metallothionein, or other sulfur-containing molecules, increasing the repair capacity of platinum-induced DNA damage at the total level. The genome and DNA sequence become specific and the failure of the apoptotic response. Increasing the delivery of platinum to the tumor, a combination of platinum drugs with targeted molecular agents, modulators of platinum resistance, and new platinum drugs that target resistance mechanisms are the most important strategies being pursued that after intensive studies by many researchers are working to circumvent the resistance of cisplatin and carboplatin [20, 21].

Mortality trends in OC show the inefficiency of current therapeutics modalities except for PARPi and anti-VEGF. Thus, it is urgent to explore novel and efficient therapeutic options for epithelial OC that have the most lethal world gynecologic malignancy.

3. Nanotechnology as a therapeutic option for ovarian cancer

3.1 Nanoparticles

Nanotechnology as a science for minimizing material with particular properties has been used in various fields and multidisciplinary sciences such as chemistry, biology and physic. NPs in medicine application is called nanomedicine and it is utilized for the profit of human health and well being. In the field of nanomedicine, NPs in diagnosis, pharmacological treatment at a molecular level, molecular imaging, tissue engineering and regenerative medicine are widely used [9, 12, 22].

Agents through surface interaction, encapsulation, or entrapping loaded into NPs, and based on their properties avail for active and passive drug delivery. NPs based on their diverse structure like branched, spherical, or shell shape offer to become suitable for drug delivery to specific diseases such as cancer. Conventional chemotherapy distributes in the whole body and destroys both normal and tumor cells, as well as, after a while cancer cells become resistant to drugs [11, 23].

Controlling drug delivery and accumulation in tumor cells caused to require lower drug concentration for improving oncotherapy and diminishing the side effect for normal cells. Released agents from NPs are controlled by external or internal stimuli like pH, electric or magnetic field, temperature, redox and sound, and it ameliorates target therapy [24].

The optimal nano-size range for increase efficiency is typically 1-100 nm. There are different types of NPs for instance polymeric NPs, quantum dots, lipid-based NPs, mesoporous silica and dendrimers. Biodistribution, circulation time, stability, bioavailability, size, shape and surface charge are common characteristics of NPs that play an important role in their functioning [25].

For experimental and clinical trials, preparing an NP requires attention to some properties for better quality. Cellular recognition by specific antibodies is necessary for target delivery to specific cells [26]. NPs shouldn't stimulate the immune system to prevent degradation of them and their agents [27].

In gen delivery NPs carrying nucleic acids containing microRNA (miRNA), short hairpin RNA (shRNA), antisense oligonucleotides (AONS) and small interfering RNA (siRNA), with the silencing or downregulation purpose of genes or proteins which related to drug-resistant, angiogenesis or metastasis are used for improving oncotherapy and resolve the conventional therapy limitation [28]. We summarize nanotechnology based therapeutics in **Figure 2**. Here, we review the pre-clinical application of NPs for OC oncotherapy.

3.2 Drug delivery

In this section, we gathered some experiments that used different types of NPs for drug delivery to overcome the common problem in the treatment of OC as a lethal gynecological cancer worldwide, which almost diagnosis in late stages with the high rate of drug resistance for diagnosis and treatment. The advantages encourage researchers to utilized NPs consist of: NPs are used for drug delivery that lead to more effective in OC treatment. Also, reduce side effects due to specificity targeted NPs to OC cells.

SKOV3 and A2780 are the most usable cells for in vitro experiments that are treated by different kinds of drug loaded NPs. NPs are modified by several ligands such as hyaluronic acid, folic acid and HER2-targeted ligand for enhancing target delivery. GSH (Glutathione)-sensitive and pH-sensitive are other properties of these NPs that improve their effectiveness. As results showed the stability and biodistribution of these NPs that encapsulate drugs are very impressive. Increasing cellular uptake and cytotoxicity by inducing apoptosis or necrosis for in vitro experiments, and tumor growth and volume inhibition in the level of in vivo are the usual results that have been obtained.

The most barrier to entrance NPs into the cells through endosomes is an endosomal escape. Transferrin (Tf) and octaarginine (R8) play role in endosomal scape and specific delivery respectively. IAR-CPP R8 and Tf linked to the surface of PEGylated liposomes, which encapsulated doxorubicin (DOX) (DOXIL®) for

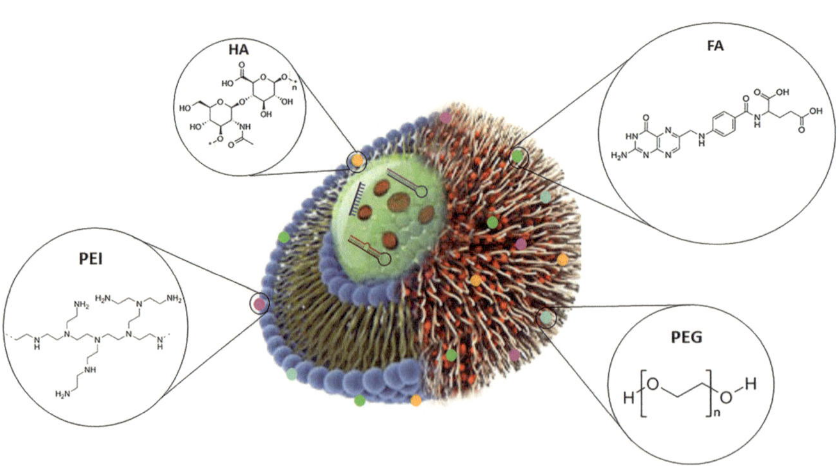

Figure 2.
Drugs or RNA interference (miRNA/siRNA/shRNA) loaded to lipid-based or polymeric nanoparticle as common nanocarriers are designed for delivery to OC cells in order to oncotherapy. Surface of these nanoparticles modified by different ligands such as hyaluronic acid (HA), folic acid (FA), Polyethylene glycol (PEG) and Polyethylenimine (PEI) for enhancing efficiency.

specific target therapy in A2780 cells. Results indicated efficiency in both entry pathways and accumulation in tumor cells increased [29].

3.2.1 Modified NPs: HA, FA, HER2 antibody for specific targeting

Adding a ligand to the surface of NPs enhances drug delivery effectiveness to OC cells. Hyaluronic acid (HA) that is linked to CD44 which is a cell-surface glycoprotein and expresses specifically in tumor cells improves target delivery [30]. In the following, we mention an example that NPs modified by HA. Cisplatin-loaded polyarginine-HA NPs (CIS-pARG-HA NPs) were produced in this study, to overcome peritoneal carcinomatosis which generally diagnosis in the late stage of OC patients. In vitro studies on SKOV-3 cells showed reduced cell viability, by cooperation CD44 in cancer cells and an increase in cellular uptake. Also, the effectiveness of CIS-pARG-HA NPs improved, when these NPs were administered by pressurized intraperitoneal aerosol chemotherapy (PIPAC) due to the penetration into the peritoneal tumor [31].

Folate receptor α (FRα) is another marker that overexpresses in OC cells, so modifying NPs surface by folic acid (FA) is another mechanism in specific target delivery. Using FA due to low immunogenic, inexpensive and stable properties, is more welcomed. Below we gather two examples in the level of in vitro and in vivo, to evaluating target delivery by FA ligand which binds to NPs [30].

PTX loaded PLGA NPs modified by FA for oncotherapy. For comparison, modified NPs with non-modified NPs, were used to treat SKOV3 cells. FA improved the effect of NPs and rise up the cytotoxicity by increasing cellular uptake, and disrupt in cell division and apoptosis process [32]. In another study, Nanoemulsion (NE) as a delivery system was used to loaded docetaxel (DTX) and FA for treating OC. Cell treatment by this nanocarrier enhanced cytotoxicity due to the DTX, while treatment transgenic mouse model of ovarian carcinoma induced inhibition in tumor growth and volume [33].

The overexpression of the HER2 receptor is another specific marker that contributes to OC. CIS and trastuzumab and HER2-targeted antibody conjugated with poly(lactic-co-glycolic) NPs target HER2 receptor. CIS via impressing on DNA conformational and by a dose-dependent manner cause cytotoxicity and apoptosis in SKOV3 cells. The effectiveness of this delivery system after modifying by trastuzumab and chitosan increased in both in vitro and in vivo experiments [34]. Cell viability in HER-2-overexpressing cell line can also decrement by treating them with poly(butylene adipate-co-butylene terephthalate) (Ecoflex®) NPs by adding an aptamer engineer to improving the efficacy and reducing the side effects of DTX. For evaluating antitumor activity and biodistribution, tumor-bearing B6 athymic mice received NPs intravenously and significant results were obtained [35].

3.2.2 Control drug released from NPs: pH and GSH sensitive NPs

pH-sensitive NPs are widely utilized for drug delivery. Drugs released from NPs are controlled by various factors like pH. A2780 as a CIS sensitive and A2780DDP as a CIS resistant OC cells treated by pH-sensitive Fe_3O_4 NPs encapsulating CIS for reducing its side effect and drug resistance. NPs@CIS cause more internalization and in the following more drug accumulation in OC cells. In both cell lines, cytotoxicity and apoptosis increased because of the drug entry into the cell nucleus. The existence of an external magnetic field for in vivo experiments enhanced the antitumor efficacy and inhibition toxicity in normal tissues [36].

In another study, Tariquidar (TQR) and DOX loaded a pH-sensitive liposome formulation (pHSL) (pHSL/TQR/DOX) was prepared to overcome multidrug resistance. pHSL made from CHEMS (cholesteryl hemisuccinate), DOPE (1,2-dioleoyl-sn-glycero-3-phosphoethanolamine) and PEGylated lipid which DOX and TQR placed in the water and lipid phases respectively and this nano vehicle prolong circulation. Cytotoxicity was investigated by treatment OVCAR8/ADR cells with pHSL/TQR/DOX (**Figure 3**) [37].

Combination of FA ligand for specific target delivery and pH-sensitive NPs proposed phenomenal nanocarrier for ovarian oncotherapy. Magnetic NPs (MNPs) and MTX through carboxylic acid groups and amino groups of chitosan linked to chitosan copolymer and prepared thermos and pH-sensitive MTX-CSC@MNPs that conjugate with erlotinib (ETB) for target delivery. Since MTX and FA are similar structurally this nano vehicle absorbed with folate receptor on OVCAR-3 cells and prompt cytotoxicity and apoptosis induced by ETB [38]. Moreover, pH-sensitive Glucose/gluconic acid-coated magnetic NPs that linked to FA in the surface, enclosed DOX. External magnetic fields improve drug release in tumor tissue. For evaluating cell viability A2780, OVCAR3 and SKOV3 cells treated by these NPs and results demonstrated an increase in internalization and cytotoxicity. Analyzing the tissues of the SKOV3-Luc cell-xenografted nude mouse model showed accumulation of the drug in tumor cells more than other parts of the body that it causes to block the tumor growth [39].

Drug released is also controlled by intracellular GSH concentration. GSH sensitive polymersomal DOX nano vehicle that modified by GE11 peptide (GE11-PS-Dox) is one of these NPs produced for treatment SKOV3 cells with a high level of epidermal growth factor receptor (EGFR). After drug delivery to tumor tissue and cancer cells, DOX enters the cell nucleus and inhibits tumor progress and increases cytotoxicity. The efficiency of this treatment is more than Lipo-Dox or Dox alone (**Figure 4**) [40].

3.2.3 Novel approaches drug delivery platform with the integration of different factors

In some cases, to ameliorate the level of treatment dual drug delivery suggests. For example, for carrying quercetin and gefitinib individually and together to PA-1 OC cells polyvinylpyrrolidone (PVP)-functionalized graphene oxide NPs (GO-PVP-NPs) as a system delivery was used. The results indicated combination delivery is more effective than individually in PA-1 cells [41].

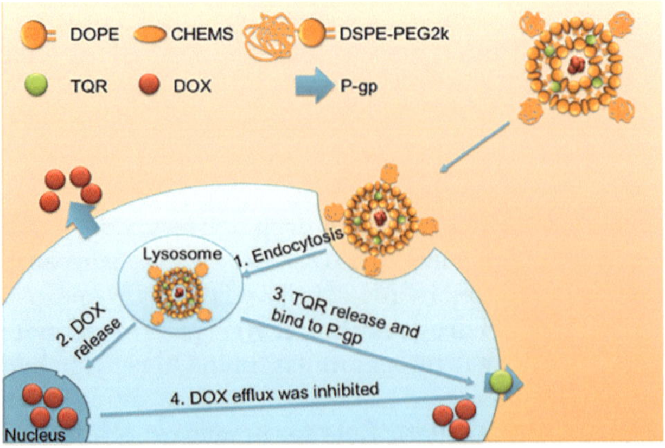

Figure 3.
Tariquidar and doxorubicin conjugated with pH sensitive liposomes to overcome multidrug resistance of OC cells. This figure was obtained with permission from [37] under the terms of creative commons CC BY license.

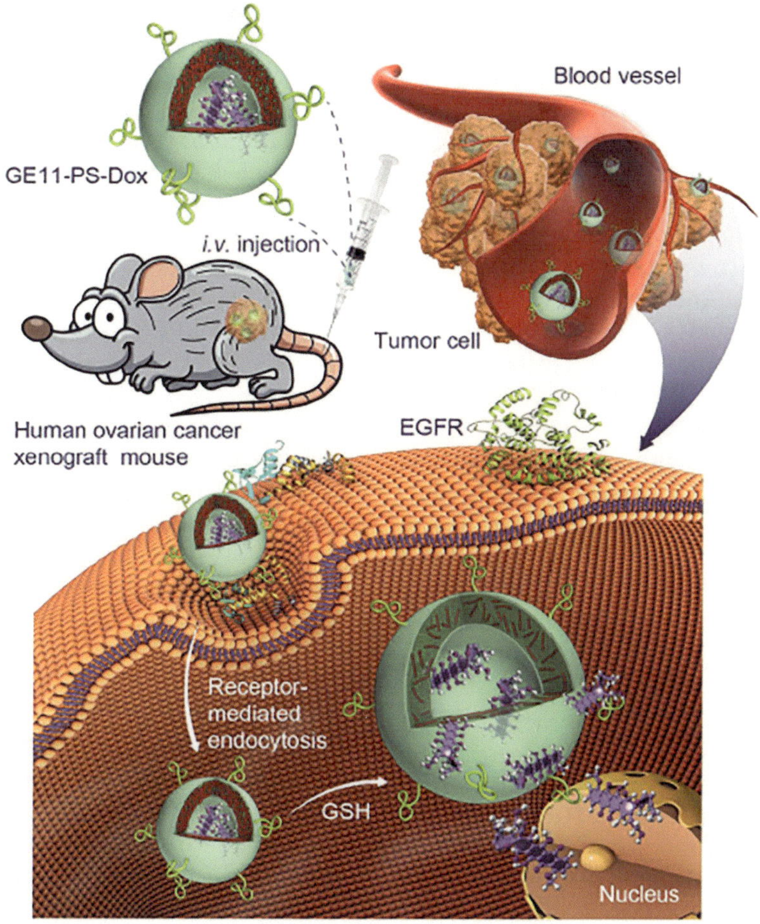

Figure 4.
Polymersomal doxorubicin with GE11peptide designed as an alternative to Clinical Liposomal Formulation for ovarian oncotherapy. This figure was obtained with permission from [40] under the terms of creative commons CC BY license.

Polymeric NPs and lipid-based NPs are the most usable nanocarriers that sometimes a combination of them make NPs suitable for drug delivery with high efficacy. In this experiment, a Pluronic F127 and a lipid-PEG stabilizer were used to generate NPs which have internal cubic phases are called cubosomes (CB) and external sponge phase. These NPs are conjugated with PTX against HEY cells and disrupt EGFR that overexpress in OC. Decreasing the cell viability and inhibiting the tumor growth are the results of this study [42].

Platinum-resistant OC (PROC) isn't possible to treat by conventional therapy for solving this problem, PROC is treated by CIS and wortmannin (Wtmn) as a DNA repair inhibitor conjugated with PEG-PLGA NPs. After treated A2780 cells, γH2AX foci as a DNA double-strand breaks marker analyzed for Wtmn activity and cytotoxicity. High solubility and stability are other properties of this dual nanocarrier. In vivo studies displayed the low concentration of drugs could inhibit tumor growth [43].

Nucleic acid-based NPs is another nanovehicle for transferring drugs to OC cells. For instance, an annexin A2 aptamer (ndo28) bind to pRNA-3WJ NPs and design a GC rich sequence in NPs for linking DOX. Treating SKOV3 cells by this NP increase cytotoxicity, and xenograft mice models showed targeting and accumulation of this NP in tumor tissues [44].

NP-drug conjugates (NDCs) are more effective than antibody-drug conjugates (ADCs) for loading monomethyl auristatin E (MMAE) in OC therapy. So, the results were very promising in the level of in vitro and in vivo, and inhibition of tumor growth and cytotoxicity in a patient-derived xenograft model of platinum-resistant OC is twice as much in comparison with CIS administration [45].

Depolarization of mitochondria and augment the level of ROS that cause apoptosis and finally, cytotoxicity in tumor cells are other results of administration NPs individually or in combination with chemotherapy drugs. So, Gold NPs encapsulate theaflavin (tea-extracted polyphenols) (AuNP@TfQ) as an apoptosis inducer in tumor cells. Anti-cancer activity of AuNP@TfQ enhanced by pristine theaflavin oxidation to its quinone derivative on the surface of gold NPs. The entrance of AuNP@TfQ into the PA-1 cells takes place through endocytosis. In this study caspase-3, Bax, Bad, BID, and BIM as pro-apoptotic markers and Bcl-2 and Bcl-was anti-apoptotic markers were evaluated [46].

But NPs individually can lead to cytotoxicity and apoptosis in tumor cells too. Gurunathan and colleagues proposed Ag NPs and ZnO NPs with a broad range of application in biomedical was used to treat OC individually and synergy with gemcitabine (GEM). Results represented a reduction in cell viability in a dose and time dependent manner and DNA double-strand break due to the overproduction of ROS and mitochondria dysfunction in both experiments [47, 48].

3.3 Gene delivery

Herein, we focused on some gene delivery based examples used for OC treatment. NPs due to their properties are used as a vehicle for delivery of different nucleic acids such as siRNA, miRNA and shRNA. Increasing cytotoxicity by inducing apoptosis and suppressing tumor growth and volume are the common results obtain via silencing or downregulating oncogenes. Modifying NPs with ligands for improving delivery is also utilized in this technique.

3.3.1 NPs for siRNA delivery

Using siRNA in oncotherapy because of low toxicity, high effectiveness and specificity is a terrific choice. To improve the efficiency and overcome the problem such as degradation by RNase and lack of the ability to penetrate the membrane cells, is better not to use naked siRNA. To facilitate the capability of siRNA and presence in proper concentration for silencing or downregulating of oncogenes, gene delivery systems play an essential role. Polymeric and lipid-based NPs are the most usable carriers for siRNA. Polymeric NPs especially PEI, PEG and chitosan with a positive charge easily bind to oligonucleotides with a negative charge through electrostatic interactions. While lipid NPs such as liposomes encapsulate siRNA in its aqueous core [30]. Polyethylenimine-graft-polycaprolactone-block-poly(ethylene glycol) modified FA (hyPEI-g-PCL-b-PEG-FA) is one of the examples polymeric NPs was used for transfer siRNA to SKOV-3/LUC cells with a high level of FRα [49].

Another protein targeted is TWIST that responsible for epithelial-mesenchymal transition and is related to angiogenesis, metastasis and drug resistance. So, using siRNA against TWIST protein conjugated with mesoporous silica nanoparticles (MSN-HAs) (siTWIST-MSN-HA) for delivery to epithelial OC (EOC) cells. HA help to specific target delivery to CD44 positive cells (A2780R cells). Moreover, due to the positive charge of PEI, the surface of MSN modified that, to improved attachment of the siRNA (negative charge) and HA to the amine groups in the PEI. By down-regulation of TWIST protein, OC cells become sensitive to drugs such as CIS. In vivo studies showed inhibition in tumor growth, and evaluating TWIST,

Vimentin, N-Cadherin, and E-Cadherin tumor mRNA as EMT markers in mice that were treated by siTWIST-MSN-HA + CIS indicated great result in combination therapy [50].

Protein kinases are a considerable target for gene delivery for cancer treatment, so knockdown of p70 S6 kinase (p70S6K) is necessary for a decrease in migration, invasion and proliferation of OC stem cells (in vitro) and reduction in tumor growth and metastasis (in vivo). In this regard, p70S6K siRNA by G6 dendriplex NPs, that protect it from degradation, transfer to OC stem cells. Also, knockdown of p70S6K via this NP complex can inhibit the stemness and self-renewal properties of cancer stem cells (**Figure 5**) [51].

Kinesin spindle protein (KSP) is another gene, that by silencing, cell cycle arrest in mitotic phase and apoptosis happened in cancer cells. So, for transfection of KSP siRNA into the SKOV3 cells, PEGylated DC-Chol/DOPE lipoplexes were prepared. These NPs are caused to enhance accumulation in tumor tissue for suppression of tumor growth and decrease damage to kidneys and liver in SKOV3 tumor-bearing mice [52].

Besides, growth and metastasis of tumor cells regulate by angiogenesis, so develop an NP with anti-angiogenesis property, plays an essential role in the treatment of OC. HA attached to chitosan NP enclose PLXDC1 siRNA for inhibition PLXDC1 as an angiogenesis gene. HUVEC and MOEC cells via expression CD44 have the potential to absorbed these nanocarriers and induced cytotoxicity and apoptosis. Administration HA-CH-NP/siRNA by A2780 tumor-bearing mice demonstrated antitumor characterization that causes to suppressing tumor growth and volume [53].

In another method for gene delivery, NPs were designed to transfer two siRNA to cancer cells to obtain the higher output. For instance, PLGA NPs loaded MDR1 and BCL2 siRNA were prepared. Silencing both genes simultaneously have an extraordinary effect on resistant OC cell sensitivity to PTX and CIS. In vitro experiments

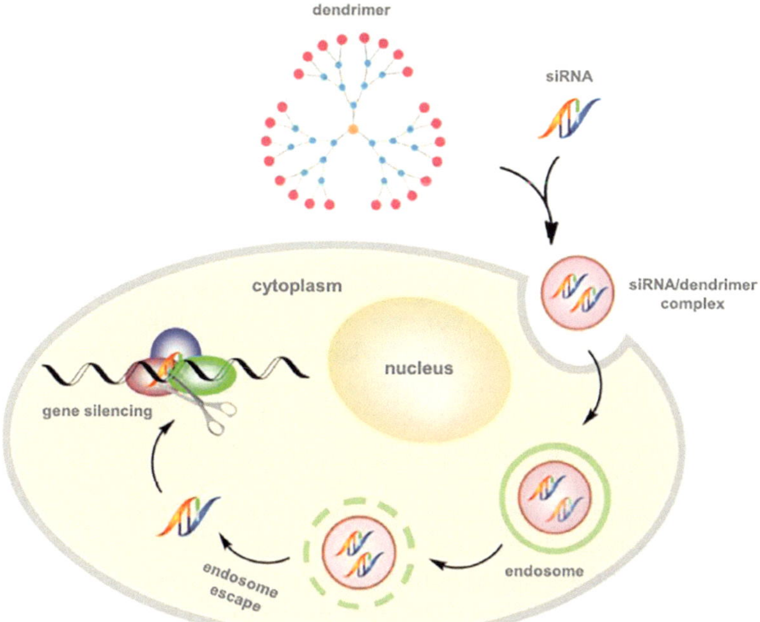

Figure 5.
Targeting p70S6K with dendriplex nanoparticles inhibit stemness and metastatic properties of OC cells. This figure was obtained with permission from [51] under the terms of creative commons CC BY license.

implement on the PTX-resistant and CIS-resistant, SKOV3-TR and A2780-CP20 cells respectively. The observations indicated an increment in cellular uptake that induces cell death by apoptosis and necrosis [54].

3.3.2 NPs for shRNA delivery

shRNA is a stem-loop RNA that in comparison with siRNA cause prolong gene silencing and highly effective. In the following, 2 examples of this procedure have been brought. PEG NPs with a peptide of FSH β 33-53 for specific target delivery encapsulate shRNA for silencing growth-regulated oncogene α (gro-α) (FSH33-G-NP). Internalization in FSHR positive cells like HEY cells is more. FSH33-G-NP decrement cell proliferation, invasion and migration and also in vivo experiments showed antitumor activity [55]. Also, overexpression of pin1 is related to cancer malignancy by regulating oncogenes and tumor suppressor genes, so silencing of pin1 can inhibit the tumor growth in a syngeneic mouse model and induce apoptosis in OC cells. Proteasome-dependent degradation of Pin1 happened via liposome-based NPs that were modified by cyclodextrins for shRNA delivery (**Figure 6**) [56].

3.3.3 NPs for miRs delivery

Micro RNAs (miRs) are short and non-coding RNAs that modulate gene expression at the level of post-transcriptional. The existence of them is necessary for the regulation of cell metabolism, differentiation, proliferation, and apoptosis. But sometimes, dysregulation and improper expression of miRs (oncomiRs) are related to the early and advanced stages of cancers, so, anti-miR delivery for downregulating oncomiR is an anticancer strategy. A high level of miR-21 is related to the incidence of many cancers including OC. In order to improve cancer therapy porous silicon NPs that were modified by MAL-PEG-SVA enclosed anti-miR-21 (LAN) to target OAW42 ovarian cells. In this study, CREK peptide as a control peptide for no targeting activity in cell culture and CGKRK peptide for displaying tumor-homing and tumor penetrating properties were analyzed for comparison. Findings illustrated a decrease in cell viability due to apoptosis by evaluating caspase-3, and also, COV-318 xenograft tumors subcutaneously transplanted into nude mice after treatment represented the higher accumulation of NPs in tumor tissue that lead to inhibition effect on tumor growth and volume [57].

3.4 Combination of gene and drug delivery

The combination of gene and drug delivery is another factor to enhance the chance of success in oncotherapy. For example, Both paclitaxel (PTX) and focal adhesion kinase (FAK) siRNA loading HA-labeled poly(d,l-lactide-co-glycolide) NPs (HA-PLGA-NP-PTX+FAK siRNA) were used for ovarian oncotherapy. Tumor cells due to the presence of CD44 obtain more HA-PLGA-NP-PTX+FAK siRNA which decreases cell viability by inducing apoptosis in both SKOV3-TR and HeyA8-MDR (multidrug resistance) cells. Knockdown of AKT pathway that has a role in metastasis and drug resistance, have occurred by FAK siRNA [58].

In another experiment, a novel combination of chemotherapy and gene therapy for A2780DDP cells and xenograft nude mice model was developed. Platinum(IV)–azide complexes (Pt(IV) prodrugs) and the siRNA of c-fos (si(c-fos)) embedded in a photoactivatable polymeric NP. Pt(IV) prodrugs are nontoxic in dark but after mild light (blue light) irradiation, it released the Pt(II) drug that has cytotoxic activity. This nano vehicle has high drug loading properties and extraordinary stability that lead to cytotoxicity and antitumor characterization (**Figure 7**) [59].

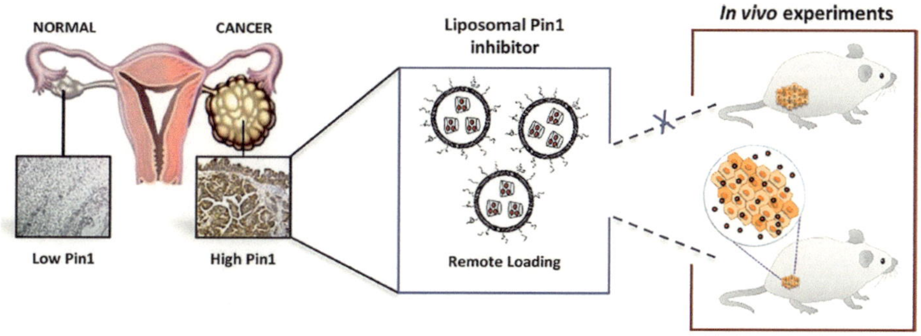

Figure 6.
Anti-Pin1 and cyclodextrins loaded to liposome as a new therapy for OC. This figure was obtained with permission from [56] under the terms of creative commons CC BY license.

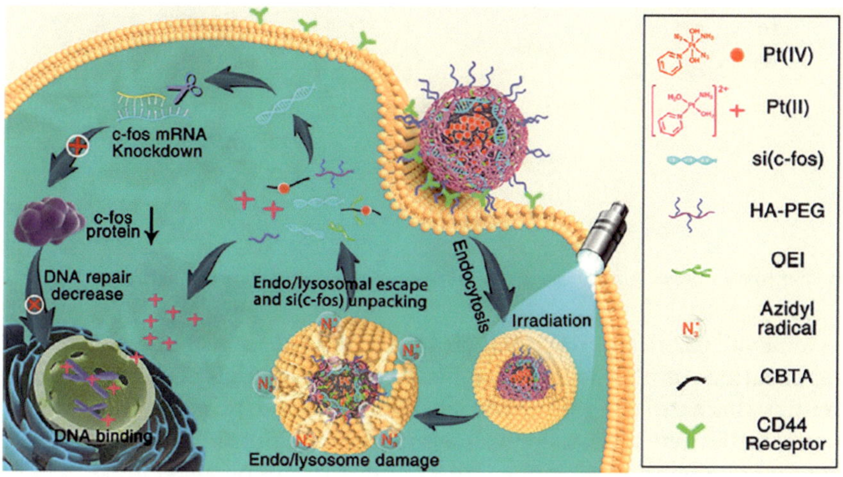

Figure 7.
Photoactivatable polymeric nanoparticles as a gene and drug delivery for platinum-resistant OC. This figure was obtained with permission from [63] under the terms of creative commons CC BY license.

Furthermore, A2780R cells treated by two separate NPs were developed for the delivery of drug and gene. CIS resistance leads from overexpression of miRNA-21 in OC. So, anti-miRNA-21 by PEGylated poly(lactic-co-glycolic acid) NPs which decorated with AS1411 antinucleolin aptamer for developing target delivery (Ap anti-miR-21-NPs) and NPs contain CIS (Ap–CIS–NPs) deliver to A2780R cells. It is caused to the reduction in drug resistance by inhibiting miRNA-21 and increased mortality via induction apoptosis [60].

4. Gas plasma based therapy for ovarian cancer oncotherapy

4.1 Gas plasma: key features and applications

Gas plasma is a novel technology with potential and actual applications ranging from energy and water to food sciences [61]. Management of gas plasma effects on biological objects is related to different factors including charged particles, electric fields, UV radiation, and RONS. These chemical and physical factors are involved in combination or multimodal forms, provide a solution for a variety of medical applications [62] (**Figure 8**). Cancer therapy, wound healing, virus inactivation,

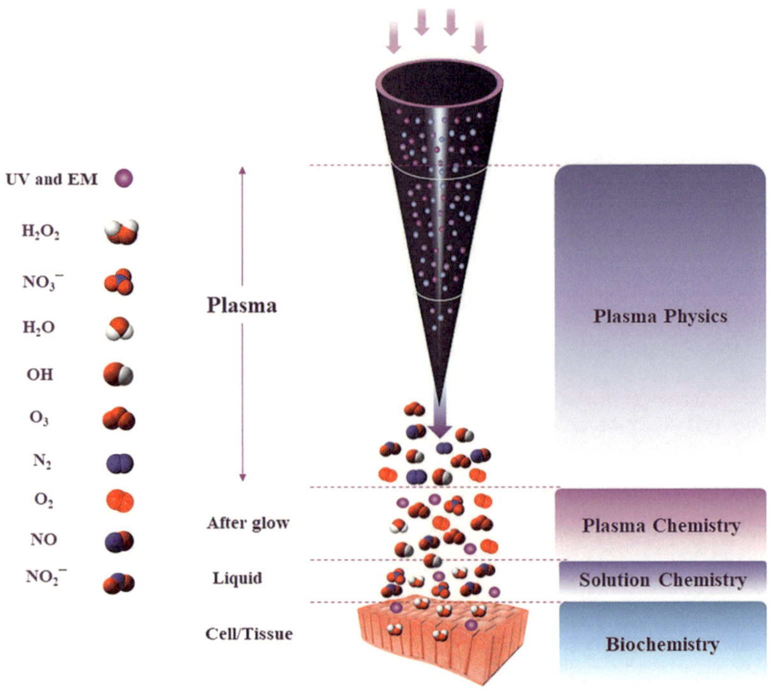

Figure 8.
The key role of reactive agents from generation in the plasma to interaction with the biological objects.

biofilm removal, dentistry, and ophthalmology, as well as cosmetic uses, are some of the applications of plasma in medicine. It is now clear that plasma is a promising therapeutic candidate for the multivariate condition of cancer [63, 64].

Recent studies revealed, gas plasma oncotherapy provides insights into the wide context challenging of cancer treatment through physical and chemical effects. Until now, the underlying mechanisms of plasma action were ascribed to RONS, but more recently, the role of physical factors (UV and EM) is also emphasized [62, 65]. These cocktails inducing dose-dependent effects, redox flux increase to cells, flexibility in use, multimodality nature, and the mild effect that are primary features of gas plasma [8]. Also, these unique physicals, chemical and biological properties have a high potential to act synergistically and will be crucial to the achievement of selectivity for cancer cells, enhancing cancer chemosensitivity, stimulation of the immune system, elimination of cancer stem cells, halting cancer metastasis as medical features of gas plasma oncotherapy [6, 63]. Thus, plasma as an alternative effective technology eliminates some of the most important undesirable consequences and side effects of common treatments. The great antitumor impact of plasma for all types of cancer have been reported [66].

4.2 Direct and indirect plasma treatment: role of the device and liquid

Plasma treatment is divided into two general direct and indirect modalities in order to offer new solutions to its increasingly diverse range of applications, as well as to cover the requirement related to them. In addition to exposing biological objects to plasma radiation, another method was developed. In the indirect treatment modality that has known as plasma activated liquid, the solution is exposed to plasma irradiation and then is added to the biological target [15, 67, 68]. It seems like the direct method is suitable for superficial tumors, but for peritoneal tumors, the indirect method or plasma-activated liquid is a good option and can be used as innovative technology. By ignoring the unknown complexities of plasma liquid interaction, the RONS play a dominant role in PAL.

Atmospheric Pressure Plasma Jets (APPJ) and volume and surface Dielectric Barrier Discharge (DBD) are three configuration types of common plasma devices used for biomedical application. Regarding the feeding gas, noble gases, air, nitrogen, or a combination of that, are utilized for the generation of plasma depending on the configuration used [69, 70]. Toward the APPJ, the DBD seems to be appropriate for the production of plasma-activated liquid due to the larger volume of exposed solution [69].

Culture mediums (DMEM, RPMI, alpha-MEM), Phosphate-buffered saline (PBS), and Ringer's solution have been reported as an exposed solution for PAL generation. Currently, all three types of solutions are used to produce PAL. As it was previously mentioned, aside from plasma device and process parameters, the compositions of the liquid have a pivotal role in the plasma action [15, 71]. It is appropriate to use solutions that have less interaction with plasma and do not change their function. However, it is well established that the sensitivity of cells to culture conditions is another limitation of this method and many cells are destroyed by changing the culture medium. Taken together, further research in this regard is very vital.

4.3 Ovarian cancer oncotherapy through gas plasma: selectivity, restores chemotherapy sensitivity, and metastasis inhibition

OC, colorectal cancer, pancreatic/appendiceal cancer, stomach cancer, peritoneal mesothelioma, and primary peritoneal cancer are the most common cancers that cause peritoneal carcinomatosis. In recent years, treatment strategies for these cancers, improved by combining several existing methods. [72]. Nevertheless, peritoneal carcinomatosis treatments are ineffective and require new multiple strategies that provide targeted drug delivery on a large scale.

OC the most important type of cancer in the cancer cells response discovering process to the plasma. Albeit the number of relevant studies examining OC with gas plasma is limited compared to other cancers. Most studies have been examined the selectivity of gas plasma oncotherapy on cancer or healthy cells. Regarding chemotherapy resistance, the impact of plasma on acquired and intrinsic resistance cells also have been investigated. Besides, various evidence suggests that gas plasma plays a crucial role in OC by mediating several genes involved in proliferation, apoptosis, migration, and metastasis.

The selectivity mechanism of gas plasma oncotherapy has been demonstrated in our previous work [73], briefly, plasma-derived H_2O_2 and NO_2^- produce primary $^1O_2$, thereby inactivating some of the catalase of cancer cells. Then, Due to the differences between healthy and cancerous cells, cell-based secondary $^1O_2$ generation is high, and therefore more catalase is inactivated. So, H_2O_2 with penetrating the cells through aquaporin causes depletes GSH or activities Hypochlorous acid (HOCl) and $^\bullet NO/ONOO^-$ signaling that leads to caspase-mediated cell death [74] (**Figure 9**).

Here, we outline the existing studies about the application of gas plasma and the mechanisms responsible for their expression strictly in OC. PAL has great potential to act as an innovative approach and overcome multiple biological barriers and treatment challenges in peritoneal cancers. Thus, PAL is a commonly used therapeutic option in this chapter. Also, it seems Ringer Lactate solution will be a proper liquid for future plasma activated liquid and has direct anti-cancer activities.

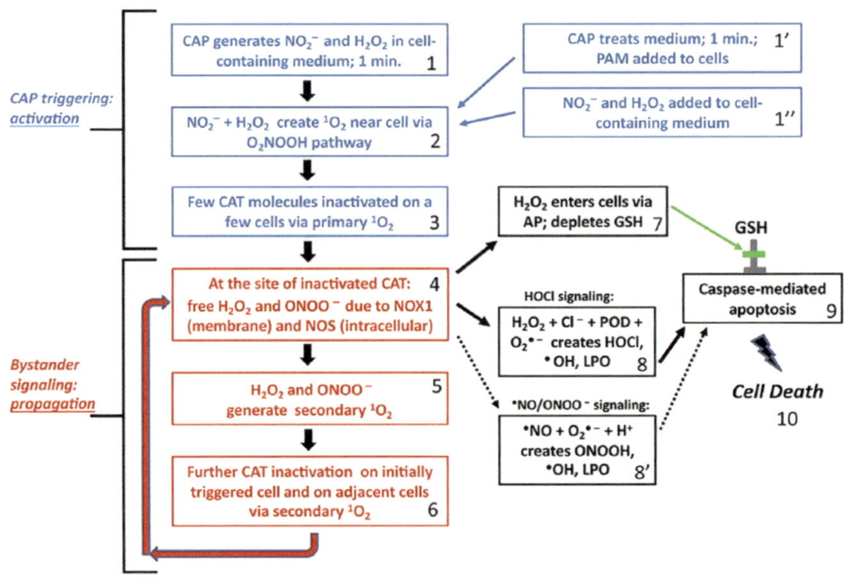

Figure 9.
Flow chart of major steps in CAP leading to selective apoptosis of tumor cells. Step 1: CAP generates NO_2^- and H_2O_2 in cell containing medium for 1 minute. Alternatively, CAP is used to treat medium, creating PAM (step 1′). Defined concentrations of NO_2^- and H_2O_2 containing medium are used in reconstitution experiments (step 1″). Step 2: NO_2^-- and H_2O_2 create primary $^1O_2$ near cells following O_2NOOH pathway, as described in reference. Step 3: Few catalase molecules on a few cells are inactivated due to primary $^1O_2$ near cells. Step 4: At the site of inactivated catalase, H_2O_2 and $ONOO^-$ (generated through NOX1 and NOS) are no longer decomposed. Step 5: The reaction between H_2O_2 and $ONOO^-$ is leading ultimately to secondary $^1O_2$. Step 6: This additional $^1O_2$ leads to further catalase inactivation and the process cycles back to step 4. Step 7: Increased H_2O_2 resulting from catalase loss from secondary $^1O_2$ leads to H_2O_2 entering cells via aquaporins, leading to antioxidant glutathione depletion. Step 8: In parallel with step 7, increased H_2O_2 resulting from catalase loss from secondary $^1O_2$ also leads to HOCl generation by peroxidase, in the presence of Cl^-. The interaction between NOX1 derived $O_2^{\bullet -}$ leads to $^\bullet OH$ formation near the cell membrane and lipid oxidation. Step 8′: If HOCl signaling is suppressed, an alternative $^\bullet NO/ONOO^-$ signaling can also lead to lipid peroxidation. Step 9: If both lipid peroxidation and glutathione depletion occur, then caspase-associated apoptosis can take place, finally leading to cell death. Steps 1–3 correspond to CAP triggering or activation of a few cells, thereby initiating propagating bystander signaling in steps 4–6. Steps 7–9 are the steps that lead to the final cell apoptosis. These steps are activated only if the repeated performance of steps 4–6 has caused a sufficiently high degree of catalase inactivation for reactivation of HOCl or $^\bullet NO/ONOO^-$ - mediated apoptosis-inducing signaling. This figure was obtained with permission from [74] under the terms of creative commons CC BY license.

Selectivity towards cancer cells, chemotherapy-resistance elimination, restore sensitivity to chemotherapy, inhibition of metastasis, and more recently the possible mechanism of plasma action has been achieved in these studies.

Gas plasma effects on OC were first examined on two human epithelial ovarian carcinoma cell lines, SKOV3 and HRA and normal human fetal lung fibroblast cell lines, WI-38 and MRC-5. Nonequilibrium atmospheric pressure plasma (NEAPP) was utilized to assess toxicity and proliferation inhibition. Cell proliferation, flow cytometry, western blot analysis along with pH, temperature, and volume of the medium before and after plasma treatments were evaluated. NEAPP selectively targets two cancer cells and induces apoptosis in them, while normal cells were not damaged. Although the authors do not address the mechanism of action, they assume a pivotal role in the process of plasma application for UV radiation, charged particles, and free radicals such as reactive oxygen species (ROS). Also, pH, temperature, and volume of culture medium did not affect by plasma irradiation [75].

Given that compositions of culture medium act as key mediators of biological responses triggered by gas plasma and can affect results. In a study by Boehm et al. hypothesized that instead of a culture medium, PBS to be used. The solution compounds used can play an important role in investigating the cytotoxic effect of plasma on HeLa and CHO-K1 cell lines. They found that the surrounding milieu and the presence of anti-oxidants such as pyruvate in PBS can change and influence the generation of H_2O_2 and related results [76].

In addition, cell proliferation and cell motility of SKOV-3, OVCAR-3, TOV-21G, and TOV-112G cells as OC cells investigated by direct and indirect exposure to gas plasma. In accordance with other studies, CAP and PAM have similar cytotoxicity effects on the mentioned cell lines. Also, dose-response effects depending on cell type and exposure time [77].

Bekeschus and colleagues attempt to insight the interaction of gas plasma with tumor microenvironment and immunomodulatory properties. Accordingly, human OC cell lines OVCAR-3 and SKOV-3 as well as human THP-1 monocytes have been used to examined gas plasma effect. The results indicate that plasma can trigger cell death in a caspase 3/7 independent and dependent manner for OVCAR-3 and SKOV-3 OC cell lines, respectively. Also, tumor cell-induced monocyte/macrophage phenotype reverted by plasma therapy [78].

Owing to clinical facts and desirability of Ringer's Lactate solution in comparison to the culture medium, Bisag et al. investigated the efficacy of plasma-activated Ringer's Lactate solution (PA-RL) on OC cell lines (SKOV-3 and OV-90) and non-cancer cells (HOSE cell line and two lines of immortalized fibroblasts (F1 and F2)). It was the first time that a multiwire plasma source without needing technical gas was used to activate a solution with a volume of 20 mL. Chemical characterization and measurement of long-lived RONS concentration in different PA-RL dilutions were performed. Results confirm that PA-RL showed selective cytotoxicity towards cancer cells, whereas normal cells remained unaffected. These observations are related to the pH and H_2O_2 and NO_2^- in the PA-RL [79].

4.3.1 Gas plasma restores chemotherapy sensitivity in chemoresistance OC cells

Improving the performance of conventional treatments is a significant part of oncotherapy. The cancer treatment new strategy requires advantages over conventional treatment methods. This is achieved by exploring new approaches to restore sensitivity to chemotherapy. Thus, gas plasma oncotherapy to introducing as an innovative oncotherapeutics agent should have been effective than conventional drugs. Besides, able to re-sensitize chemotherapy resistance cells to chemotherapeutic agents while maintaining selective effect toward normal and cancer cells.

Combination effects of CAP and PAL with conventional therapy like chemotherapy, radiation therapy, pulsed electric fields, nanoparticles, and plant origin have been discussed in recent years to improve the effectiveness of these methods. Here we also report the last work about the combination of chemotherapy drugs with gas plasma that has been conducted for OC treatment.

In a most recent research, to develop an innovative strategy for OC treatment, Rasouli et al. focused on the selective effect of gas plasma oncotherapy and eliminating chemotherapy resistance. For this purpose, hypodiploid human cell line, A2780 CP, SKOV-3 as OC cell lines, and Granulosa cells (GCs) as normal primary cells were used. As shown in **Figure 10**, we further utilized several treatment modalities including chemotherapeutic agents (carboplatin (CAR), PTX, a combination of CAR and PTX), gas plasma (direct exposure (CAP), plasma activated medium (PAM)), and combination of PAM whit chemotherapy drugs. IC_{50} of mentioned cells and selectivity index of cancer cell lines were obtained. Our results demonstrated the calculated selectivity indices of the CAR and PAM for A2780 CP, SKOV-3 smaller than the three that specified for the interesting selectivity index. Among all plasma treatment methods, PAM 10% FBS induced high selectivity

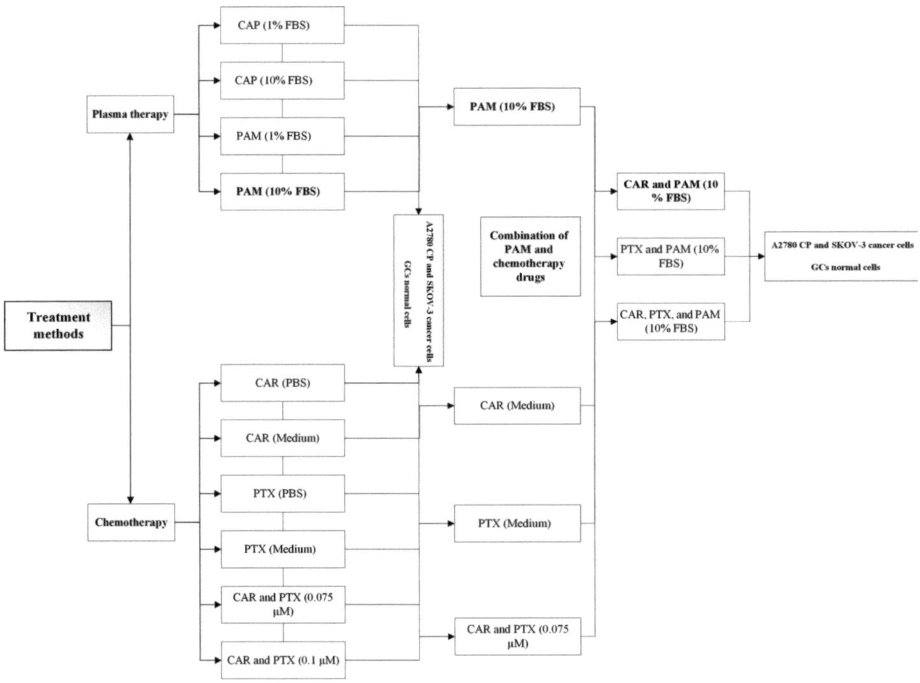

Figure 10.
Diagram of treatment methods in this study. CAP (cold atmospheric plasma), PAM (plasma activated medium), PTX (paclitaxel), CAR (carboplatin). All treatment methods were performed on three A2780 CP, SKOV-3, and GCs cells.

towards OC cells. Also, selectivity performance of other plasma therapies such as CAP 1% FBS, CAP 10% FBS, and PAM 1% FBS compared with chemotherapy drugs were desirable. According to the carboplatin resistance of cancer cells, it was a very interesting result [19].

In another part of this study, to improve the performance of chemotherapy drugs, co-treatment of these agents with PAM was investigated. Although PAM improves efficacy and selectivity indices of CAR and PTX but induces high selectivity in conjunction with CAR. In general, we concluded that PAM alone and simultaneous with CAR selectively induced apoptosis in chemotherapy-resistant OC cells accompanied with high expression of P53, BAX, and CASP-3. The novelty of PAM and combination treatment led to developing a new trend in OC oncotherapy associated with produced RONS (H_2O_2, NO_2^-, NO_3^-), reduced pH in plasma activated medium and physical factors such as UV and electric field [19].

Assuming gas plasma oncotherapy is closer to the therapeutic facts, Utsumi et al. used NEAPP-activated medium (NEAPP-AM) as an intraperitoneal (IP) treatment modality. To this end, for the first time, NOS2 and NOS3 as chronic paclitaxel/cisplatin-resistant OC cells and xenografted tumors in a mouse model were investigated by NEAPP-AM. Also, they assessed the role of ROS or their scavengers in NOS2 and NOS3 OC cells. Given fact that NOS2 and NOS3 are acquired resistance to paclitaxel, the study was a very crucial role in plasma oncotherapy research. The results revealed PAM has an interesting cytotoxicity effect on chemo-resistant OC cells. Besides, PAM can induce an anti-tumor effect on the xenograft model. There is no difference between direct and indirect treatment, but due to the benefits that PAM creates the authors suggested it as future intraperitoneal administration [80].

Clear cell carcinoma (CCC) of the ovary is a rare histological subtype of epithelial OC (EOC), has the worst prognosis and exhibits high rates of recurrence and low chemosensitivity. Therefore, developed a novel approach to combat CCC is critical. Hence, Utsumi et al investigated the influence of gas plasma on TOV21G as a CCC cell line by NEAPP-AM. The ES-2, SKOV3, and NOS2 as other EOC cell lines and omentum derived human fibroblastic cells (OHFC) and human peritoneal mesothelial cells (HPMC) as normal cells were examined. The study demonstrated that PAM with high selectivity induces apoptosis in CCC cells which is resistant to chemotherapy. Also, ROS produced by PAM in cancer cells were considered as a selectivity factor [81].

E-cadherin has pivotal roles in epithelial cell behavior, tissue formation, and suppression of cancer and is a critical part of epithelial cell adhesion and epithelial-to-mesenchymal transition (EMT). Furthermore, transforming growth factor-β1 (TGF-β1) is a multifunctional growth factor that plays a crucial role in chronic inflammation in various tissues and regulates several cellular processes, including cell cycle arrest, differentiation, morphogenesis, and apoptosis. From this viewpoint, Wang et al. focused on various factors such as cell numbers and the morphological characteristics of cells, that are thought to be effective in the interaction of plasma and cells. Four human OC cell lines, OVCAR-3, TOV21G, NOS2, and ES-2 used to examine differences in responses to gas plasma oncotherapy through direct and indirect irradiation. The point to consider was the different sensitivities of the used cancer cells to conventional chemotherapy drugs. They concluded compared with the other two cell lines, TOV21G and ES-2 cells were drastically sensitive to PAM treatment, as well as, sensitivity to PAM therapy in OC cells is related to their number and morphology. Having a negative impact of cell density on cell proliferation inhibition rate (PIR) is more evident in OVCAR-3 and NOS2 cells. Regarding cell morphology and PAM sensitivity, low E-cadherin expression was suggested as a factor for more PAM sensitivity. Also, TGF-β1 with inducing mesenchymal morphologic change can sensitize cancer cells to PAM [82].

OC is one of the gynecological malignancies that penetrates the peritoneum. That means cancer developed a spread of largest volume and treatment of it is challenging. Intraperitoneal therapy is a concept utilized in these cases to focused

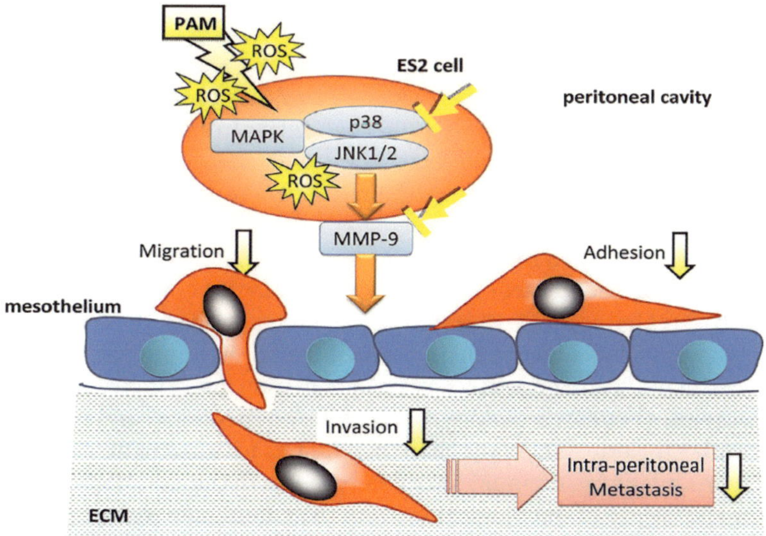

Figure 11.
Mechanisms of the anti-metastatic effect of PAM. ROS in PAM diffuses into ES2 cells and down-regulates MMP-9 expression via inhibiting of MAPK pathway, suppressing cancer cell adhesion, migration and invasion onto mesothelial cells lining the peritoneal cavity. Finally, PAM prevents intraperitoneal metastasis. This figure was obtained with permission from [83] under the terms of creative commons CC BY license.

on local delivery. For this purpose, Nakamura et al. introducing PAM intraperitoneal therapy as an innovative option for OC oncotherapy. The experiments were designed to assess the inhibit metastasis effectiveness of PAM on OC ES2, SKOV3, and WI-38 cell lines in vitro and ES2 in in-vivo levels. They mentioned that PAM treatment suppressed ES2 cell migration, invasion, and adhesion while cell viability changes were negligible [83].

Most importantly, PAM inhibited peritoneal dissemination of ES2 cells, resulting in prolonged survival in an in-vivo mouse model of intraperitoneal metastasis. Furthermore, the evaluated underlying mechanism revealed PAM inhibited the phosphorylation of JNK1/2 and p38 MAPK and prevented the MAPK pathway activation. Besides, PAM was decreased MMP-9 expression [83] (**Figure 11**).

5. Conclusion and perspective

Despite rapid advancements for OC oncotherapy, our understanding of the cause and management of OC is limited. Cancer cells become resistant to conventional chemotherapy and increasing the concentration of drugs just enhances the side effects, and does not cause any improvement in recovery. Besides, approved oncotherapy drugs for clinical and preclinical administration, faces several obstacles to treatment. Introducing combined therapeutic strategies such as nanoparticle and gas plasma that used the synergizing advantage of these approaches holds great potential for future combination or multimodal OC treatment.

The bioavailability property of NPs enhances their efficacy in drug loading and protects them from physiological barriers. To provide a suitable platform for clinical trials, it is very crucial to analyze the NPs safety at the level of in vitro and in vivo. Therefore, the reviewed NPs need more experiments in the level of in vivo for entrance into the clinical arena. Furthermore, gas plasma is not considered as the therapeutic strategy for modern medicine unless focused studies are performed on the design and manufacturing of simple, accurate, standard, and low-cost plasma devices.

While the identification of the underlying mechanism of each gas plasma and nanocarriers technology is under debate, promising observations open up interesting avenues for them as an emerging candidate in future oncotherapy. Independently from action mechanisms of gas plasma and nanoparticles, these therapies rely on the selective ability of them to discriminate between healthy cells and cancerous ones.

Indeed, gas plasma and nanoparticles as novel biomedical fields need funding from a wide range of government agencies and international research centers to be specifically targeted towards research at the intersection of these disciplines and resolve modern challenges such as cancer. Finally, we hope that this chapter will enhance collaboration between researchers in interdisciplinary research fields including physics, chemistry, biology, oncology, and medicine, and provide the needed interplay to address current challenges in OC management. Aside from providing new knowledge on molecular mechanisms in the mentioned modalities, to overcome the failure of oncological ovarian treatment, synergizing of innovative therapeutic approaches can be useful.

Collectively, our strategy potentially opens a new and accessible approach and led to addresses several cancer challenges. As a future direction, we hope to combine new approaches with conventional treatments to obtain finer modalities, improve the efficiency of each of them, and resolve oncotherapy challenges.

Conflict of interest

The authors have no conflict of interest to declare.

Acronyms and abbreviations

RONS	Reactive Oxygen and Nitrogen Species
DDS	Drug delivery system
GDS	Gene delivery system
CTX	Chemotherapy
ECT	Electrochemotherapy
RT	Radiotherapy
PDT	Photodynamic Therapy
HT	Hyperthermia
UV	Ultraviolet
NPs	Nanoparticles
miRNA	microRNA
shRNA	Short Hairpin RNA
AONS	Antisense Oligonucleotides
siRNA	Small interfering RNA
Tf	Transferrin
R8	Octaarginine
DOX	Doxorubicin
HA	Hyaluronic acid
CIS-pARG-HA NPs	Cisplatin-loaded polyarginine-HA NPs
PIPAC	Pressurized Intraperitoneal Aerosol Chemotherapy
FRα	Folate Receptor α
FA	Folic Acid
NE	Nanoemulsion
DTX	Docetaxel
TQR	Tariquidar
pHSL	pH-Sensitive Liposome
CHEMS	Cholesteryl Hemisuccinate
DOPE	1,2-dioleoyl-sn-glycero-3-phosphoethanolamine
MNPs	Magnetic NPs
ETB	Erlotinib
MRI	Magnetic Resonance Image
GO-PVP-NPs	Polyvinylpyrrolidone functionalized Graphene Oxide NPs
CB	Cubosomes
EGFR	Growth Factor Receptor
PROC	Platinum-Resistant Ovarian Cancer
Wtmn	Wortmannin
CIS	Cisplatin
NDCs	NP-Drug Conjugates
ADCs	Antibody-Drug Conjugates
MMAE	Monomethyl Auristatin E
GEM	Gemcitabine
PEI-g-PCL-b-PEG-FA	Polyethylenimine-graft-polycaprolactone-block-poly(ethyleneglycol) modified FA
EOC	Epithelial Ovarian Cancer
p70S6K	p70 S6 kinase
KSP	Kinesin Spindle Protein

gro-α	Growth-Regulated Oncogene α
miRs	Micro RNAs
PTX	Paclitaxel
FAK	Focal Adhesion Kinase
MDR	Multidrug Resistance
DBD	Dielectric Barrier Discharge
PBS	Phosphate-buffered saline
HOCl	Hypochlorous acid
NEAPP	Nonequilibrium atmospheric pressure plasma
ROS	Reactive Oxygen Species
PA-RL	Plasma-Activated Ringer's Lactate solution
GCs	Granulosa Cells
CAR	Carboplatin
PAM	Plasma Activated Medium
NEAPP-AM	NEAPP-Activated Medium
IP	Intraperitoneal
CCC	Clear Cell Carcinoma
EOC	Epithelial Ovarian Cancer
OHFC	Omentum Derived Human Fibroblastic Cells
HPMC	Human Peritoneal Mesothelial Cells
EMT	Epithelial-to-Mesenchymal Transition
TGF-β1	Transforming Growth Factor-β1
PIR	Proliferation Inhibition Rate

Author details

Milad Rasouli[1]*, Nadia Fallah[2] and Kostya (Ken) Ostrikov[3]

1 Department of Physics, Institute for Plasma Research, Kharazmi University, Tehran, Iran

2 Department of Cellular and Molecular Biology, Faculty of Biological Science, Kharazmi University, Tehran, Iran

3 School of Chemistry and Physics and Institute for Health and Biomedical Innovation, Queensland University of Technology, Brisbane, QLD, Australia

*Address all correspondence to: miladrasouli@outlook.com

References

[1] Kurman, Robert J. MD; Shih, Ie-Ming MD, PhD The Origin and Pathogenesis of Epithelial Ovarian Cancer: A Proposed Unifying Theory, The American Journal of Surgical Pathology: March 2010 - Volume 34 - Issue 3 - p 433-443 doi: 10.1097/PAS.0b013e3181cf3d79

[2] Wiegand KC, Shah SP, Al-Agha OM, Zhao Y, Tse K, Zeng T, Senz J, McConechy MK, Anglesio MS, Kalloger SE, Yang W. ARID1A mutations in endometriosis-associated ovarian carcinomas. New England Journal of Medicine. 2010 Oct 14;363(16):1532-43. doi.org/10.1056/NEJMoa1008433

[3] Galluzzi, L., Senovilla, L., Vitale, I. et al. Molecular mechanisms of cisplatin resistance. Oncogene 31, 1869-1883 (2012). doi.org/10.1038/onc.2011.384

[4] Ishaq, M., Evans, M., and Ostrikov, K., (2014), Effect of atmospheric gas plasmas on cancer cell signaling. Int. J. Cancer, 134: 1517-1528. doi.org/10.1002/ijc.28323

[5] Peer, D., Karp, J., Hong, S. et al. Nanocarriers as an emerging platform for cancer therapy. Nature Nanotech 2, 751-760 (2007). doi.org/10.1038/nnano.2007.387

[6] Dai X, Bazaka K, Richard DJ, Thompson ER, Ostrikov KK. The emerging role of gas plasma in oncotherapy. Trends in biotechnology. 2018 Nov 1;36(11):1183-98. doi.org/10.1016/j.tibtech.2018.06.010.

[7] Dai X, Yu L, Zhao X, Ostrikov KK. Nanomaterials for oncotherapies targeting the hallmarks of cancer. Nanotechnology. 2020 Sep;31(39):392001. doi.org/10.1088/1361-6528/ab99f1.

[8] Levy-Nissenbaum E, Radovic-Moreno AF, Wang AZ, Langer R, Farokhzad OC. Nanotechnology and aptamers: applications in drug delivery. Trends in biotechnology. 2008 Aug 1;26(8):442-9. doi.org/10.1016/j.tibtech.2008.04.006.

[9] Bertrand N, Wu J, Xu X, Kamaly N, Farokhzad OC. Cancer nanotechnology: the impact of passive and active targeting in the era of modern cancer biology. Advanced drug delivery reviews. 2014 Feb 1;66:2-5. doi.org/10.1016/j.addr.2013.11.009

[10] Uma Prabhakar, Hiroshi Maeda, Rakesh K. Jain, Eva M. Sevick-Muraca, William Zamboni, Omid C. Farokhzad, et al., Cancer Res April 15 2013 (73) (8) 2412-2417; DOI: 10.1158/0008-5472.CAN-12-4561

[11] Tibbitt MW, Dahlman JE, Langer R. Emerging frontiers in drug delivery. Journal of the American Chemical Society. 2016 Jan 27;138(3):704-17. DOI: 10.1021/jacs.5b09974

[12] Shi J, Kantoff PW, Wooster R, Farokhzad OC. Cancer nanomedicine: progress, challenges and opportunities. Nature Reviews Cancer. 2017 Jan;17(1):20. doi:10.1038/nrc.2016.108

[13] Metclmann HR, Von Woedtke T, Weltmann KD, editors. Comprehensive clinical plasma medicine: cold physical plasma for medical application. Springer; 2018 May 4.

[14] Dai X, Bazaka K, Thompson E, Ostrikov K. Cold Atmospheric Plasma: A Promising Controller of Cancer Cell States, Cancers. MDPI AG; 2020 Nov 13;12(11):3360. doi.org/10.3390/cancers12113360

[15] Zhou R, Zhou R, Wang P, Xian Y, Mai-Prochnow A, Lu X, Cullen PJ, Ostrikov KK, Bazaka K. Plasma-activated water: generation, origin of reactive species and

biological applications. Journal of Physics D: Applied Physics. 2020 May 19;53(30):303001. doi.org/10.1088/1361-6463/ab81cf

[16] Lu X, Naidis GV, Laroussi M, Reuter S, Graves DB, Ostrikov K. Reactive species in non-equilibrium atmospheric-pressure plasmas: Generation, transport, and biological effects. Physics Reports. 2016 May 4;630:1-84. doi.org/10.1016/j.physrep.2016.03.003

[17] Kong MG, Keidar M, Ostrikov K. Plasmas meet nanoparticles—where synergies can advance the frontier of medicine. Journal of Physics D: Applied Physics. 2011 Apr 14;44(17):174018. doi.org/10.1088/0022-3727/44/17/174018

[18] Parmakhtiar, B., Burger, R. A., Kim, J. & Fruehauf, J. P. HIF Inactivation of p53 in Ovarian Cancer Can Be Reversed by Topotecan , Restoring Cisplatin and Paclitaxel Sensitivity HIF Inactivation of p53 in Ovarian Cancer Can Be Reversed by Topotecan , Restoring Cisplatin and Paclitaxel Sensitivity. (2019) doi:10.1158/1541-7786.MCR-18-1109.

[19] Rasouli M, Mehdian H, Hajisharifi K, et al. Plasma Activated Medium Induces Apoptosis in Chemotherapy-resistant Ovarian Cancer Cells: High Selectivity and Synergy with Carboplatin. Research Square; 2020. DOI: 10.21203/rs.3.rs-123386/v1.

[20] Kelland, L. The resurgence of platinum-based cancer chemotherapy. Nat Rev Cancer 7, 573-584 (2007). doi.org/10.1038/nrc2167

[21] Michelle McMullen, Ainhoa Madariaga, Stephanie Lheureux, New approaches for targeting platinum-resistant ovarian cancer, Seminars in Cancer Biology, 2020, doi.org/10.1016/j.semcancer.2020.08.013.

[22] Bhatia S. Nanoparticles types, classification, characterization, fabrication methods and drug delivery applications. Natural polymer drug delivery systems 2016 (pp. 33-93). Springer, Cham. doi.org/10.1007/978-3-319-41129-3_2

[23] Yih TC, Al-Fandi M. Engineered nanoparticles as precise drug delivery systems. Journal of cellular biochemistry. 2006 Apr 15;97(6):1184-90. doi.org/10.1002/jcb.20796

[24] Lee JH, Yeo Y. Controlled drug release from pharmaceutical nanocarriers. Chemical engineering science. 2015 Mar 24;125:75-84. doi.org/10.1016/j.ces.2014.08.046

[25] Salvioni L, Rizzuto MA, Bertolini JA, Pandolfi L, Colombo M, Prosperi D. Thirty years of cancer nanomedicine: Success, frustration, and hope. Cancers. 2019 Dec;11(12):1855. doi.org/10.3390/cancers11121855

[26] Hans ML, Lowman AM. Biodegradable nanoparticles for drug delivery and targeting. Current Opinion in Solid State and Materials Science. 2002 Aug 1;6(4):319-27. doi.org/10.1016/S1359-0286(02)00117-1

[27] La-Beck NM, Gabizon AA. Nanoparticle interactions with the immune system: clinical implications for liposome-based cancer chemotherapy. Frontiers in immunology. 2017 Apr 6;8:416. doi.org/10.3389/fimmu.2017.00416

[28] Riley MK, Vermerris W. Recent advances in nanomaterials for gene delivery—a review. Nanomaterials. 2017 May;7(5):94. doi.org/10.3390/nano7050094

[29] Deshpande P, Jhaveri A, Pattni B, Biswas S, Torchilin V. Transferrin and octaarginine modified dual-functional liposomes with improved cancer cell targeting and enhanced intracellular delivery for the treatment of ovarian cancer. Drug delivery. 2018 Jan

1;25(1):517-32. doi.org/10.1080/1071754 4.2018.1435747

[30] van den Brand D, Mertens V, Massuger LF, Brock R. siRNA in ovarian cancer–Delivery strategies and targets for therapy. Journal of Controlled Release. 2018 Aug 10;283:45-58. doi.org/10.1016/j.jconrel.2018.05.012

[31] Shariati M, Lollo G, Matha K, Descamps B, Vanhove C, Van de Sande L, Willaert W, Balcaen L, Vanhaecke F, Benoit JP, Ceelen W. Synergy between intraperitoneal aerosolization (PIPAC) and cancer nanomedicine: cisplatin-loaded polyarginine-hyaluronic acid nanocarriers efficiently eradicate peritoneal metastasis of advanced human ovarian cancer. ACS Applied Materials & Interfaces. 2020 Jun 8. doi.org/10.1021/acsami.0c05554

[32] Luiz MT, Abriata JP, Raspantini GL, Tofani LB, Fumagalli F, de Melo SM, da Silva Emery F, Swiech K, Marcato PD, Lee R, Marchetti JM. In vitro evaluation of folate-modified PLGA nanoparticles containing paclitaxel for ovarian cancer therapy. Materials Science and Engineering: C. 2019 Dec 1;105:110038. doi.org/10.1016/j.msec.2019.110038

[33] Patel NR, Piroyan A, Ganta S, Morse AB, Candiloro KM, Solon AL, Nack AH, Galati CA, Bora C, Maglaty MA, O'Brien SW. In Vitro and In Vivo evaluation of a novel folate-targeted theranostic nanoemulsion of docetaxel for imaging and improved anticancer activity against ovarian cancers. Cancer biology & therapy. 2018 Jul 3;19(7):554-64. doi.org/10.1080/1538 4047.2017.1395118

[34] Domínguez-Ríos R, Sánchez-Ramírez DR, Ruiz-Saray K, Oceguera-Basurto PE, Almada M, Juárez J, Zepeda-Moreno A, del Toro-Arreola A, Topete A, Daneri-Navarro A. Cisplatin-loaded PLGA nanoparticles for HER2 targeted ovarian cancer therapy. Colloids and Surfaces B: Biointerfaces. 2019 Jun 1;178:199-207. doi.org/10.1016/j.colsurfb.2019.03.011

[35] Ghassami E, Varshosaz J, Jahanian-Najafabadi A, Minaiyan M, Rajabi P, Hayati E. Pharmacokinetics and in vitro/in vivo antitumor efficacy of aptamer-targeted Ecoflex® nanoparticles for docetaxel delivery in ovarian cancer. International journal of nanomedicine. 2018;13:493. doi.org/10.2147%2FIJN.S152474

[36] Song H, Quan F, Yu Z, Zheng M, Ma Y, Xiao H, Ding F. Carboplatin prodrug conjugated Fe3O 4 nanoparticles for magnetically targeted drug delivery in ovarian cancer cells. Journal of Materials Chemistry B. 2019;7(3):433-42. doi.org/10.1039/C8TB02574F

[37] Xia Y, Fang M, Dong J, Xu C, Liao Z, Ning P, Zeng Q. pH sensitive liposomes delivering tariquidar and doxorubicin to overcome multidrug resistance of resistant ovarian cancer cells. Colloids and Surfaces B: Biointerfaces. 2018 Oct 1;170:514-20. doi.org/10.1016/j.colsurfb.2018.06.055

[38] Fathi M, Barar J, Erfan-Niya H, Omidi Y. Methotrexate-conjugated chitosan-grafted pH-and thermo-responsive magnetic nanoparticles for targeted therapy of ovarian cancer. International journal of biological macromolecules. 2020 Jul 1;154:1175-84. doi.org/10.1016/j.ijbiomac.2019.10.272

[39] Ak G, Yilmaz H, Güneş A, Hamarat Sanlier S. In vitro and in vivo evaluation of folate receptor-targeted a novel magnetic drug delivery system for ovarian cancer therapy. Artificial Cells, Nanomedicine, and Biotechnology. 2018 Oct 31;46(sup1):926-37. doi.org/10.1080/21691401.2018.1439838

[40] Zou Y, Xia Y, Meng F, Zhang J, Zhong Z. GE11-directed functional polymersomal doxorubicin as an advanced alternative to

clinical liposomal formulation for ovarian cancer treatment. Molecular Pharmaceutics. 2018 Mar 23;15(9):3664-71. doi.org/10.1021/acs.molpharmaceut.8b00024

[41] Tiwari H, Karki N, Pal M, Basak S, Verma RK, Bal R, Kandpal ND, Bisht G, Sahoo NG. Functionalized graphene oxide as a nanocarrier for dual drug delivery applications: The synergistic effect of quercetin and gefitinib against ovarian cancer cells. Colloids and Surfaces B: Biointerfaces. 2019 Jun 1;178:452-9. doi.org/10.1016/j.colsurfb.2019.03.037

[42] Zhai J, Luwor RB, Ahmed N, Escalona R, Tan FH, Fong C, Ratcliffe J, Scoble JA, Drummond CJ, Tran N. Paclitaxel-loaded self-assembled lipid nanoparticles as targeted drug delivery systems for the treatment of aggressive ovarian cancer. ACS applied materials & interfaces. 2018 Jul 2;10(30):25174-85. doi.org/10.1021/acsami.8b08125

[43] Zhang M, Hagan IV CT, Min Y, Foley H, Tian X, Yang F, Mi Y, Au KM, Medik Y, Roche K, Wagner K. Nanoparticle co-delivery of wortmannin and cisplatin synergistically enhances chemoradiotherapy and reverses platinum resistance in ovarian cancer models. Biomaterials. 2018 Jul 1;169:1-0. doi.org/10.1016/j.biomaterials.2018.03.055

[44] Pi F, Zhang H, Li H, Thiviyanathan V, Gorenstein DG, Sood AK, Guo P. RNA nanoparticles harboring annexin A2 aptamer can target ovarian cancer for tumor-specific doxorubicin delivery. Nanomedicine: Nanotechnology, Biology and Medicine. 2017 Apr 1;13(3):1183-93. doi.org/10.1016/j.nano.2016.11.015

[45] Qi R, Wang Y, Bruno PM, Xiao H, Yu Y, Li T, Lauffer S, Wei W, Chen Q, Kang X, Song H. Nanoparticle conjugates of a highly potent toxin enhance safety and circumvent platinum resistance in ovarian cancer. Nature communications. 2017 Dec 18;8(1):1-2. doi.org/10.1038/s41467-017-02390-7

[46] Maity R, Chatterjee M, Banerjee A, Das A, Mishra R, Mazumder S, Chanda N. Gold nanoparticle-assisted enhancement in the anti-cancer properties of theaflavin against human ovarian cancer cells. Materials Science and Engineering: C. 2019 Nov 1;104:109909. doi.org/10.1016/j.msec.2019.109909

[47] Yuan YG, Peng QL, Gurunathan S. Silver nanoparticles enhance the apoptotic potential of gemcitabine in human ovarian cancer cells: combination therapy for effective cancer treatment. International journal of nanomedicine. 2017;12:6487. doi.org/10.2147%2FIJN.S135482

[48] Bai DP, Zhang XF, Zhang GL, Huang YF, Gurunathan S. Zinc oxide nanoparticles induce apoptosis and autophagy in human ovarian cancer cells. International journal of nanomedicine. 2017;12:6521. doi.org/10.2147%2FIJN.S140071

[49] Jones SK, Douglas K, Shields AF, Merkel OM. Correlating quantitative tumor accumulation and gene knockdown using SPECT/CT and bioluminescence imaging within an orthotopic ovarian cancer model. Biomaterials. 2018 Sep 1;178:183-92. doi.org/10.1016/j.biomaterials.2018.06.014

[50] Shahin SA, Wang R, Simargi SI, Contreras A, Echavarria LP, Qu L, Wen W, Dellinger T, Unternaehrer J, Tamanoi F, Zink JI. Hyaluronic acid conjugated nanoparticle delivery of siRNA against TWIST reduces tumor burden and enhances sensitivity to cisplatin in ovarian cancer. Nanomedicine: Nanotechnology, Biology and Medicine. 2018 Jun 1;14(4):1381-94. doi.org/10.1016/j.nano.2018.04.008

[51] Ma J, Kala S, Yung S, Chan TM, Cao Y, Jiang Y, Liu X, Giorgio S, Peng L, Wong AS. Blocking Stemness and Metastatic Properties of Ovarian Cancer Cells by Targeting p70S6K with Dendrimer Nanovector-Based siRNA Delivery. Molecular Therapy. 2018 Jan 3;26(1):70-83. doi.org/10.1016/j.ymthe.2017.11.006

[52] Lee J, Ahn HJ. PEGylated DC-Chol/DOPE cationic liposomes containing KSP siRNA as a systemic siRNA delivery Carrier for ovarian cancer therapy. Biochemical and biophysical research communications. 2018 Sep 10;503(3):1716-22. doi.org/10.1016/j.bbrc.2018.07.104

[53] Kim GH, Won JE, Byeon Y, Kim MG, Wi TI, Lee JM, Park YY, Lee JW, Kang TH, Jung ID, Shin BC. Selective delivery of PLXDC1 small interfering RNA to endothelial cells for anti-angiogenesis tumor therapy using CD44-targeted chitosan nanoparticles for epithelial ovarian cancer. Drug delivery. 2018 Jan 1;25(1):1394-402. doi.org/10.1080/10717544.2018.1480672

[54] Risnayanti C, Jang YS, Lee J, Ahn HJ. PLGA nanoparticles co-delivering MDR1 and BCL2 siRNA for overcoming resistance of paclitaxel and cisplatin in recurrent or advanced ovarian cancer. Scientific reports. 2018 May 14;8(1):1-2. doi.org/10.1038/s41598-018-25930-7

[55] Hong SS, Zhang MX, Zhang M, Yu Y, Chen J, Zhang XY, Xu CJ. Follicle-stimulating hormone peptide-conjugated nanoparticles for targeted shRNA delivery lead to effective gro-α silencing and antitumor activity against ovarian cancer. Drug delivery. 2018 Jan 1;25(1):576-84. doi.org/10.1080/10717544.2018.1440667

[56] Spena CR, De Stefano L, Palazzolo S, Salis B, Granchi C, Minutolo F, Tuccinardi T, Fratamico R, Crotti S, D'Aronco S, Agostini M. Liposomal delivery of a Pin1 inhibitor complexed with cyclodextrins as new therapy for high-grade serous ovarian cancer. Journal of Controlled Release. 2018 Jul 10;281:1-10. doi.org/10.1016/j.jconrel.2018.04.055

[57] Bertucci A, Kim KH, Kang J, Zuidema JM, Lee SH, Kwon EJ, Kim D, Howell SB, Ricci F, Ruoslahti E, Jang HJ. Tumor-targeting, microRNA-silencing porous silicon nanoparticles for ovarian cancer therapy. ACS applied materials & interfaces. 2019 Jun 17;11(27):23926-37. doi.org/10.1021/acsami.9b07980

[58] Byeon Y, Lee JW, Choi WS, Won JE, Kim GH, Kim MG, Wi TI, Lee JM, Kang TH, Jung ID, Cho YJ. CD44-targeting PLGA nanoparticles incorporating paclitaxel and FAK siRNA overcome chemoresistance in epithelial ovarian cancer. Cancer Research. 2018 Nov 1;78(21):6247-6256. DOI: 10.1158/0008-5472.CAN-17-3871

[59] Zhang Q, Kuang G, He S, Lu H, Cheng Y, Zhou D, Huang Y. Photoactivatable Prodrug-Backboned Polymeric Nanoparticles for Efficient Light-Controlled Gene Delivery and Synergistic Treatment of Platinum-Resistant Ovarian Cancer. Nano Letters. 2020 Apr 6;20(5):3039-49. doi.org/10.1021/acs.nanolett.9b04981

[60] Vandghanooni S, Eskandani M, Barar J, Omidi Y. AS1411 aptamer-decorated cisplatin-loaded poly (lactic-co-glycolic acid) nanoparticles for targeted therapy of miR-21-inhibited ovarian cancer cells. Nanomedicine. 2018 Nov;13(21):2729-58. doi.org/10.2217/nnm-2018-0205

[61] Weltmann, K-D, Kolb, JF, Holub, M, et al. The future for plasma science and technology. Plasma Process Polym. 2019;16:e1800118, doi.org/10.1002/ppap.201800118

[62] Yan D, Wang Q, Adhikari M, Malyavko A, Lin L, Zolotukhin DB, Yao X, Kirschner M, Sherman JH,

Keidar M. A physically triggered cell death via transbarrier cold atmospheric plasma cancer treatment. ACS Applied Materials & Interfaces. 2020 Jul 10;12(31):34548-34563. DOI: 10.1021/acsami.0c06500

[63] Liu, D, Szili, EJ, Ostrikov, K(K). Plasma medicine: Opportunities for nanotechnology in a digital age. Plasma Process Polym. 2020; 17:e2000097. doi.org/10.1002/ppap.202000097

[64] Mirpour, S., Fathollah, S., Mansouri, P. et al. Cold atmospheric plasma as an effective method to treat diabetic foot ulcers: A randomized clinical trial. Sci Rep 10, 10440 (2020). doi.org/10.1038/s41598-020-67232-x

[65] Wang Q, Malyavko A, Yan D, Lamanna OK, Hsieh MH, Sherman J, Keidar M. A comparative study of cold atmospheric plasma treatment, chemical versus physical strategy. Journal of Physics D: Applied Physics. 2020 Nov 2. doi.org/10.1088/1361-6463/abc6d5

[66] Keidar M, Shashurin A, Volotskova O, Ann Stepp M, Srinivasan P, Sandler A, Trink B. Cold atmospheric plasma in cancer therapy. Physics of Plasmas. 2013 May 15;20(5):057101. doi.org/10.1063/1.4801516

[67] Dai, X, Zhang, Z, Zhang, J, Ostrikov, K. Dosing: The key to precision plasma oncology. Plasma Process Polym. 2020; 17:e1900178. doi.org/10.1002/ppap.201900178

[68] Lu X, Keidar M, Laroussi M, Choi E, Szili EJ, Ostrikov K. Transcutaneous plasma stress: From soft-matter models to living tissues. Materials Science and Engineering: R: Reports. 2019 Oct 1;138:36-59. doi.org/10.1016/j.mser.2019.04.002

[69] Liu, D, Zhang, Y, Xu, M, Chen, H, Lu, X, Ostrikov, K. Cold atmospheric pressure plasmas in dermatology: Sources, reactive agents, and therapeutic effects. Plasma Process Polym. 2020; 17:e1900218. doi.org/10.1002/ppap.201900218

[70] Lu P, Cullen PJ, Ostrikov K. Atmospheric pressure nonthermal plasma sources. In Cold plasma in food and agriculture 2016 Jan 1 (pp. 83-116). Academic Press. doi.org/10.1016/B978-0-12-801365-6.00004-4

[71] Wende, K., von Woedtke, T., Weltmann, K., & Bekeschus, S. (2019). Chemistry and biochemistry of cold physical plasma derived reactive species in liquids, Biological Chemistry, 400(1), 19-38. doi.org/10.1515/hsz-2018-0242

[72] Coccolini F, Gheza F, Lotti M, Virzì S, Iusco D, Ghermandi C, Melotti R, Baiocchi G, Giulini SM, Ansaloni L, Catena F. Peritoneal carcinomatosis. World journal of gastroenterology: WJG. 2013 Nov 7;19(41):6979. doi: 10.3748/wjg.v19.i41.6979

[73] Milad Rasouli, Nadia Fallah and Kostya (Ken) Ostrikov (December 28th 2020). Lung Cancer Oncotherapy through Novel Modalities: Gas Plasma and Nanoparticle Technologies, IntechOpen, DOI: 10.5772/intechopen.95494.

[74] Bauer, G., Sersenová, D., Graves, D.B. et al. Dynamics of Singlet Oxygen-Triggered, RONS-Based Apoptosis Induction after Treatment of Tumor Cells with Cold Atmospheric Plasma or Plasma-Activated Medium. Sci Rep 9, 13931 (2019). doi.org/10.1038/s41598-019-50329-3

[75] Iseki S, Nakamura K, Hayashi M, Tanaka H, Kondo H, Kajiyama H, Kano H, Kikkawa F, Hori M. Selective killing of ovarian cancer cells through induction of apoptosis by nonequilibrium atmospheric pressure plasma. Applied Physics Letters. 2012 Mar 12;100(11):113702. doi.org/10.1063/1.3694928

[76] Boehm, D., Heslin, C., Cullen, P. et al. Cytotoxic and mutagenic potential of solutions exposed to cold atmospheric plasma. Sci Rep 6, 21464 (2016). doi.org/10.1038/srep21464

[77] Koensgen D, Besic I, Guembel D, Kaul A, Weiss M, Diesing K, Kramer A, Bekeschus S, Mustea A, Stope MB. Cold atmospheric plasma (CAP) and CAP-stimulated cell culture media suppress ovarian cancer cell growth–a putative treatment option in ovarian cancer therapy. Anticancer Research. 2017 Dec 1;37(12):6739-6744.

[78] Bekeschus S, Wulf CP, Freund E, Koensgen D, Mustea A, Weltmann KD, Stope MB. Plasma treatment of ovarian cancer cells mitigates their immuno-modulatory products active on THP-1 monocytes. Plasma. 2018 Sep;1(1):201-17. doi.org/10.3390/plasma1010018

[79] Bisag A, Bucci C, Coluccelli S, Girolimetti G, Laurita R, De Iaco P, Perrone AM, Gherardi M, Marchio L, Porcelli AM, Colombo V. Plasma-activated Ringer's Lactate Solution Displays a Selective Cytotoxic Effect on Ovarian Cancer Cells. Cancers. 2020 Feb;12(2):476. doi.org/10.3390/cancers12020476

[80] Utsumi F, Kajiyama H, Nakamura K, Tanaka H, Mizuno M, Ishikawa K, Kondo H, Kano H, Hori M, Kikkawa F. Effect of indirect nonequilibrium atmospheric pressure plasma on anti-proliferative activity against chronic chemo-resistant ovarian cancer cells in vitro and in vivo. PloS one. 2013 Dec 18;8(12):e81576. doi.org/10.1371/journal.pone.0081576

[81] Utsumi, F., Kajiyama, H., Nakamura, K. et al. Selective cytotoxicity of indirect nonequilibrium atmospheric pressure plasma against ovarian clear-cell carcinoma. SpringerPlus 3, 398 (2014). doi.org/10.1186/2193-1801-3-398

[82] Utsumi F, Kajiyama H, Nakamura K, Tanaka H, Mizuno M, Toyokuni S, Hori M, Kikkawa F. Variable susceptibility of ovarian cancer cells to non-thermal plasma-activated medium. Oncology reports. 2016 Jun 1;35(6):3169-77. doi.org/10.3892/or.2016.4726

[83] Nakamura, K., Peng, Y., Utsumi, F. et al. Novel Intraperitoneal Treatment with Non-Thermal Plasma-Activated Medium Inhibits Metastatic Potential of Ovarian Cancer Cells. Sci Rep 7, 6085 (2017). doi.org/10.1038/s41598-017-05620-6

Chapter 12

The Anti-Cancer Effects of Anti-Parasite Drug Ivermectin in Ovarian Cancer

Xianquan Zhan and Na Li

Abstract

Ivermectin is an old, common, and classic anti-parasite drug, which has been found to have a broad-spectrum anti-cancer effect on multiple human cancers. This chapter will focus on the anti-cancer effects of ivermectin on ovarian cancer. First, ivermectin was found to suppress cell proliferation and growth, block cell cycle progression, and promote cell apoptosis in ovarian cancer. Second, drug pathway network, qRT-PCR, and immunoaffinity blot analyses found that ivermectin acts through molecular networks to target the key molecules in energy metabolism pathways, including PFKP in glycolysis, IDH2 and IDH3B in Kreb's cycle, ND2, ND5, CYTB, and UQCRH in oxidative phosphorylation, and MCT1 and MCT4 in lactate shuttle, to inhibit ovarian cancer growth. Third, the integrative analysis of TCGA transcriptomics and mitochondrial proteomics in ovarian cancer revealed that 16 survival-related lncRNAs were mediated by ivermectin, SILAC quantitative proteomics analysis revealed that ivermectin extensively inhibited the expressions of RNA-binding protein EIF4A3 and 116 EIF4A3-interacted genes including those key molecules in energy metabolism pathways, and also those lncRNAs regulated EIF4A3-mRNA axes. Thus, ivermectin mediated lncRNA-EIF4A3-mRNA axes in ovarian cancer to exert its anticancer capability. Further, lasso regression identified the prognostic model of ivermectin-related three-lncRNA signature (ZNRF3-AS1, SOS1-IT1, and LINC00565), which is significantly associated with overall survival and clinicopathologic characteristics in ovarian cancer patients. These ivermectin-related molecular pattern alterations benefit for prognostic assessment and personalized drug therapy toward 3P medicine practice in ovarian cancer.

Keywords: ovarian cancer, ivermectin, anti-cancer effect, therapeutic targets, prognostic assessment, biomarker, predictive preventive personalized medicine

1. Introduction

Ivermectin is chemically derived from avermectin that was discovered and isolated from soil in Jan by Omura in 1973 [1]. It was approved by Federal Drug Administration (FDA) to use for anti-parasite drug in 1987, which has significantly improved global public health as an antiparasite medicine [2]. In 2015, its discovers Drs. Omura and Campbell earned the Nobel Prize in physiology or medicine [2]. Recent years, many studies have demonstrated that ivermectin has extensive roles in anti-bacteria, anti-virus, and anticancer, except for its anti-parasite effects [3–5].

Its anticancer effect has been shown by many *in vitro* and *in vivo* experiments in multiple cancers, including ovarian cancer, breast cancer, triple-negative breast cancer, cervical cancer, lung cancer, gastric cancer, colon cancer, glioblastoma, melanoma, and leukemia [4, 6], with a wide safe and clinically reachable drug concentration of anticancer according to its pharmacokinetic range in treatment of a parasite-infected patient [7]. It offers a promising opportunity to develop a new anticancer drug via drug repositioning of this existing compound with confirmed clinical safety [8].

Ovarian cancer, a very common cancer with high mortality and poor survival in women [9, 10], are involved in multiple signaling pathway network changes [11, 12]. Many intracellular molecules and signaling pathways would be the targets of ivermectin [13]. Ivermectin have shown a potential addition role for ovarian cancer treatment. For example, ivermectin can improve the chemosensitivity of overran cancer via targeting Akt/mTOR signaling pathway [14], and can inhibit PAK1-dependent growth of ovarian cancer cells via blocking the oncogenic kinase PAK1 [15]. Ivermectin also acts as a PAK1 inhibitor to induce autophagy in breast cancer [16]. Ivermectin can enhance p53 expression and cytochrome C release, and reduce the expression levels of CDK2, CDK4, CDK6, Bcl-2, cyclin E, and cyclin D1 in glioblastoma, those promoted the cancer cell apoptosis [17]. Ivermectin can inhibit cancer cell proliferation via decreasing YAP1 protein expression in the Hippo pathway [18]. Ivermectin represses WNT-TCF pathway in WNT-TCF-dependent disease [19]. Ivermectin can promote TFE3 (Ser321) dephosphorylation to block the binding between TFE3 and 14-3-3, and induce TFE3 accumulation in the nucleus of human melanoma cells [20]. Moreover, ivermectin also affects other signaling pathway network in human cancers, including oxidative stress, mitochondrial dysfunction, angiogenesis, epithelial-mesenchymal transition, drug resistance, and stemness in tumor [6]. Thereby, ivermectin demonstrates the potential therapeutic efficiency in multiple malignant tumors.

This book chapter discussed the anti-cancer effects of ivermectin on ovarian cancer in the following aspects: (i) ivermectin inhibited cell proliferation and growth, blocked cell cycle progression, and promoted cell apoptosis in ovarian cancer [4, 21]; (ii) ivermectin inhibited ovarian cancer growth through molecular networks to target the key molecules in energy metabolism pathways, including glycolysis, Kreb's cycle, oxidative phosphorylation, and lactate shuttle pathways [21]; (iii) Integrated omics revealed that ivermectin mediated lncRNA-EIF4A3-mRNA axes in ovarian cancer to exert its anticancer capability [4, 13]; and (iv) lasso regression identified the prognostic model of ivermectin-related three-lncRNA signature (ZNRF3-AS1, SOS1-IT1, and LINC00565) that is significantly related to overall survival and clinicopathologic characteristics of ovarian cancers [4].

2. Methods

2.1 Ovarian cancer cell biological behaviors affected by ivermectin

The normal ovarian cells IOSE80 and ovarian cancer cells TOV-21 and SKOV3 were treated with ivermectin to measure ivermectin-mediated ovarian cancer cell biological behavior changes. (i) IOSE80, TOV-21G, and SKOV3 were treated with ivermectin (0–60 μM) for 24 h, followed by the use of CCK8 to measure the IC50 of ivermectin in each cell. (ii) TOV-21G and SKOV3 were treated with ivermectin (0 μM, 10 μM, 20 μM, and 30 μM) for 24 h, followed by the use of EdU assay to measure DNA synthesis in each cell. (iii) TOV-21G and SKOV3 were treated with ivermectin (0 μM, 10 μM, 20 μM, and 30 μM) for 48 h, followed by clonogenic assay to measure the *in vitro* effects of ivermectin in each cell. (iv)TOV-21G and SKOV3 were treated with ivermectin (0 μM, 10 μM, 20 μM, and 30 μM) for 24 h, followed by flow cytometry to measure cell cycle and cell apoptosis changes in each cell. (v) When A2780 and TOV-21G seeded in 6-well plates were grown to approximately 90% confluency, followed by the use of 10-μl pipette tip to make an artificial wound, and then treated with ivermectin (0 μM, 10 μM, 20 μM, and 30 μM) for 24 h, and measure the wound healing. The relative percentage of wound healing = (the width of wound at 0 h − the width of wound at 24 h)/the width of wound at 0 h. The detailed procedure was described previously [4, 21].

2.2 Ivermectin-mediated pathway network predicted by ingenuity pathway analysis

The classical pathway network analysis software, Ingenuity Pathway Analysis (IPA) (http://www.ingenuity.com) [5] was used to predict ivermectin-related potential target molecules in three energy metabolism pathways. For this analysis, ivermectin and target genes in three energy metabolism pathways are all input into the IPA tool. The detailed procedure was described previously [21]. The predicted ivermectin-mediated targets in energy metabolism pathways were the basis for further experiment verification.

2.3 Ivermectin-mediated target molecule changes in energy metabolism pathways verified at the mRNA and protein levels

TOV-21G and SKOV3 were treated with ivermectin (0 μM, 10 μM, 20 μM, and 30 μM) for 24 h, and 48 h. At the 24 h time point, the RNAs were extracted for quantitative real-time PCR (qRT-PCR) analysis to measure the mRNA expression of target molecules (CS, PDHB, IDH2, IDH3A, IDH3B, PFKP, PKM, MCT1, MCT4, OGDHL, ND2, ND5, CYTB, and UQCRH) in energy metabolism pathways. At the 48 h time point, the proteins were extracted for Western blot analysis to measure the protein expression of target molecules (CS, PDHB, IDH2, IDH3A, IDH3B, PFKP, PKM, MCT1, MCT4, OGDHL, ND2, ND5, CYTB, and UQCRH) in energy metabolism pathways. The detailed procedure was described previously [21].

2.4 Ivermectin-mediated proteome changes in ovarian cancer identified by SILAC-based quantitative proteomics

SILAC (stable isotope labeling with amino acids in cell culture)-based quantitative proteomics was used to identified differentially expressed proteins in ovarian cancer TOV-21G treated with and without 20 μM ivermectin [13]. The identified differentially expressed proteins were used for molecular network and signaling pathway analyses to obtain ivermectin-related signaling pathway networks [13]. The detailed procedure was described previously [13].

2.5 Transcriptomics and clinical data of ovarian cancer patients extracted from TCGA database

Level 3 RNA-seq V2 transcriptomics data of 411 OC patients were extracted from The Cancer Genome Atlas (TCGA) data portal (http://cancergenome.nih.gov/) with the corresponding clinical data, including cancer status (with tumor or tumor-free), clinical stage (stages IIA, IIB, IIC, IIIA, IIIB, IIIC, and IV), neoplasm histologic grade (G1, G2, G3, G4, and GX), anatomic neoplasm subdivision (right, left, and bilateral), age at initial pathologic diagnosis (aged from 30 to 87), lymphatic invasion (yes/no), primary therapy outcome success (complete remission/response, partial remission/response, progressive disease, and stable disease), additional radiation therapy (yes/no), survival time (days), tumor residual disease (no macroscopic disease, 1–10 mm, 11–20 mm, and > 20 mm), survival status (0 = alive, and 1 = dead), and PANCAN (Pan-Cancer Atlas). TANRIC (http://ibl.mdanderson.org/tanric/design/basic/index.html) was used for survival analysis of lncRNAs in ovarian cancer. The large-scale CLIP-Seq data with starBasev 2.0 (http://starbase.sysu.edu.cn/mirCircRNA.php) was used to predict the EIF4A3-binding mRNAs. The Kaplan–Meier method relative to the log-rank test was used for survival analysis of mRNAs in ovarian cancers. Statistical significance was set as p value <0.05. GenCLiP 3 (http://ci.smu.edu.cn/genclip3/analysis.php) was used for pathway enrichment analysis of the association of EIF4A3-binding mRNAs and patient survival rates. The detailed procedure was described previously [4].

2.6 Ivermectin-related lncRNAs verified with qRT-PCR

TRizol® Reagent (Invitrogen, CA, USA) was used to extract total RNAs of cells TOV21G and A2780 treated with different concentration of ivermectin (0 μM, 10 μM, 20 μM, and 30 μM). The extracted total RNAs was reversely transcribed into cDNAs for qRT-PCR analysis of each lncRNA expression, including KIF9-AS1, HCG15, PDCD4-AS1, ZNRF3-AS1, ZNF674-AS1, LINC00565, SOS1-IT1, WWTR1-AS1, PLCH1-AS1, LINC00517, SNHG3, STARD13-IT1, AL109767.1, HOXC-AS3, LEMD1-AS1, and LBX2-AS1. Beta-actin was set as internal control for qRT-PCR analysis. The detailed procedure was described previously [4].

2.7 LncRNA-based prognostic signature optimized with lasso regression for ovarian cancers

Lasso regression means least absolute shrinkage and selection operator regression, which was used to optimize and construct lncRNA-based prognostic signature, and the glmnet R package was used to measure the association between survival risk and lncRNA signature in ovarian cancers. Moreover, univariate and multivariate Cox regression, and Kaplan–Meier method were used to identify overall survival-related clinical characteristics described above in ovarian cancers to confirm the established lncRNA-based prognostic model. The detailed procedure was described previously [4].

2.8 Statistical significance

Benjamini–Hochberg (FDR) for multiple testing was used to correct the p values of IPA, GO, and KEGG analyses. Student's t test was used for qRT-PCR and western blot data ($p < 0.05$) with data expression of mean ± SD ($n = 3$).

3. Results and discussion

3.1 Effects of ivermectin on biological behaviors of ovarian cancers

First, CCK8 experiments were used to measure cell proliferation changes between ovarian cancer cells (SKOV3; TOV-21G) and control cells (IOSE80), treated with and without ivermectin (**Figure 1**). Each type of cells was significantly inhibited by ivermectin with a dose-dependent relationship. The IC50 (half maximal inhibitory concentration) was 29.46 μM for IOSE80 cells, 20.85 μM for SKOV3,

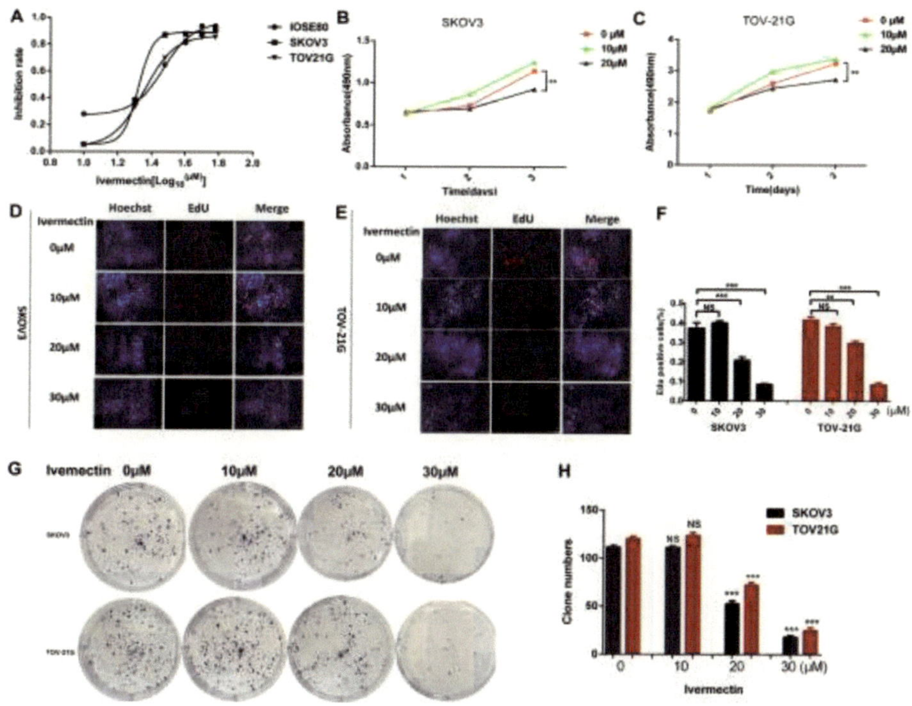

Figure 1.
Ivermectin suppressed ovarian cancer cell proliferation in vitro, *measured with CCK8 (A-C), EdU (D-F), and clonogenic experiments (G, H). Reproduced from Li et al. [21], with copyright permission from nature springer publisher, copyright 2020.*

and 22.54 μM for TOV-21G (**Figure 1A**). The IC50 of ovarian cancers were significantly lower than the normal controls. Further, 20 μM ivermectin - slightly lower than IC50 – can effectively inhibit ovarian cancer proliferation (**Figure 1B** and **C**) [21]. For *in vivo* human trial, the highest FDA-approved ivermectin dose was 200 μg/kg for human use in anti-parasite; however, a study on 68 human subjects found that the dose up to 2,000 μg/kg still worked well without CNS toxicity. The mean area under the curve ratios for the 30 and 60 mg doses were 1.24 and 1.40, indicating a minimal accumulation of ivermectin [5, 22]. These data demonstrate that ivermectin was a well-tolerated safe drug. Second, EdU cell proliferation experiments also confirmed that ivermectin significantly suppressed cell proliferation of ovarian cancers with a time-dependent relationship (**Figure 1D-F**) [21]. Third, Clonogenic survival experiments confirmed that ivermectin effectively inhibited the formation of cell clones with a time-dependent relationship (**Figure 1G-H**) [21]. Moreover, 10 μM ivermectin cannot effectively inhibit cell proliferation of ovarian cancers, 30 μM ivermectin caused cell death of ovarian cancers, and 20 μM ivermectin was a suitable dose to significantly suppress growth and proliferation of ovarian cancer cells.

3.2 Effects of ivermectin on cell cycle and apoptosis in ovarian cancers

Flow cytometry was used to measure cell cycle and apoptosis of ovarian cancer cells treated with and without ivermectin (**Figure 2**) [21]. First, the cell proportion was significantly increased in G0/G phase, decreased in S phase, and no change in G2/M phase in the high concentration (20- and 30-μM) compared to the low concentration (0- and 10-μM) of ivermectin groups (**Figure 2A-C**). Second, compared to control group, the proportion of apoptosis cells was significantly increased

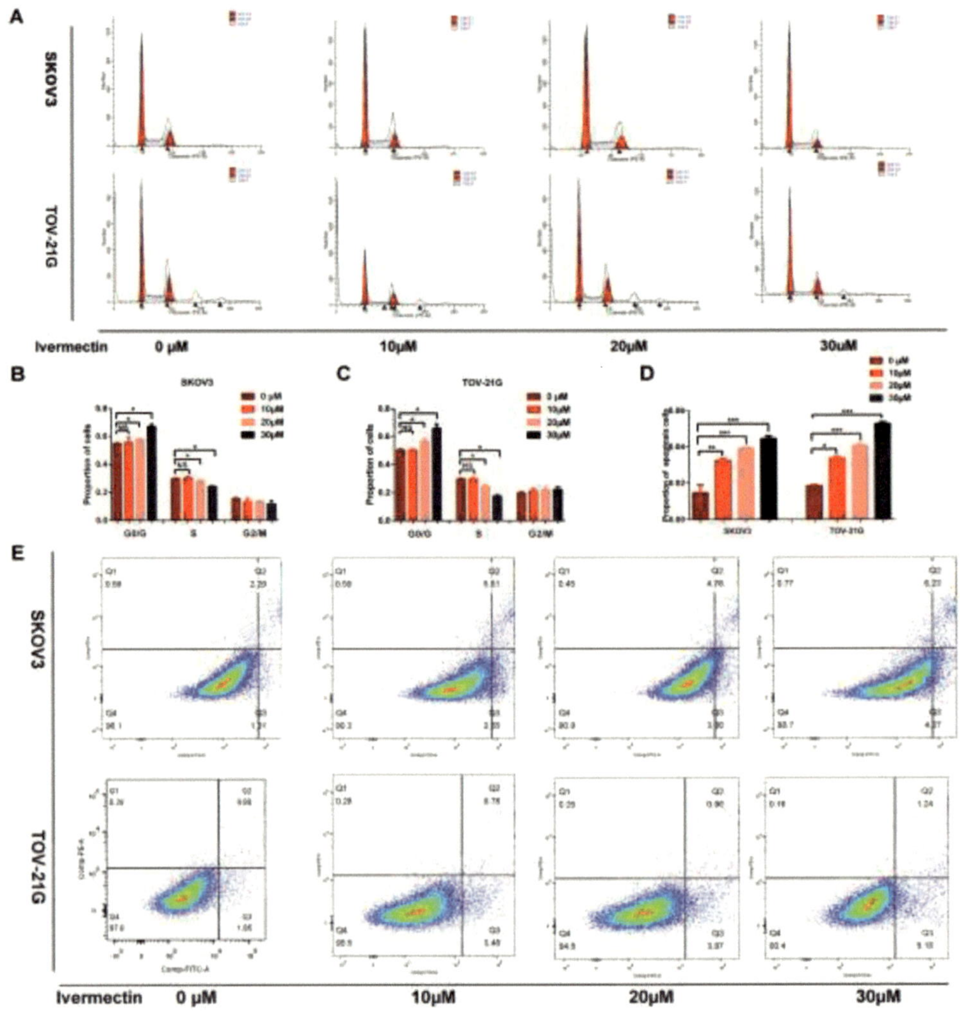

Figure 2.
Ivermectin blocked cell cycle progression (A, B, C) and promoted cell apoptosis (D, E) of ovarian cancer cells. Reproduced from Li et al. [21], with copyright permission from nature springer publisher, copyright 2020.

in different concentration of ivermectin groups, with a dose-dependent relationship (**Figure 2D** and **E**).

3.3 Effect of ivermectin on cell migration in ovarian cancers

Wound healing experiment was used to test the effect of ivermectin on cell migration of ovarian cancer cells. The results showed that cell migration was significantly inhibited in cells A2780 and TOV-21G after treatment of 20 μM and 30 μM ivermectin (**Figure 3**) [4].

3.4 Pharmaceutic molecular network predicted the association of ivermectin with ROS and energy metabolism

Ingenuity Pathway Analysis (IPA) was used for pharmaceutic molecular network analysis of ivermectin. The results showed that ivermectin was significantly

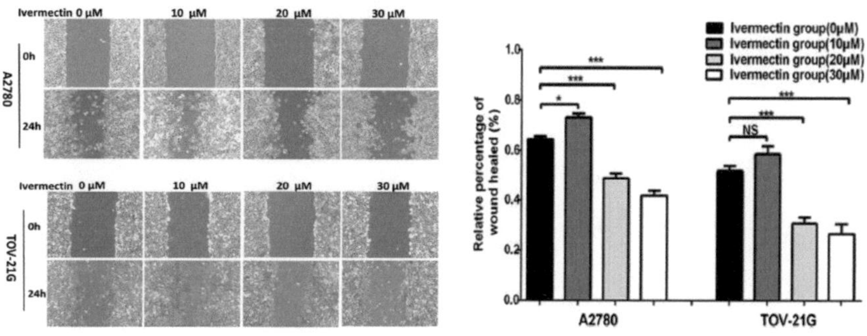

Figure 3.
Ivermectin inhibited cell migration of ovarian cancer cells TOV-21G relative to control cells A2780, analyzed with wound healing experiments. Reproduced from Li et al. [4], with copyright permission from nature springer publisher, copyright 2020.

associated with reactive oxygen species (ROS) and energy metabolism pathways, including pyruvate kinase muscle (PKM), oxoglutarate dehydrogenase L (OGDHL), mitochondrially encoded NADH dehydrogenase 2 (ND2), mitochondrially encoded NADH dehydrogenase 5 (ND5), CytB, and ubiquinolcytochrome c reductase hinge protein (UQCRH) (**Figure 4**) [21]. Moreover, ivermectin directly regulated Rbp, CYP3A4, P2RX7, ABCB1, GLRB, ABCG2, P2RX4, P glycoprotein, Abcb1b, strychnine, cytokine, and insulin; and indirectly regulated TNF, APP, MAPK1, ERK1/2, MAPK3, MAPK13, ROS, NFKBIA, testosterone, and STAT3 [21].

3.5 SILAC quantitative proteomics revealed the effects of ivermectin on key proteins in energy metabolism pathways in ovarian cancer cells

SILAC quantitative proteomics was used to detect, identify, and quantify the key protein alterations in energy metabolic pathways in ovarian cancer cells treated with (SILAC: H) and without (SILAC: L) 20 μM ivermectin for 24 h (**Table 1**) [21]. This study found that ivermectin significantly reduced (i) the expression levels of glycolysis-related enzymes, including ADH5, ENO1, GPI, GAPDH, LDHA, LDHB, PFKP, and PKM; (ii) the Kreb's cycle-related enzymes, including ACON, PCK2, PDHB, MDH2, CS, IDH2, IDH3A, IDH3B, SUCLG2, and OGDHL; (iii) the OXPHOS-related enzymes, including CYTB, UQCRH, COX17, COX1, COX6C, COX4I1, COX2, COX7A2L, COX7A2, ATP6V0C, and ATP6; and (iv) the lactate shuttle proteins MCT1 and MCT4, in ovarian cancer cells.

3.6 RT-qPCR and Western blot confirmed the effects of ivermectin on the key molecules in energy metabolism pathways at the mRNA and protein levels

RT-qPCR analysis confirmed the mRNA expression alterations of key molecules in energy metabolism pathways in ovarian cancer cells treated with ivermectin (0 μM, 10 μM, 20 μM, and 30 μM) (**Figure 5**), and further western blot analysis confirmed the protein expression alterations of those corresponding key molecules (**Figure 6**) [21]. These key molecules included PFKP, and PKM in glycolysis pathway, PDHB, CS, IDH2, IDH3A, IDH3B, and OGDHL in Kreb's cycle pathway, ND2, ND5, CYTB, and UQCRH in oxidative phosphorylation pathway, MCT1, and MCT4 in lactate shuttle. These results clearly showed that ivermectin regulated energy metabolism pathways in ovarian cancer cells.

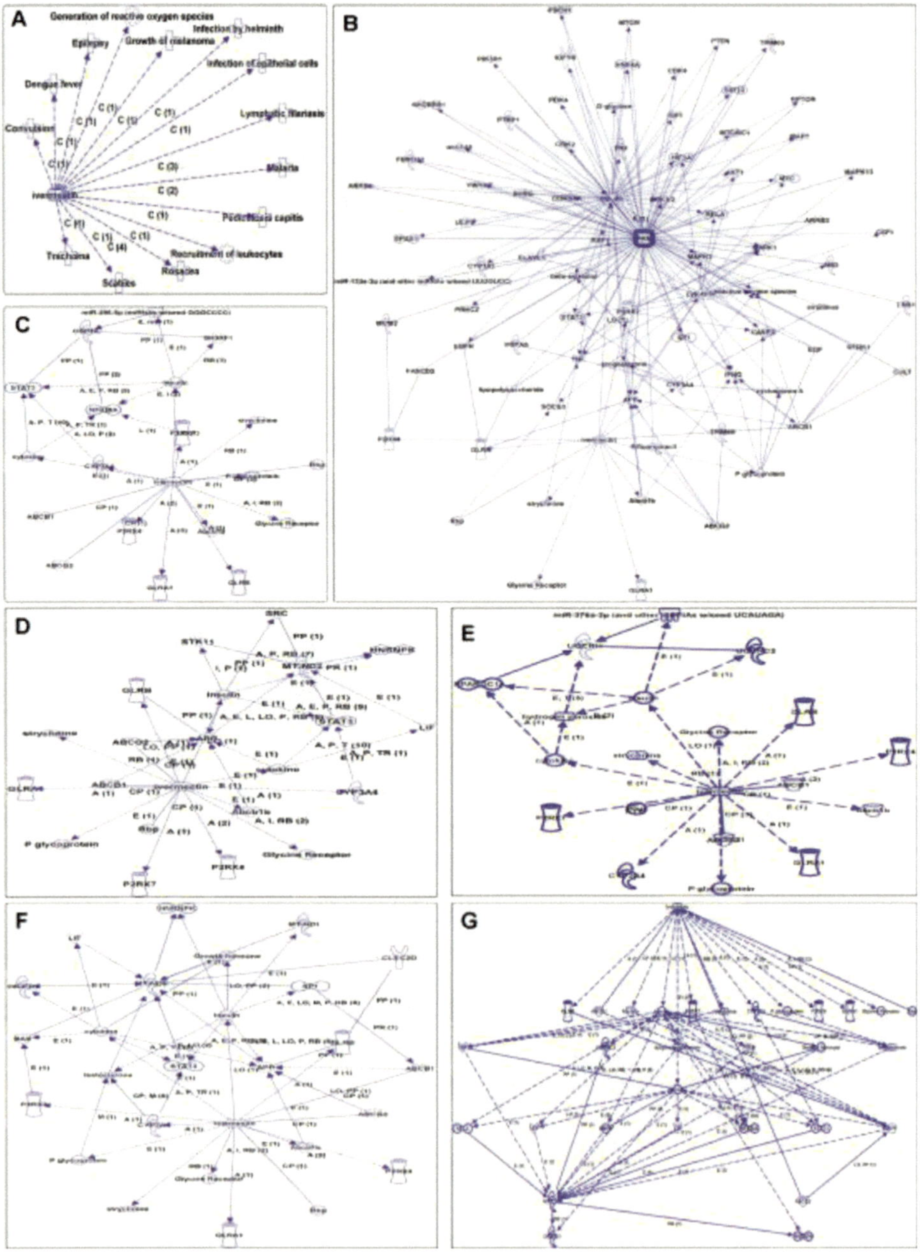

Figure 4.
Pharmaceutic molecular network predicted the associations of ivermectin with reactive oxygen species (ROS) and energy metabolism pathways (A) Disease and functional analysis of ivermectin based on IPA database (B-G). The association of ivermectin with PKM (B), OGDHL (C), ND2 (D), UQCRH (E), ND5 (F), and CYTB (G). Reproduced from Li et al. [21], with copyright permission from nature springer publisher, copyright 2020.

3.7 Ivermectin regulated lncRNA-EIF4A3-mRNA axis in ovarian cancer cells

Our quantitative mitochondrial proteomics data identified 1198 differentially mitochondrial proteins (mtDEPs) in human ovarian cancer tissues relative to control ovary tissues [11, 23]. Six RNA-binding proteins among those 1198 mtDEPs were identified, including EIF4A3, SFRS1, IGF2BP2, UPF1, C22ORF28, and EWSR1. Of them, only EIF4A3 was predicted to bind to the mRNA of key molecules in energy metabolism pathways. Further, Starbase predicted 3636 EIF4A3-biding mRNAs in various cancer; and of them, 306 EIF4A3-binding mRNAs was associated

Pathway	Protein ID	Gene name	Protein name	Q-value	Intensity H	Intensity L	Ratio H/L
Glycolysis pathway	PFKAP	PFKP	ATP-dependent 6-phosphofructokinase, platelet type	0.00E+00	14226000000	25587000000	0.54
	H3BQ34	PKM	Pyruvate kinase	7.46E-03	10727000	0	+
	ODPB	PDHB	Pyruvate dehydrogenase E1 component subunit beta, mitochondrial	0.00E+00	407280000	1649500000	0.46
	K4EN11	GAPDH	GAPDH (Fragment)	0.00E+00	0	0	/
	ENOA	ENO1	Alpha-enolase	0.00E+00	54687000000	125660000000	0.44
	F5GXY2	LDHA	L-lactate dehydrogenase A chain (Fragment)	1.00E+00	10379000	29470000	0.34
	Q5U077	LDHB	L-lactate dehydrogenase	0.00E+00	27852000000	66990000000	0.42
	A0A0A0MTS2	GPI	Glucose-6-phosphate isomerase (Fragment)	1.00E+00	56685000	138520000	0.44
	Q6IRT1	ADH5	S-(hydroxymethyl)glutathione dehydrogenase	0.00E+00	1308100000	3513700000	0.45
	B3KUV2	ACSS2	cDNA FLJ40707 fis, clone THYMU2026835, highly similar to Acetyl-coenzyme A synthetase, cytoplasmic	9.53E-03	9455200	25758000	0.73
	H3BRS6	ADPGK	ADP-dependent glucokinase (Fragment)	5.31E-04	11465000	18413000	0.69
	AL1B1	ALDH1B1	Aldehyde dehydrogenase X, mitochondrial	0.00E+00	69821000	196750000	0.45
	ALDH2	ALDH2	Aldehyde dehydrogenase, mitochondrial	0.00E+00	812240000	1822600000	0.44

Pathway	Protein ID	Gene name	Protein name	Q-value	Intensity H	Intensity L	Ratio H/L
	AL3A2	ALDH3A2	Aldehyde dehydrogenase family 3 member A2	0.00E+00	225000000	394360000	0.55
	AL9A1	ALDH9A1	4-trimethylaminobutyraldehyde dehydrogenase	0.00E+00	529020000	1322400000	0.48
	A0A024QZ64	ALDOC	Fructose-bisphosphate aldolase	0.00E+00	1104800000	2650700000	0.43
	H0YDD4	DLAT	Acetyltransferase component of pyruvate dehydrogenase complex (Fragment)	0.00E+00	530720000	1251100000	0.46
	A0A024R713	DLD	Dihydrolipoyl dehydrogenase	0.00E+00	632170000	1843800000	0.52
	Q6FHV6	ENO2	ENO2 protein	0.00E+00	618190000	2887100000	0.26
	ENOB	ENO3	Beta-enolase	0.00E+00	215810000	482340000	0.59
	B4DG62	HK1	cDNA FLJ56506, highly similar to Hexokinase-1	0.00E+00	1617000000	4075800000	0.53
	HKDC1	HKDC1	Hexokinase HKDC1	0.00E+00	132850000	568430000	0.30
	PCKGC	PCK1	Phosphoenolpyruvate carboxykinase, cytosolic [GTP]	0.00E+00	1267700	160370000	0.07
	A0A384MTT2	PCK2	Epididymis secretory sperm binding protein	0.00E+00	403190000	1032500000	0.56
	A0A024RBX9	PDHA1	Pyruvate dehydrogenase E1 component subunit alpha	0.00E+00	457490000	1353000000	0.49
	PFKAL	PFKL	ATP-dependent 6-phosphofructokinase, liver type	0.00E+00	1242500000	2567300000	0.52

Pathway	Protein ID	Gene name	Protein name	Q-value	Intensity H	Intensity L	Ratio H/L
	A0A024R0Y5	PFKM	ATP-dependent 6-phosphofructokinase	0.00E+00	1677600000	3768800000	0.47
	Q6P6D7	PGAM1	Phosphoglycerate mutase	0.00E+00	11906000000	30409000000	0.36
	A0A3B3ITK7	PGM1	Phosphoglucomutase-1	0.00E+00	721450000	1641900000	0.43
	PGM2	PGM2	Phosphoglucomutase-2	0.00E+00	144180000	423580000	0.40
	A0A024R5Z9	PKM2	Pyruvate kinase	1.00E+00	35541000	125430000	0.54
Kreb's cycle	ODPB	PDHB	Pyruvate dehydrogenase E1 component subunit beta, mitochondrial	0.00E+00	407280000	1649500000	0.46
	B4DJV2	CS	Citrate synthase	0.00E+00	2428500000	5338700000	0.45
	IDHP	IDH2	Isocitrate dehydrogenase [NADP], mitochondrial	0.00E+00	1281200000	2994300000	0.46
	IDH3A	IDH3A	Isocitrate dehydrogenase [NAD] subunit alpha, mitochondrial	0.00E+00	268600000	1119300000	0.40
	A0A087WZN1	IDH3B	Isocitrate dehydrogenase [NAD] subunit, mitochondrial	0.00E+00	142630000	477180000	0.41
	OGDHL	OGDHL	2-oxoglutarate dehydrogenase-like, mitochondrial	0.00E+00	17707000	119970000	0.56
	O75944	ACON	Aconitase (Fragment)	0.00E+00	0	48304000	—
	A0A384MTT2	PCK2	Epididymis secretory sperm binding protein	0.00E+00	403190000	1032500000	0.56

Pathway	Protein ID	Gene name	Protein name	Q-value	Intensity H	Intensity L	Ratio H/L
	Q0QF37	MDH2	Malate dehydrogenase (Fragment)	0.00E+00	5856200000	14406000000	0.42
	A0A024R325	SUCLG2	Succinate–CoA ligase [GDP-forming] subunit beta, mitochondrial	0.00E+00	232210000	779800000	0.41
	Q71UF1	ACO2	Aconitate hydratase, mitochondrial	1.00E+00	0	12950000	—
	A0A024R1Y2	ACLY	ATP-citrate synthase	0.00E+00	2033900000	4490700000	0.46
	H0YDD4	DLAT	Acetyltransferase component of pyruvate dehydrogenase complex (Fragment)	0.00E+00	530720000	1251100000	0.46
	A0A024R713	DLD	Dihydrolipoyl dehydrogenase	0.00E+00	632170000	1843800000	0.52
	Q6IBS5	DLST	DLST protein	0.00E+00	601540000	1338700000	0.53
	A0A0S2Z4C3	FH	Epididymis secretory sperm binding protein (Fragment)	0.00E+00	1498700000	3849500000	0.43
	IDH3G	IDH3G	Isocitrate dehydrogenase [NAD] subunit gamma, mitochondrial	0.00E+00	55446000	230380000	0.54
	ODO1	OGDH	2-oxoglutarate dehydrogenase, mitochondrial	0.00E+00	325090000	949610000	0.43
	A0A494C101	PC	Pyruvate carboxylase, mitochondrial (Fragment)	7.83E-04	3454600	19685000	0.28
	PCKGC	PCK1	Phosphoenolpyruvate carboxykinase, cytosolic [GTP]	0.00E+00	1267700	160370000	0.07
	A0A024RBX9	PDHA1	Pyruvate dehydrogenase E1 component subunit alpha	0.00E+00	457490000	1353000000	0.49

Pathway	Protein ID	Gene name	Protein name	Q-value	Intensity H	Intensity L	Ratio H/L
	A0A024QZ30	SDHA	Succinate dehydrogenase [ubiquinone] flavoprotein subunit, mitochondrial	0.00E+00	1096500000	2950800000	0.44
	SDHB	SDHB	Succinate dehydrogenase [ubiquinone] iron–sulfur subunit, mitochondrial	0.00E+00	143030000	516360000	0.37
	D3DVH1	SDHC	Succinate dehydrogenase complex, subunit C, integral membrane protein, 15 kDa, isoform CRAa	0.00E+00	68060000	130150000	0.46
	B7ZAF6	SUCLA2	Succinate–CoA ligase [ADP-forming] subunit beta, mitochondrial	0.00E+00	114900000	726200000	0.33
	Q6IAL5	SUCLG1	Succinate–CoA ligase [ADP/GDP-forming] subunit alpha, mitochondrial	0.00E+00	261580000	1105700000	0.34
Oxidative phosphorylation	D2Y6X2	ND5	NADH dehydrogenase subunit 5 (Fragment)	5.33E-04	4125200	24591000	0.41
	A0A1B0TCA9	CYTB	Cytochrome b (Fragment)	3.59E-03	53396000	59765000	0.55
	Q567R0	UQCRH	UQCRH protein	0.00E+00	252050000	546900000	0.51
	C9J8T6	COX17	Cytochrome c oxidase copper chaperone	0.00E+00	7643200	53020000	0.36
	Q6FGA0	COX7A2L	COX7A2L protein	5.34E-04	22802000	1280400	17.81
	U3L4G0	ATP6	ATP synthase subunit a	0.00E+00	193600000	355900000	0.73
	X2C5C9	COX1	Cytochrome c oxidase subunit 1	7.89E-04	21347000	57543000	0.38
	A0A346M047	COX2	Cytochrome c oxidase subunit II (Fragment)	0.00E+00	1046600000	2406000000	0.38

Pathway	Protein ID	Gene name	Protein name	Q-value	Intensity H	Intensity L	Ratio H/L
	H3BNI4	ATP6V0C	V-type proton ATPase proteolipid subunit	1.00E+00	11819000	33788000	0.47
	Q496I0	COX7A2	COX7A2 protein	0.00E+00	223550000	687660000	0.32
	COX6C	COX6C	Cytochrome c oxidase subunit 6C	0.00E+00	24314000	57899000	0.34
	COX41	COX4I1	Cytochrome c oxidase subunit 4 isoform 1, mitochondrial	0.00E+00	1057000000	2524600000	0.40
	AT12A	ATP12A	Potassium-transporting ATPase alpha chain 2	1.00E+00	25608000	48153000	0.50
	ATPG	ATP5F1C	ATP synthase subunit gamma, mitochondrial	0.00E+00	610730000	1752800000	0.61
	ATPD	ATP5F1D	ATP synthase subunit delta, mitochondrial	0.00E+00	173290000	378660000	0.59
	ATP5I	ATP5ME	ATP synthase subunit e, mitochondrial	0.00E+00	139860000	416580000	0.28
	ATPK	ATP5MF	ATP synthase subunit f, mitochondrial	0.00E+00	146600000	369660000	0.57
	E9PN17	ATP5MG	ATP synthase subunit g, mitochondrial	0.00E+00	501810000	1039800000	0.45
	Q5QNZ2	ATP5PB	ATP synthase F(0) complex subunit B1, mitochondrial	0.00E+00	1074900000	2486300000	0.46
	ATP5H	ATP5PD	ATP synthase subunit d, mitochondrial	0.00E+00	525070000	965510000	0.39
	ATPO	ATP5PO	ATP synthase subunit O, mitochondrial	0.00E+00	1495600000	3024300000	0.56

Pathway	Protein ID	Gene name	Protein name	Q-value	Intensity H	Intensity L	Ratio H/L
	VPP1	ATP6V0A1	V-type proton ATPase 116 kDa subunit a isoform 1	0.00E+00	98038000	557300000	0.35
	R4GN72	ATP6V0D1	V-type proton ATPase subunit d 1	0.00E+00	258530000	806720000	0.31
	VATA	ATP6V1A	V-type proton ATPase catalytic subunit A	0.00E+00	1191800000	3218800000	0.37
	VATB2	ATP6V1B2	V-type proton ATPase subunit B, brain isoform	0.00E+00	583390000	2310600000	0.35
	A0A024R9I0	ATP6V1C1	V-type proton ATPase subunit C	0.00E+00	105790000	524300000	0.36
	Q53Y06	ATP6V1E1	ATPase, H+ transporting, lysosomal 31 kDa, V1 subunit E isoform 1	0.00E+00	226190000	457540000	0.46
	A4D1K0	ATP6V1F	V-type proton ATPase subunit F	0.00E+00	72747000	287010000	0.62
	A0A024R883	ATP6V1G1	V-type proton ATPase subunit G	0.00E+00	121660000	150890000	0.58
	A0A024R7X3	ATP6V1H	V-type proton ATPase subunit H	0.00E+00	33783000	166330000	0.37
	COX15	COX15	Cytochrome c oxidase assembly protein COX15 homolog	0.00E+00	52507000	160350000	0.47
	A0A343FH12	COX3	Cytochrome c oxidase subunit 3	0.00E+00	251800000	620670000	0.40
	H3BNX8	COX5A	Cytochrome c oxidase subunit 5A, mitochondrial	0.00E+00	489640000	1451700000	0.67
	COX5B	COX5B	Cytochrome c oxidase subunit 5B, mitochondrial	0.00E+00	237370000	754990000	0.33

Pathway	Protein ID	Gene name	Protein name	Q-value	Intensity H	Intensity L	Ratio H/L
	CX6B1	COX6B1	Cytochrome c oxidase subunit 6B1	0.00E+00	278190000	1028600000	0.28
	CY1	CYC1	Cytochrome c1, heme protein, mitochondrial	0.00E+00	426190000	876770000	0.51
	Q5T1Z0	LHPP	Phospholysine phosphohistidine inorganic pyrophosphate phosphatase	9.74E-03	0	20832000	—
	D8VCQ0	ND4	NADH–ubiquinone oxidoreductase chain 4 (Fragment)	3.36E-03	3604800	7493900	0.44
	Q7Z518	NDUFA10	NADH dehydrogenase [ubiquinone] 1 alpha subcomplex subunit 10, mitochondrial	0.00E+00	46879000	194320000	0.31
	NDUAD	NDUFA13	NADH dehydrogenase [ubiquinone] 1 alpha subcomplex subunit 13	0.00E+00	43461000	261780000	0.34
	NDUA2	NDUFA2	NADH dehydrogenase [ubiquinone] 1 alpha subcomplex subunit 2	0.00E+00	35677000	165030000	0.24
	NDUA4	NDUFA4	Cytochrome c oxidase subunit NDUFA4	0.00E+00	99542000	1041400000	0.28
	NDUA5	NDUFA5	NADH dehydrogenase [ubiquinone] 1 alpha subcomplex subunit 5	0.00E+00	126370000	440540000	0.46
	NDUA8	NDUFA8	NADH dehydrogenase [ubiquinone] 1 alpha subcomplex subunit 8	0.00E+00	75771000	226560000	0.33
	NDUA9	NDUFA9	NADH dehydrogenase [ubiquinone] 1 alpha subcomplex subunit 9, mitochondrial	0.00E+00	38134000	212250000	0.38
	H3BNK3	NDUFAB1	Acyl carrier protein (Fragment)	0.00E+00	91383000	220140000	0.41
	NDUB1	NDUFB1	NADH dehydrogenase [ubiquinone] 1 beta subcomplex subunit 1	0.00E+00	52572000	104780000	0.46

Pathway	Protein ID	Gene name	Protein name	Q-value	Intensity H	Intensity L	Ratio H/L
	H3BPJ9	NDUFB10	NADH dehydrogenase [ubiquinone] 1 beta subcomplex subunit 10	0.00E+00	68400000	353550000	0.41
	NDUBB	NDUFB11	NADH dehydrogenase [ubiquinone] 1 beta subcomplex subunit 11, mitochondrial	0.00E+00	40408000	192110000	0.31
	C9JKQ2	NDUFB3	NADH dehydrogenase [ubiquinone] 1 beta subcomplex subunit 3 (Fragment)	7.84E-04	19660000	91217000	0.33
	NDUB4	NDUFB4	NADH dehydrogenase [ubiquinone] 1 beta subcomplex subunit 4	0.00E+00	15764000	129660000	0.40
	NDUB8	NDUFB8	NADH dehydrogenase [ubiquinone] 1 beta subcomplex subunit 8, mitochondrial	0.00E+00	38897000	134110000	0.34
	A0A3B3IT57	NDUFB9	NADH dehydrogenase [ubiquinone] 1 beta subcomplex subunit 9	0.00E+00	47909000	178250000	0.26
	E5KRK5	NDUFS1	Mitochondrial NADH–ubiquinone oxidoreductase 75 kDa subunit	0.00E+00	87635000	1424000000	0.27
	NDUS2	NDUFS2	NADH dehydrogenase [ubiquinone] iron–sulfur protein 2, mitochondrial	0.00E+00	255210000	555800000	0.40
	NDUS3	NDUFS3	NADH dehydrogenase [ubiquinone] iron–sulfur protein 3, mitochondrial	0.00E+00	303550000	1007100000	0.38
	H0Y9M8	NDUFS4	NADH dehydrogenase [ubiquinone] iron–sulfur protein 4, mitochondrial (Fragment)	0.00E+00	22776000	124620000	0.20
	Q6IBA0	NDUFS5	NADH dehydrogenase (Ubiquinone) Fe-S protein 5, 15 kDa (NADH-coenzyme Q reductase)	0.00E+00	13539000	83631000	0.36
	B7Z4P1	NDUFS7	cDNA FLJ58024, highly similar to NADH–ubiquinone oxidoreductase 20 kDa subunit, mitochondrial	3.38E-03	89666000	146530000	1.06
	E9PKH6	NDUFS8	NADH dehydrogenase [ubiquinone] iron–sulfur protein 8, mitochondrial (Fragment)	0.00E+00	25384000	70988000	0.38

Pathway	Protein ID	Gene name	Protein name	Q-value	Intensity H	Intensity L	Ratio H/L
	G3V0I5	NDUFV1	NADH dehydrogenase [ubiquinone] flavoprotein 1, mitochondrial	0.00E+00	25550000	98424000	0.34
	Q9UEH5	NDUFV2	24-kDa subunit of complex I (Fragment)	0.00E+00	120810000	407130000	0.33
	IPYR2	PPA2	Inorganic pyrophosphatase 2, mitochondrial	0.00E+00	815730000	1743800000	0.42
	A0A024QZ30	SDHA	Succinate dehydrogenase [ubiquinone] flavoprotein subunit, mitochondrial	0.00E+00	1096500000	2950800000	0.44
	SDHB	SDHB	Succinate dehydrogenase [ubiquinone] iron–sulfur subunit, mitochondrial	0.00E+00	143030000	516360000	0.37
	D3DVH1	SDHC	Succinate dehydrogenase complex, subunit C, integral membrane protein, 15 kDa, isoform CRAa	0.00E+00	68060000	130150000	0.46
	A0A024R5E5	TCIRG1	V-type proton ATPase subunit a	0.00E+00	139450000	227300000	0.73
	QCR9	UQCR10	Cytochrome b-c1 complex subunit 9	0.00E+00	260330000	491890000	0.52
	QCR7	UQCRB	Cytochrome b-c1 complex subunit 7	0.00E+00	208330000	523300000	0.37
	QCR1	UQCRC1	Cytochrome b-c1 complex subunit 1, mitochondrial	0.00E+00	1326400000	3772100000	0.43
	QCR2	UQCRC2	Cytochrome b-c1 complex subunit 2, mitochondrial	0.00E+00	1718400000	3636100000	0.43
	A0A384NPX8	UQCRFS1	Cytochrome b-c1 complex subunit Rieske, mitochondrial	0.00E+00	79904000	211540000	0.34
	QCR8	UQCRQ	Cytochrome b-c1 complex subunit 8	0.00E+00	88536000	237890000	0.57

DOI: http://dx.doi.org/10.5772/intechopen.95556

Pathway	Protein ID	Gene name	Protein name	Q-value	Intensity H	Intensity L	Ratio H/L
Lactate shuttle	B4E106	MCT1	cDNA FLJ53399, highly similar to Monocarboxylate transporter 1	0.00E+00	23799000	115420000	0.53
	MOT4	MCT4	Monocarboxylate transporter 4	0.00E+00	818320000	2103700000	0.38

Table 1.
SILAC quantitative proteomics revealed the protein expression changes of key molecules in energy metabolic pathways in ovarian cancer cells TOV-21G treated with (SILAC: H) and without (SILAC: L) 20 μM ivermectin for 24 h. - means the protein expressed in L group but not in H group. + means the protein expressed in H group but not in L group. /means the protein with expressed value 0 in both H and L groups. Ratio H/L means the ratio of the ivermectin-treated group (SILAC: H) to the no ivermectin-treated group (SILAC: L). Reproduced from Li et al. [21], with copyright permission from nature springer publisher, copyright 2020.

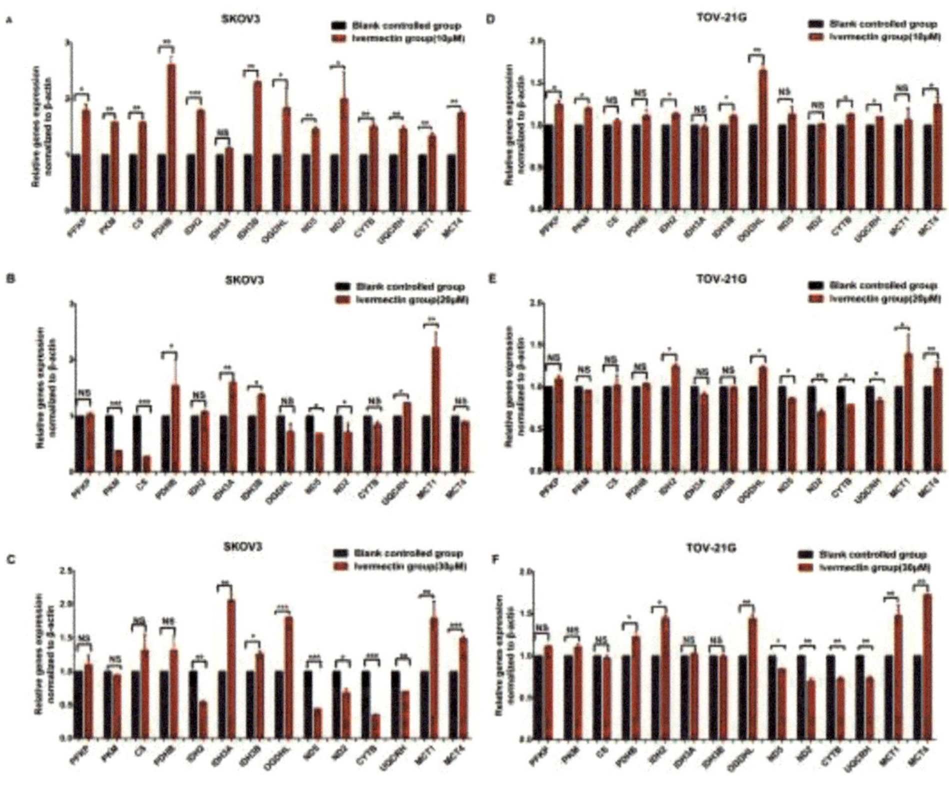

Figure 5.
*RT-qPCR confirmed the effects of ivermectin on the mRNA expressions of key molecules in the energy metabolism pathways in ovarian cancer cells (a-f). The effects of different concentration of ivermectin (0, 10, 20, and 30 μM) on mRNA expressions of PFKP, PKM, CS, PDHB, IDH2, IDH3A, IDH3B, OGDHL, ND5, ND2, CYTB, UQCRH, MCT1, and MCT4. n = 3. *p < 0.05, **p < 0.01, ***p < 0.001. Reproduced from Li et al. [21], with copyright permission from nature springer publisher, copyright 2020.*

with ovarian cancer survival rate. Among 306 EIF4A3-binding mRNAs, the protein expressions of 116 EIF4A3-binding mRNAs and EIF4A3 were found to be inhibited by ivermectin, identified by SILAC quantitative proteomics in ovarian cancer cells treated with and without ivermectin (**Table 2**) [4].

Moreover, TCGA transcriptomics analysis found that 16 lncRNAs had binding sites with EIF4A3 and associated with ovarian cancer survival rate, including SNHG3, HCG15, PDCD4-AS1, KIF9-AS1, ZNRF3-AS1, ZNF674-AS1, LINC00565, SOS1-IT1, WWTR1-AS1, PLCH1-AS1, LINC00517, STARD13-IT1, LEMD1-AS1, AL109767.1, HOXC-AS3, and LBX2-AS1 [23]. Further, RT-qPCR analysis of these 16 lncRNA expressions in ovarian cancer cells treated with ivermectin (0 μM, 10 μM, 20 μM, and 30 μM) compared to control cells, which found 9 lncRNAs (PDCD4-AS1, ZNRF3-AS1, HCG15, KIF9-AS1, LINC00565, ZNF674-AS1, AL109767.1, SOS1-IT1, and LBX2-AS1) were significantly affected by ivermectin (**Figure** 7) [4].

These findings clearly demonstrated that ivermectin regulated lncRNA-EIF4A3-mRNA axis in ovarian cancer cells, and these mRNAs included the key molecules in energy metabolism pathways in ovarian cancer cells.

3.8 The prognostic model of ivermectin-related three-lncRNA signature for ovarian cancers identified and optimized by lasso regression

Based on those nine ivermectin-mediated lncRNAs in ovarian cancers, survival analysis and lasso regression were used to identify and optimize the prognostic model of ivermectin-related three-lncRNA signature (ZNRF3-AS1,

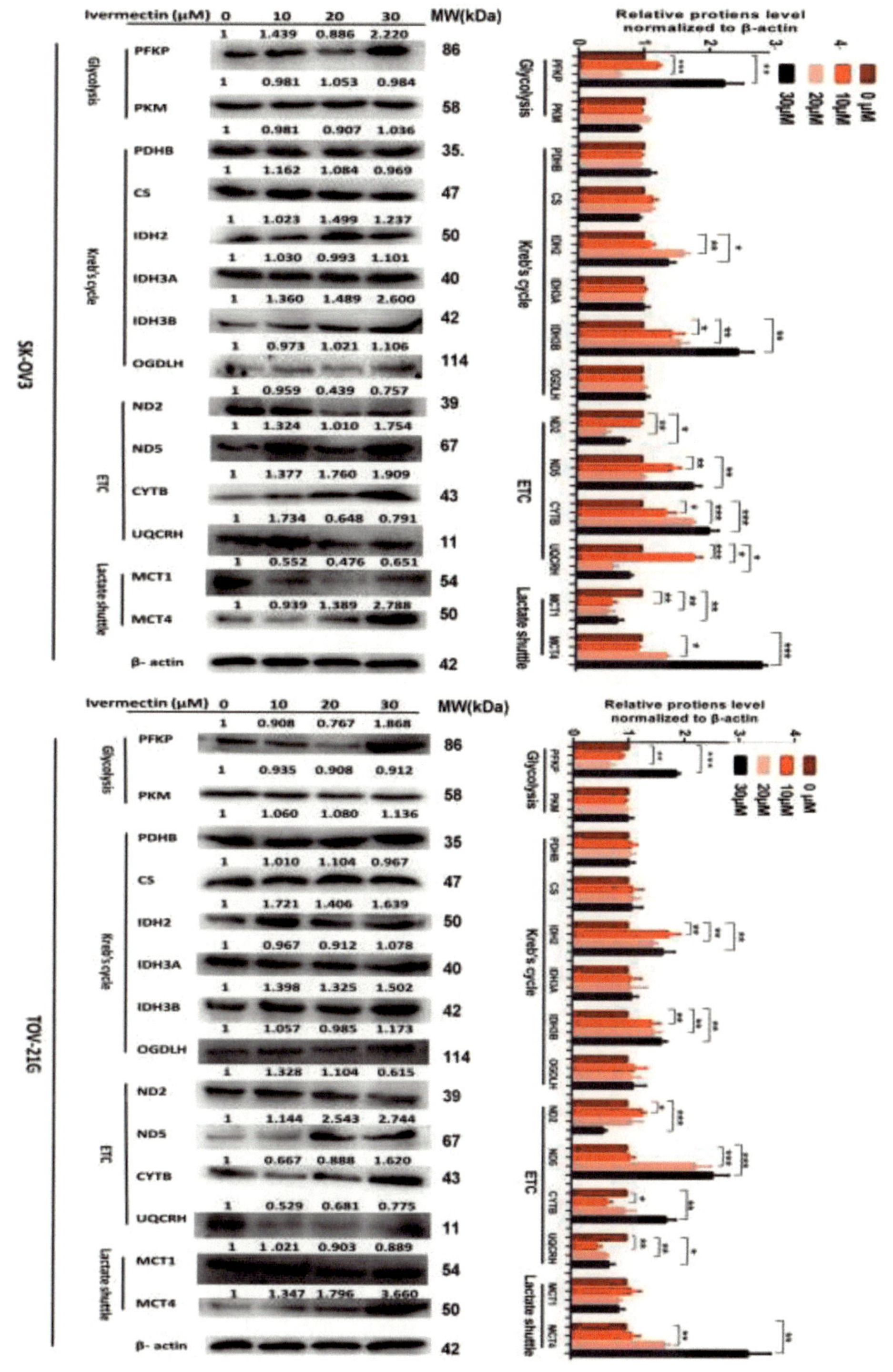

Figure 6.
*Western blot confirmed the effects of ivermectin on the protein expressions of key molecules in the energy metabolism pathways in ovarian cancer cells. n = 3. *p < 0.05, **p < 0.01, ***p < 0.001. Reproduced from Li et al. [21], with copyright permission from nature springer publisher, copyright 2020.*

SOS1-IT1, and LINC00565) (**Figure 8**) [4]. This prognostic model was significantly related to overall survival and clinicopathologic characteristics in ovarian cancer patients [4], which might benefit for prognostic assessment and personalized drug therapy toward 3P medicine practice in ovarian cancer.

Protein IDs	Protein names	Gene names	Q-value	Score	Intensity H	Intensity L	Ratio H/L
A0A0S2Z4C6	Serine/threonine-protein phosphatase 2B catalytic subunit alpha isoform	PPP3CA	0	106	450040000	2.321E+09	0.17
A0A024R7B0	Ubiquitin-like protein 5	UBL5	0	3	33400000	156360000	0.20
A0A024R9A9	Ubiquitin-conjugating enzyme E2 T	UBE2T	0	7	54580000	216150000	0.22
A0A494C101	Pyruvate carboxylase;Pyruvate carboxylase, mitochondrial	PC	0	3	3454600	19685000	0.28
A0A1W2PNM1	Hydroxyacyl-coenzyme A dehydrogenase, mitochondrial	HADH	0	11	85389000	332200000	0.30
Q496I0	Cytochrome c oxidase subunit 7A2, mitochondrial	COX7A2	0	10	223550000	687660000	0.32
Q149N6	Dedicator of cytokinesis protein 4	DOCK4	0	4	2402200	12153000	0.33
Q15036	Sorting nexin-17	SNX17	0	9	2545600	64295000	0.33
J3KN67	Tropomyosin alpha-3 chain	TPM3	0	3	44208000	225430000	0.34
Q8WZ82	Ovarian cancer-associated gene 2 protein	OVCA2	0	8	22175000	92294000	0.34
G3V0I5	NADH dehydrogenase [ubiquinone] flavoprotein 1, mitochondrial	NDUFV1	0	9	25550000	98424000	0.34
J3QLR8	28S ribosomal protein S23, mitochondrial	MRPS23	0	8	59957000	127510000	0.35
J3KSI8	28S ribosomal protein S7, mitochondrial	MRPS7	0	9	56198000	98108000	0.35
B4DP80	NAD(P)H-hydrate epimerase	APOA1BP	0	47	81014000	347980000	0.37
C9JFE4	COP9 signalosome complex subunit 1	GPS1	0	25	189930000	447320000	0.38
Q9Y3B7	39S ribosomal protein L11, mitochondrial	MRPL11	0	5	17279000	5213500	0.38
Q9Y333	U6 snRNA-associated Sm-like protein LSm2	LSM2	0	23	188570000	423780000	0.38
P63261	Actin	ACTG1	0	212	3.864E+09	1.674E+10	0.38
Q07954	Prolow-density lipoprotein receptor-related protein 1	LRP1	0	5	3971000	52428000	0.38
Q68E01	Integrator complex subunit 3	INTS3	0	11	32873000	113610000	0.38
K7EKI4	39S ribosomal protein L4, mitochondrial	MRPL4	0	9	41947000	121900000	0.39
V9GZ56	U6 snRNA-associated Sm-like protein LSm4	LSM4	0	4	89988000	217330000	0.39

Protein IDs	Protein names	Gene names	Q-value	Score	Intensity H	Intensity L	Ratio H/L
A0A0S2Z4T1	DNA replication licensing factor MCM3	MCM3	0	187	1.033E+09	3.186E+09	0.40
A0A0S2Z3L0	Electron transfer flavoprotein subunit alpha, mitochondrial	ETFA	0	44	623280000	1.382E+09	0.40
Q8NFH5	Nucleoporin NUP53	NUP35	0	81	206630000	398870000	0.40
Q5T7C4	High mobility group protein B1	HMGB1	0	98	2.916E+09	1.141E+10	0.40
A0A024R8M4	Phosphoribosyl pyrophosphate synthase-associated protein 1	PRPSAP1	0	20	88227000	200670000	0.41
G3V2D5	Zinc finger protein 36, C3H1 type-like 1	ZFP36L1	0	18	6238500	15019000	0.41
A6NMQ3	Alpha-endosulfine	ENSA	0	5	80231000	206330000	0.41
A0A0J9YYL3	Poly(U)-binding-splicing factor PUF60	PUF60	0	135	468910000	1.281E+09	0.42
A0A481SVJ4	Matrix-remodeling-associated protein 7	MXRA7	0	2	4184200	24167000	0.42
J3KTF8	Rho GDP-dissociation inhibitor 1	ARHGDIA	0	56	1.44E+09	3.59E+09	0.42
P49736	DNA replication licensing factor MCM2	MCM2	0	90	937140000	2.544E+09	0.43
K7EJH0	Kinetochore protein Spc24	SPC24	0	7	91278000	196000000	0.43
Q9BRA2	Thioredoxin domain-containing protein 17	TXNDC17	0	38	745240000	1.838E+09	0.43
P15531	Nucleoside diphosphate kinase A	NME1	0	20	312380000	966090000	0.43
D3DVA5	Rho guanine nucleotide exchange factor 2	ARHGEF2	0	16	26979000	80246000	0.44
B7ZM10	Exportin-6	XPO6	0	7	7924200	14822000	0.44
G8JLD3	ELKS/Rab6-interacting/CAST family member 1	ERC1	0	44	179630000	428430000	0.44
B2R7W3	Breast carcinoma amplified sequence 2	BCAS2	0	15	38190000	177190000	0.44
C9JJ19	28S ribosomal protein S34, mitochondrial	MRPS34	0	10	69862000	158490000	0.44
A0A0S2Z4Q4	Hepatocyte growth factor-regulated tyrosine kinase substrate	HGS	0	10	52165000	121060000	0.44
Q53Y51	D-dopachrome decarboxylase	DDT	0	36	259770000	672160000	0.45
A0A024R8U9	Pyrroline-5-carboxylate reductase 1, mitochondrial	PYCR1	0	20	72360000	265100000	0.45

Protein IDs	Protein names	Gene names	Q-value	Score	Intensity H	Intensity L	Ratio H/L
Q6FHQ0	Histone-binding protein RBBP7	RBBP7	0	160	2.134E+09	4.792E+09	0.45
P29144	Tripeptidyl-peptidase 2	TPP2	0	173	523060000	1.368E+09	0.45
Q9UP83	Conserved oligomeric Golgi complex subunit 5	COG5	0	5	14333000	32372000	0.46
E9PID8	Cleavage stimulation factor subunit 2	CSTF2	0	39	128240000	239460000	0.46
A0A024R496	Calcium-binding protein 39	CAB39	0	24	198430000	418650000	0.46
Q6IAP9	U4/U6 small nuclear ribonucleoprotein Prp4	PRPF4	0	42	168190000	621480000	0.46
A0A024RB32	Prostaglandin E synthase 3	PTGES3	0	110	2.02E+09	5.058E+09	0.46
E9PMG1	RalBP1-associated Eps domain-containing protein 1	REPS1	0	8	13894000	28102000	0.46
P28066	Proteasome subunit alpha type-5	PSMA5	0	107	1.677E+09	4.011E+09	0.46
I3L2G3	Ketosamine-3-kinase	FN3KRP	0	7	16246000	54477000	0.46
A0A0S2Z4Z0	RNA-binding protein 14	RBM14	0	83	606470000	1.446E+09	0.46
A8K651	Complement component 1 Q subcomponent-binding protein, mitochondrial	C1QBP	0	109	3.184E+09	7.587E+09	0.47
O60506	Heterogeneous nuclear ribonucleoprotein Q	SYNCRIP	0	121	3.657E+09	8.092E+09	0.47
P42345	Serine/threonine-protein kinase mTOR	MTOR	0	14	52206000	144780000	0.47
A8K878	Mesencephalic astrocyte-derived neurotrophic factor	MANF	0	38	604460000	1.613E+09	0.47
A0MNN4	Shwachman-Bodian-Diamond syndrome isoform 1	SMU1	0	60	321320000	679840000	0.47
A0A024R8B1	TBC1 domain family member 13	TBC1D13	0	4	20484000	74249000	0.47
Q9UHR4	Brain-specific angiogenesis inhibitor 1-associated protein 2-like protein 1	BAIAP2L1	0	6	21391000	41855000	0.47
Q5SRT3	Chloride intracellular channel protein 1	CLIC1	0	299	1.295E+10	2.924E+10	0.47
A0A0S2Z5I7	Ribosome maturation protein SBDS	SBDS	0	16	344540000	808860000	0.48
Q13505	Metaxin-1	MTX1	0	10	45737000	109770000	0.49
J3KS15	Peptidyl-tRNA hydrolase ICT1, mitochondrial	ICT1	0.01	2	29017000	45629000	0.50

Protein IDs	Protein names	Gene names	Q-value	Score	Intensity H	Intensity L	Ratio H/L
Q53HN4	DNA fragmentation factor subunit alpha	DFFA	0	31	272390000	539710000	0.50
P38919	Eukaryotic initiation factor 4A-III	EIF4A3	0	77	1.57E+09	3.534E+09	0.50
B4DY09	Interleukin enhancer-binding factor 2	ILF2	0	96	2.642E+09	6.06E+09	0.50
E9PF19	Transducin beta-like protein 2	TBL2	0	28	109400000	213970000	0.50
A0A087WXS7	ATPase ASNA1	ASNA1	0	63	850190000	1.755E+09	0.51
O43324	Eukaryotic translation elongation factor 1 epsilon-1	EEF1E1	0	29	662460000	1.236E+09	0.51
Q15717	ELAV-like protein 1	ELAVL1	0	92	2.093E+09	4.32E+09	0.51
Q9UMS4	Pre-mRNA-processing factor 19	PRPF19	0	127	897150000	2.364E+09	0.52
P14324	Farnesyl pyrophosphate synthase	FDPS	0	26	1.03E+09	2.078E+09	0.52
P28070	Proteasome subunit beta type-4	PSMB4	0	25	512090000	1E+09	0.52
Q0VGA5	SARS protein	SARS	0	149	1.216E+09	2.647E+09	0.53
A0A024RCX8	Peptidyl-prolyl cis-trans isomerase-like 1	PPIL1	0	10	122810000	365070000	0.53
Q9H8H0	Nucleolar protein 11	NOL11	0	5	22443000	80063000	0.54
E7EX90	Dynactin subunit 1	DCTN1	0	131	823150000	1.803E+09	0.54
Q05D78	Double-strand break repair protein MRE11A	MRE11A	0	3	24064000	56350000	0.54
H7C440	DIS3-like exonuclease 2	DIS3L2	0	4	13696000	21117000	0.54
Q9Y3U8	60S ribosomal protein L36	RPL36	0	34	544540000	770200000	0.55
Q9UJZ1	Stomatin-like protein 2, mitochondrial	STOML2	0	119	866230000	1.683E+09	0.55
Q567R6	Single-stranded DNA-binding protein, mitochondrial	SSBP1	0	60	561820000	1.077E+09	0.55
Q15084	Protein disulfide-isomerase A6	PDIA6	0	323	1.201E+10	2.023E+10	0.56
Q15645	Pachytene checkpoint protein 2 homolog	TRIP13	0	27	276670000	492930000	0.56
A0A024R6K8	Epididymis secretory sperm binding protein	WARS	0	80	1.769E+09	2.803E+09	0.56

Protein IDs	Protein names	Gene names	Q-value	Score	Intensity H	Intensity L	Ratio H/L
Q9NPD3	Exosome complex component RRP41	EXOSC4	0	25	239980000	490570000	0.57
Q9UHB9	Signal recognition particle subunit SRP68	SRP68	0	68	343910000	687640000	0.57
F5H0P4	Porphobilinogen deaminase	HMBS	0	9	38322000	129490000	0.57
Q96SB4	SRSF protein kinase 1	SRPK1	0	49	123510000	199050000	0.57
Q9Y6W5	Wiskott-Aldrich syndrome protein family member 2	WASF2	0	22	69082000	151250000	0.57
A0A024R8S5	Protein disulfide-isomerase	P4HB	0	300	1.656E+10	2.799E+10	0.57
A0A2X0SF71	Rho GTPase-activating protein 17	ARHGAP17	0	28	59467000	116590000	0.58
P09496	Clathrin light chain A	CLTA	0	7	508650000	765700000	0.58
R4GMU1	GDH/6PGL endoplasmic bifunctional protein	H6PD	0	4	20789000	34525000	0.60
Q8NCN5	Pyruvate dehydrogenase phosphatase regulatory subunit, mitochondrial	PDPR	0	3	10312000	28116000	0.60
Q8WY22	BRI3-binding protein	BRI3BP	0.01	2	5099700	6146700	0.62
Q6IB29	Probable rRNA-processing protein EBP2	EBNA1BP2	0	6	30468000	61825000	0.62
O15031	Plexin-B2	PLXNB2	0	18	30986000	221240000	0.62
C9JYQ9	60S ribosomal protein L22-like 1	RPL22L1	0	6	616860000	1.011E+09	0.66
Q9UNS2	COP9 signalosome complex subunit 3	COPS3	0	56	157900000	294180000	0.66
A0A0G2JNZ5	Glucosylceramidase	GBA	0	6	118570000	187510000	0.67
A0A140VK17	EH domain-binding protein 1	EHBP1	0	4	6547700	17018000	0.71
F5GWG3	Retinoic acid-induced protein 3	GPRC5A	0	11	149190000	185790000	0.76
S4R3V8	Lipolysis-stimulated lipoprotein receptor	LSR	0	4	26182000	34332000	1.05
Q9NWT6	Hypoxia-inducible factor 1-alpha inhibitor	HIF1AN	0	17	0	46940000	NaN
B7ZBQ1	Mediator of RNA polymerase II transcription subunit 20	MED20	0.01	2	0	18220000	NaN
H3BR38	Target of rapamycin complex subunit LST8	MLST8	0	3	0	13473000	NaN

Protein IDs	Protein names	Gene names	Q-value	Score	Intensity H	Intensity L	Ratio H/L
P52815	39S ribosomal protein L12, mitochondrial	MRPL12	0.01	2	0	0	NaN
A0A024R1I3	Pyridoxal phosphate phosphatase	PDXP	0	6	0	40714000	NaN
A0A2R8YDS2	Ras/Rap GTPase-activating protein SynGAP	SYNGAP1	0	2	0	18400000	NaN
J3KQA0	Synaptotagmin-1	SYT1	0	26	0	339450000	NaN
Q5W0C6	Torsin-3A	TOR3A	0	3	0	16493000	NaN
B4DSK7	Mediator of RNA polymerase II transcription subunit 1	MED1	0	2	0	14356000	NaN
Q99549	M-phase phosphoprotein 8	MPHOSPH8	0	12	0	15782000	NaN

Table 2.
The proteins of 116 EIF4A3-biding mRNAs and EIF4A3 were inhibited by ivermectin, identified with SILAC quantitative proteomics in ovarian cancer cells treated with (H) and without (L) ivermectin. Reproduced from Li et al. [4], with copyright permission from nature springer publisher, copyright 2020.

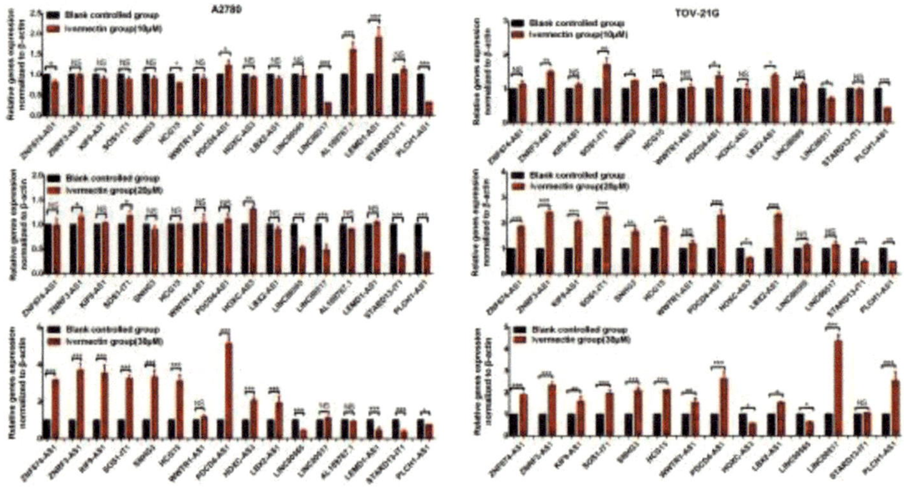

Figure 7.
RT-qPCR analysis revealed the effects of ivermectin on lncRNAs in ovarian cancers relative to control cells. Reproduced from Li et al. [4], with copyright permission from nature springer publisher, copyright 2020.

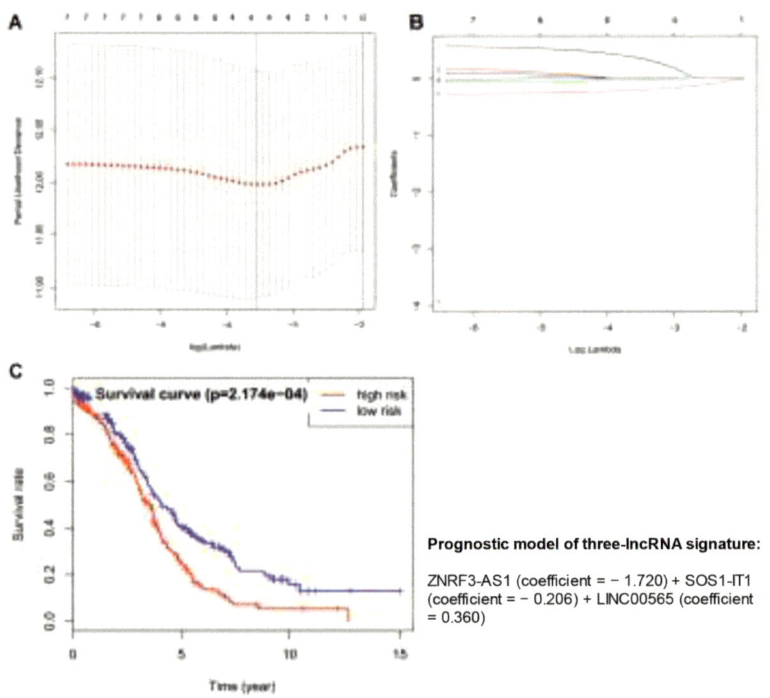

Figure 8.
Lasso regression identified and optimized the prognostic model of ivermectin-related three-lncRNA signature in ovarian cancers. (A and B). Lasso regression complexity is controlled by lambda using the glmnet R package. (C). Overall survival analysis of three-lncRNA signature between high-risk and low-risk groups. Reproduced from Li et al. [4], with copyright permission from nature springer publisher, copyright 2020.

4. Conclusions

Ivermectin, as an old, common, and classic anti-parasite drug, has demonstrated its effective *in vitro* anti-cancer efficiency for ovarian cancer. Ivermectin significantly inhibited cell proliferation, growth and migration, blocked cell cycle progression, and promoted cell apoptosis of human ovarian cancer cells. Drug pathway network analysis of ivermectin revealed that it was significantly related to the key molecules of four energy metabolism pathways, and RT-qPCR and immunoaffinity blot analyses found that ivermectin significantly regulated these key molecules for those energy metabolism pathways, including PFKP in glycolysis, IDH2 and IDH3B in Kreb's cycle, ND2, ND5, CYTB, and UQCRH in oxidative phosphorylation, and MCT1 and MCT4 in lactate shuttle. The integrative analysis of TCGA transcriptomics and mitochondrial proteomics in ovarian cancer revealed that 16 survival-related lncRNAs were mediated by ivermectin, which were further confirmed with RT-qPRC in human ovarian cancer cells. SILAC quantitative proteomics analysis revealed that the expressions of RNA-binding protein EIF4A3 and 116 EIF4A3-interacted genes were extensively inhibited by ivermectin. Those 116 EIF4A3-interacted proteins included those key molecules in four energy metabolism pathways, and those lncRNAs regulated EIF4A3-mRNA axes. Thus, ivermectin mediated lncRNA-EIF4A3-mRNA axes in ovarian cancer to exert its anticancer activities. Moreover, lasso regression identified the prognostic model of ivermectin-related three-lncRNA signature (ZNRF3-AS1, SOS1-IT1, and LINC00565), which was significantly associated with overall survival and clinicopathologic characteristics of ovarian cancer patients. These ivermectin-related molecular pattern alterations benefit for prognostic assessment and personalized drug therapy in the context of 3P medicine practice in ovarian cancer.

Moreover, one must realize that these achieved data about the anti-cancer activities of ivermectin in ovarian cancers are derived from the *in vitro* cell models. It is necessary to expand it into the *in vivo* animal experiments and pre-clinical and clinical experiments for its real application in ovarian cancers.

Acknowledgements

The authors acknowledge the financial supports from the Shandong First Medical University Talent Introduction Funds (to X.Z.), the Hunan Provincial Hundred Talent Plan (to X.Z.), and the grants from China "863" Plan Project (Grant No. 2014AA020610-1 to XZ).

Conflict of interest

We declare that we have no financial and personal relationships with other people or organizations.

Author's contributions

X.Z. conceived the concept, designed the manuscript, wrote and critically revised the manuscript, coordinated and was responsible for the correspondence work and financial support. N.L. participated in preparing figures, and partial literature analysis.

Acronyms and abbreviations

FDA	Federal Drug Administration
mtDEPs	differentially mitochondrial proteins
RT-qPCR	quantitative real-time PCR
SILAC	stable isotope labeling with amino acids in cell culture
TCGA	The Cancer Genome Atlas

Author details

Xianquan Zhan[1,2]* and Na Li[1,2]

1 University Creative Research Initiatives Center, Shandong First Medical University, Jinan, Shandong, China

2 Key Laboratory of Cancer Proteomics of Chinese Ministry of Health, Xiangya Hospital, Central South University, Changsha, China

*Address all correspondence to: yjzhan2011@gmail.com

References

[1] Burg RW, Miller BM, Baker EE, et al. Avermectins, new family of potent anthelmintic agents: producing organism and fermentation. Antimicrob Agents Chemother 1979; 15(3): 361–367.

[2] Crump A. Ivermectin: enigmatic multifaceted 'wonder' drug continues to surprise and exceed expectations. J Antibiot (Tokyo) 2017; 70(5): 495–505.

[3] Laing R, Gillan V, Devaney E. Ivermectin—old drug, new tricks? Trends Parasitol 2017; 33(6): 463–472.

[4] Li N, Zhan X. Anti-parasite drug ivermectin can suppress ovarian cancer by regulating lncRNA-EIF4A3-mRNA axes. EPMA J 2020; 11(2): 289–309.

[5] Li N, Zhao L, Zhan X. Quantitative proteomics reveals a broad-spectrum antiviral property of ivermectin, benefiting for COVID-19 treatment. J Cell Physiol 2020. DOI: 10.1002/jcp.30055.

[6] Liu J, Zhang K, Cheng L, Zhu H, Xu T. Progress in understanding the molecular mechanisms underlying the antitumour effects of ivermectin. Drug Des Devel Ther 2020; 14: 285–296.

[7] Juarez M, Schcolnik-Cabrera A, Duenas-Gonzalez A. The multitargeted drug ivermectin: from an antiparasitic agent to a repositioned cancer drug. Am J Cancer Res 2018; 8(2): 317–331.

[8] Kobayashi Y, Banno K, Kunitomi H, Tominaga E, Aoki D. Current state and outlook for drug repositioning anticipated in the field of ovarian cancer. J Gynecol Oncol 2019; 30(1): e10.

[9] Triarico S, Capozza MA, Mastrangelo S, Attinà G, Maurizi P, Ruggiero A. Gynecological cancer among adolescents and young adults (AYA). Ann Transl Med 2020; 8(6): 397.

[10] Li N, Zhan X. Mass spectrometry-based mitochondrial proteomics in human ovarian cancer. Mass Spectrom Rev 2020; 39(5–6): 471–498.

[11] Li N, Zhan X. Signaling pathway network alterations in human ovarian cancers identified with quantitative mitochondrial proteomics. EPMA J 2019; 10(2): 153–172.

[12] Li N, Li H, Cao L, Zhan X. Quantitative analysis of the mitochondrial proteome in human ovarian carcinomas. Endocr Relat Cancer 2018; 25(10): 909–931.

[13] Li N, Li J, Desiderio DM, Zhan X. SILAC quantitative proteomics analysis of vermectin-related proteomic profiling and molecular network alterations in human ovarian cancer cells. J Mass Spectrom 2020; e4659. DOI: 10.1002/jms.4659.

[14] Zhang X, Qin T, Zhu Z, et al. Ivermectin augments the in vitro and in vivo efficacy of cisplatin in epithelial ovarian cancer by suppressing Akt/mTOR signaling. Am J Med Sci 2020; 359(2): 123–129.

[15] Hashimoto H, Messerli SM, Sudo T, Maruta H. Ivermectin inactivates the kinase PAK1 and blocks the PAK1-dependent growth of human ovarian cancer and NF2 tumor cell lines. Drug Discov Ther 2009; 3(6): 243–246.

[16] Dou Q, Chen HN, Wang K, et al. Ivermectin induces cytostatic autophagy by blocking the PAK1/Akt axis in breast cancer. Cancer Res 2016; 76(15): 4457–4469.

[17] Song D, Liang H, Qu B, et al. Ivermectin inhibits the growth of glioma cells by inducing cell cycle arrest and apoptosis in vitro and in vivo. J Cell Biochem 2019; 120(1): 622–633.

[18] Nambara S, Masuda T, Nishio M, et al. Antitumor effects of the antiparasitic agent ivermectin via inhibition of Yes-associated protein 1 expression in gastric cancer. Oncotarget 2017; 8(64): 107666–107677.

[19] Melotti A, Mas C, Kuciak M, Lorente-Trigos A, Borges I, Ruiz i Altaba A. The river blindness drug ivermectin and related macrocyclic lactones inhibit WNT-TCF pathway responses in human cancer. EMBO Mol Med 2014; 6(10): 1263–1278.

[20] Slade L, Pulinilkunnil T. The MiTF/TFE family of transcription tactors: master regulators of organelle signaling, metabolism, and stress adaptation. Mol Cancer Res 2017; 15(12):1637–1643.

[21] Li N, Li H, Wang Y, Cao L, Zhan X. Quantitative proteomics revealed energy metabolism pathway alterations in human epithelial ovarian carcinoma and their regulation by the antiparasite drug ivermectin: data interpretation in the context of 3P medicine. EPMA J 2020; 11: 661–694.

[22] Guzzo CA, Furtek CI, Porras AG, Chen C, Tipping R, Clineschmidt CM, Lasseter KC. Safety, tolerability, and pharmacokinetics of escalating high doses of ivermectin in healthy adult subjects. J Clin Pharmacol. 2002; 42(10): 1122–1133.

[23] Li N, Zhan X, Zhan X. The lncRNA SNHG3 regulates energy metabolism of ovarian cancer by an analysis of mitochondrial proteomes. Gynecol Oncol. 2018; 150: 343–354.

Chapter 13

Novel Indications of Epigenetic Therapy in Ovarian Cancer

Courtney Griffiths, Michelle Bilbao, Lauren Krill and Olga Ostrovsky

Abstract

Early diagnosis and intervention are some of the longstanding challenges associated with ovarian cancer, which is the leading cause of gynecologic cancer mortality. While the majority of patients who present with advanced stage disease at time of diagnosis will initially respond to traditional combination platinum and taxane-based chemotherapy in conjunction with cytoreductive surgery, approximately 70% will ultimately recur due to chemoresistance within the first two years. Intratumor heterogeneity is proposed to be a leading factor in the development of chemoresistance and resultant poorer outcomes for those with recurrent or advanced stage disease. Both inherent and acquired mechanisms of chemoresistance are postulated to be a result of alterations in gene expression, also known as epigenetic modifications. Therefore, epigenetic therapy is a pivotal avenue which allows for reversal of chemoresistance in cancer through the targeting of aberrant mutations. In this chapter, we discuss how these epigenetic modifications prove to be promising targets in cancer therapy leading to heightened drug sensitivity and improved patient survival outcomes.

Keywords: cancer therapy, epigenetics, histone deacetylase inhibitors (HDACis), DNA methyltransferase inhibitors (DNMTis), tumor microenvironment

1. Introduction

1.1 Chemoresistance causes failure of classic ovarian cancer treatment

Ovarian cancer, similar to other malignancies, is characterized by molecular changes in cells which result in unregulated proliferation and spread to other organs [1]. Normal regulatory processes are disrupted and therefore aberrant cells are able to bypass checkpoints and lead to widespread metastatic potential [2]. Malignant ovarian neoplasms contribute to the highest mortality rates among women with gynecologic cancers [3]. Among them, high grade serous histologic subtypes are the most aggressive with an estimated 21,410 new cases and 13,770 ovarian cancer deaths in the United States in 2021 according to the American Cancer Society [4]. Due to limited feasibility of screening modalities in low risk patients and vague generalized symptoms, many patients are diagnosed at advanced stages contributing to a higher rate of treatment failures and poorer prognosis [5]. Traditional initial therapy consists of a combination of cytoreductive surgical management and platinum/taxane based chemotherapy [6]. The recommended surgical procedure includes a total hysterectomy with removal of bilateral fallopian tubes and ovaries, lymph node evaluation as well as evaluation and removal of all visible disease along the omentum and any peritoneal surfaces with full exploration of the abdomen and pelvis [7]. Despite the frequent initial success with the aforementioned approach, approximately 70% of patients develop recurrent disease either secondary to intrinsic or extrinsic causes of chemoresistance [8, 9]. Once the tumor is able to evade standard therapy, treatment options then become limited and the disease process is incurable [10]. As a result, chemoresistance is one of the leading causes of mortality among advanced stage and recurrent ovarian cancer patients. Multiple mechanisms are responsible for inducing chemoresistance, and a better understanding of these processes may lead to better treatment outcomes for patients with progressive disease [11].

1.2 Histologic subtypes and tumorigenesis

Ovarian cancer can arise from several different cell types including epithelial, germ cell and mesenchymal (stromal) origins. These histological classifications vary widely with regard to treatment options and prognosis likely secondary to unique molecular and biologic features among each subtype [12, 13]. Epithelial ovarian cancer (EOC) accounts for 90% of ovarian cancer and can be subdivided into high grade serous, low grade serous, endometrioid, clear cell, mucinous, transitional cell, among several other subtypes with over two-thirds comprising high grade serous histology [14, 15]. Among high grade serous lesions, p53 mutations are typically omnipresent as well as other important germline and somatic mutations (BRCA 1, BRCA 2, and additional homologous recombinant genes), and tend to lead to more favorable treatment outcomes [16]. Although these gene mutations may induce chemoresistant disease, it is predominantly epimutations and their associated changes in gene expression which are thought to drive tumorigenesis. As chemoresistance may be innate or acquired even after an initial positive response to platinum therapy, it is plausible that genes involved in epigenetic reprogramming are controlled by specific transcription factors, and therefore may serve as a potential target for treatment [17, 18].

As with most malignancies, the staging of ovarian cancer and concurrent optimal cytoreduction plays a pertinent role in determining prognosis [19]. Ovarian neoplasms are staged surgically and according to the International Federation of Gynecology and Obstetrics (FIGO) classification. The 5-year overall survival rate differs significantly between early and advanced stage disease at 90% for Stage I disease and approximately 15–40% for Stage III/IV disease [20]. As most ovarian cancers are diagnosed in advanced stages, an individual's response to standard platinum chemotherapeutic agents becomes a major prognosticator in determining outcomes [21, 22].

1.3 Can epigenetic therapy overcome ovarian cancer chemoresistance?

The mainstay approach to treatment of high grade serous carcinomas is with a platinum based chemotherapeutic agent whereas other histologic subtypes prove to be more chemoresistant [23]. As primary treatments involve a platinum and taxane chemotherapeutic agent, an important predictor of progression free and overall survival is the platinum-free interval [24]. Patients are classified as platinum sensitive should disease recurrence occur greater than 6 months from completion of therapy, platinum resistant if less than 6 months and refractory if progression occurs through therapy [25]. This subclassification is imperative to predicting which patients will likely recur after initial therapy and will require molecular analyses in order to determine a more targeted treatment approach. Unfortunately, only 15% of patients who develop chemoresistance respond to subsequent therapies and many ultimately will succumb to their disease within one year [26]. Multiple mechanisms have been suggested for acquired chemoresistance such as mutations in the cancer cells themselves, DNA repair failures as well as epigenetic changes [27–29].

For example, cancer stem cells (CSCs) which are capable of self-renewal, differentiation and tumorigenicity have been indicated in the development of platinum resistance disease [30, 31]. One particular study demonstrated upregulated expression of stem cell markers CD44, CD133, and ALDH1A1 in recurrent ovarian cancer in comparison to primary tumors [32]. DNA repair failures may also occur in nucleotide excision, recombination, and mismatch repair pathways enabling cancer cells to exploit repair mechanisms and therefore induce an acquired chemoresistance [33]. Point of nonsense mutations in oncogenes such as Ras or ERK signaling and/or DNA repair genes such as p53, PARP, BRCA 1 and 2 have been evidenced to cause chemoresistance and subsequent failure in standard oncologic treatments [34]. All in all, cancer renewal and heterogeneity are the main reasons for the development of chemoresistance and subsequent failure in standard oncologic treatments [35].

Another important component includes epigenetic modifications which result in silencing as well as activation of gene expression without DNA sequence alteration [36]. The majority of cancers, including ovarian cancer, have aberrant epigenetic modifications which result in the promotion of cancer growth, metastasis and chemoresistance [37].

1.4 Epigenetics

The field of epigenetics has gained heightened interest in the field of oncology over the years. This new concept of study was first described by Conrad Waddington in 1942 where he demonstrated the inheritance of an acquired characteristic in a particular population [38]. Although the definition has evolved over the years, the overall essence of epigenetics involves the alterations in gene expression without modification of the DNA sequence itself [39]. In other words, these aberrant changes are maintained through cell division without producing a change in the overall genetic information [40]. As stated previously, epigenetic alterations affect chromatin structure through a variety of mechanisms, altering patterns of gene expression. Disruptions in these epigenetic processes can in turn lead to altered gene function and further, malignant transformation through oncogene activation or tumor suppressor gene silencing [41]. As human cancer cells harbor aberrant epigenetic abnormalities, cancer progression is then enabled and mechanisms of resistance develop, which creates an opportunity for targeted therapy using epigenetic inhibitors.

Promoter hypermethylation silences crucial genes including but not limited to p16, SPARC, CTGF, CDH1 and ICAM-1. Other genes involved in methylation dysregulation include PTEN (seen in type 1 ovarian cancers), and those involved with suppression of metastasis [42]. Several studies have utilized DNA methylation assays in order to identify potential epigenetic biomarkers in cell free DNA for ovarian cancer in order to improve on early screening challenges [43–45]. This method of identification and targeting of differentially methylated regions (DMRs) has the potential to identify populations of at-risk patients for the development of epithelial ovarian cancers.

Moreover, epigenetic agents have already proved effective in acting as chemotherapy sensitizers by essentially improving or re-establishing tumor sensitivity as well as reversing resistant disease in a multitude of studies [46–48]. Where patients may ultimately be classified as platinum resistant, the use of epigenetic agents have the potential to reinvoke a response to platinum agents with one study demonstrating a 35% objective response rate after administration of decitabine followed by carboplatin among platinum resistant ovarian cancer patients [48]. Therefore, current research is concentrated on the development of treatment methodologies involving the use of classic chemotherapy in combination or sequentially with epigenetic regimens in order to overcome chemoresistance and improve outcomes.

2. Epigenetic aberrations in ovarian cancer

2.1 DNA methylation

One of the most common methods of epigenetic modulation is through DNA methylation. Modification of cytosine residues in CpG dinucleotides or CpG islands by methylation leads to transcriptional silencing in vertebrates, however, non-CpG methylation has also been identified in stem cells [49]. Typically, small amounts of CpG island promoters are methylated in normal cells, however, in the presence of hypermethylation, tumorigenesis is often incited [50]. The particular enzymes that are responsible for DNA methylation are DNA methyltransferases (DNMTs) which include DNMT1, DNMT3A, DNMT3A, DNMT3B, and DNMT3C. These enzymes are classified as either *de novo* or maintenance groups, of which *de novo* are more specific to stem cell expression (DNMT3s) whereas DNTM1 is involved in maintenance of DNA methylation during cell division [51].

Both DNA hypomethylation and gene promoter DNA hypermethylation are major oncogenic driving factors. Specifically, hypermethylation of promoters on tumor suppressor genes BRCA 1 and BRCA 2 lead to their silencing and subsequent inactivation of DNA repair driving the development of malignancies such as breast and ovarian cancers [51, 52]. However, the earliest methylation errors were of reduced activity resulting in increased mutation rates. Notably, transcription of repeats, transposable elements (TEs) and oncogenes occurred secondary to changes from hypomethylation through the loss of DNMT1 function [41, 53].

2.2 Histone acetylation

DNA is packaged as chromatin which is composed of nucleosomes. In turn, the nucleosome is comprised of histone proteins (H3, H4, H2A, H2B) which can similarly undergo many modifications and affect DNA transcription, replication and repair [54]. A "histone code" exists in order to regulate chromatin structure through several different histone modifications, which can lead to either activation or repression dependent on the residues and type of modification such as acetylation, ubiquitylation, sumoylation and phosphorylation [40, 55] (**Figure 1**). Dysregulation of any of these functions can lead to oncogenic activation or even the silencing of tumor suppressor genes.

In comparison to DNA methylation, errors in chromatin modification in the development of epithelial ovarian cancers is less understood but also pertinent. The overexpression of class I histone deacetylases (HDACs) has been identified in several cancers, with a prominent association identified in high risk ovarian of serous and clear cell subtypes. In addition, an unfavorable prognostic correlation was seen in patients with endometrioid histologies [56].

2.3 MicroRNA dysregulation

Along with histone modification and methylation dysregulation, cancer cells are prone to errors in microRNA (miRNA) regulation. MiRNAs are small non-coding

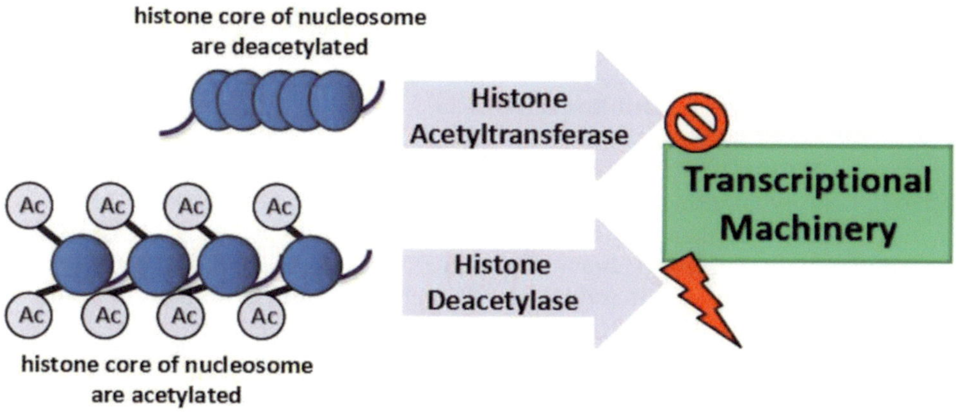

Figure 1.
The effect of histone acetylation and deacetylation on DNA transcription.

RNAs of 19–22 nucleotides in length which regulate the expression of certain genes either through degradation or inhibition of target mRNA [57]. The expression of epigenetic regulators (DNMTs and HDACs) are controlled by these miRNAs in a feedback loop of which when dysregulated, can lead to carcinogenic potential [58]. Genome analysis reveals condensed areas of miRNAs in cancer-associated genomic regions signifying that dysregulation of these particular areas could lead to aberrant expression [59]. With regard to epithelial ovarian cancer development, the aberrant expression of miRNAs can emulate oncogenic or tumor suppressor activity [60]. The overexpression of some types of miRNA as well as decreased activity of others were more closely correlated with ovarian cancer cells in comparison to healthy ovarian epithelial cells in several studies [61, 62], indicating another potential for early diagnostic screening and opportunity for intervention.

3. The clinical application of epigenetic therapies

3.1 DNA methylation inhibitors (DNMTis)

DNA methylation inhibitors (DNMTis) are deoxycytosine analogs. DNMTis prevent methyl group transfer by covalently binding to and trapping methyltransferases [63]. The simplest way to understand the effect of DNMTis is through their effect on oncogenes and tumor suppressor genes [64]. BRCA1 and BRCA2 are oncogenes that when hypermethylated, can lead to a variety of cancers including ovarian cancer [65]. In a similar way, demethylation of tumor suppressor genes like p53, MLH1, H1C1, p16, E-cadherin and APC, can also play a role in the genetic instability that leads to the development of ovarian cancer, its propagation and chemoresistance [64]. Indeed, both demethylation and hypermethylation of the genome have been associated with the development of platinum resistance in ovarian cancer [64]. Consequently, DNMTis have been shown in preclinical models to restore chemosensitivity and restore normal epigenetics [66].

The most commonly utilized DNA methyltransferase inhibitors are 5-azacitidine (AZA) and decitabine (5-aza-2'deoxycytidine) [63]. Both were developed in the 1960s for the treatment of hematologic malignancies and are currently FDA approved for myelodysplastic syndromes. Both AZA and decitabine have demonstrated some efficacy in clinical and pre-clinical ovarian cancer studies, however, their dose-limiting myelotoxicity limits their practical use. As they can be toxic, other DNMTis are currently under investigation: zebularine, procaine epigallocatechin-3-gallate (EGCG) (from green tea extracts), and RG 108 [64].

3.2 Histone deacetylase inhibitors (HDACis)

Histone deacetylase inhibitors (HDACis) act by targeting the zinc ion required for the catalytic function of the class I, II and IV HDACs [64]. The class III HDACs are not zinc dependent and are not inhibited by any of the current HDACis. HDACis are stratified by activity and chemical structure. There are pan-HDAC inhibitors, which affect classes I, II and IV, as well as class-specific inhibitors [67]. The chemical structure of HDACis include: hydroxamic acids, cyclic tetrapeptides, benzamides, and short-chain aliphatic acids [67]. They act on ovarian cancer in the alteration of gene transcription and chromatin remodeling [64]. In doing so, HDACis arrest cell growth, promote apoptosis, and inhibit angiogenesis [64].

The largest group of HDACis are the hydroxamic acids: vorinostat (suberanilohydroxamic acid or SAHA), belinostat, and panobinostat, all of which are pan-HDAC inhibitors FDA approved for hematologic malignancies [64]. Romidepsin, a tetrapeptide, has specific activity against Class I HDAC and is currently FDA approved for the treatment of cutaneous t-cell lymphoma [64]. Another HDACi in this group is etinostat [64]. Valproic acid is a short-chain aliphatic acid and is overall a weak HDACi with little clinical utility [64].

Since aberrant DNA methylation and histone acetylation contribute to the progression, metastasis and chemoresistance of high grade serous ovarian cancer, epigenetic drugs are thought to have the capability of reversing these effects (**Figure 2**).

3.3 Other epigenetic therapies

While DNMTis and HDACis have been more extensively studied, other epigenetic therapies are on the horizon. These drugs target methylation and

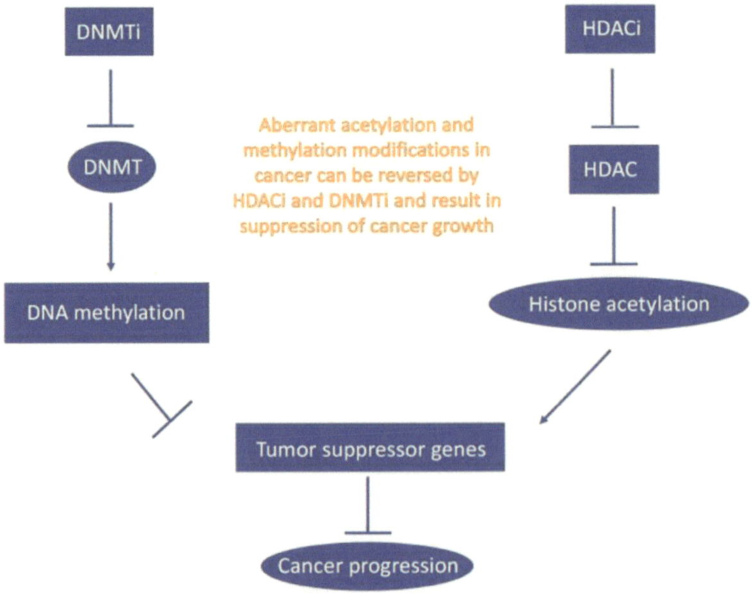

Figure 2.
The Role of DNA methyltransferase inhibitors (DNMTis) and histone deacetylase inhibitors (HDACis) in halting tumorigenesis.

phosphorylation of the cancer genome. Examples are small molecule inhibitors targeting the histone lysine methyltransferases EZH2 and inhibitors of bromodomain proteins, BET inhibitors [64]. G9A is one such target. It is a histone methyltransferase that demethylates H3K9 and is detected in 71.6% of metastatic high grade serous cancers [68]. JQ1 is an agent that targets the bromodomain and extraterminal (BET) protein BRD4 [68]. In preclinical models, JQ1 has suppressed BRD4 and restored cisplatin sensitivity in ovarian cancer [68]. Furthermore, JQ1 has been shown by other researchers to synergize with PARP inhibitors in ovarian cancer cells that are proficient in homologous recombination [68, 69]. These newer epigenetic therapies hold promise, but still need further investigation.

3.4 Efficacy of different inhibitors

It is important to note that in pre-clinical models, epigenetic therapies are more active against tumor cells, while normal cells appear to be resistant to their effects. [64] Yet, this is a double-edge sword. Because epigenetic regulators have a broad impact over the entire genome, there will be great anti-tumor effects, but also unintended nonspecific consequences [68]. These nonspecific effects explain the toxicities seen in the clinical trials done with epigenetic therapies.

4. Relevant clinical trials using epigenetic therapy in ovarian cancer

4.1 Success and failures

Clinical translation studies with epigenetic therapy have had mixed results, but the most success with epigenetic therapy appears to be when it is used in combination with other agents and at the lowest effective dose [64]. This was discovered with one of the first epigenetic clinical trials in 2008, when the Gynecologic Oncology Group learned that as a single agent, SAHA is not very effective. They conducted a phase II study of vorinostat (SAHA) in the treatment of 27 platinum resistant patients. While 9 of 27 patients had stabilization of their disease, only 1 of 27 had a partial response and only 2 patients had a progression free survival of greater than 6 months [70]. In 2013, Mendivil and colleagues conducted a study where vorinostat was given in combination with paclitaxel and carboplatin to 18 patients as upfront therapy. The investigators reported a 50 percent total response rate, however, the study was closed prematurely due to safety concerns. Patients suffered grade 3 and 4 neutropenia. Additionally, three bowel perforations effected closure of the study [71]. Matulonis et al. in 2015 conducted a phase 1 trial of platinum sensitive patients at their first recurrence again using vorinostat. In this trial, vorinostat was given with gemcitabine and carboplatin. This combination has also demonstrated some efficacy in the recurrent setting but had significant hematologic toxicity, namely, thrombocytopenia and neutropenia [72].

Fu and colleagues used azacitidine (AZA) to re-sensitize 17 platinum resistant patients to carboplatin in a phase Ib-II trial [73]. While the numbers were small, a partial response was noted in 70 percent of patients with an overall response rate of 22 percent [73]. Notably, these investigators gave their patients 5 days of AZA prior to carboplatin [73]. As it appears, epigenetic therapies may be most advantageous when used to augment classic chemotherapy and even immunotherapy, as opposed to being given in isolation or in combination with an existing regimen.

Oza and colleages recently conducted a larger study with 103 patients [74]. It randomized patients to guadecitabine and carboplatin versus investigator's choice (topotecan, pegylated liposomal doxorubicin, paclitaxel or gemcitabine) until disease progression or unacceptable toxicity. Cross-over was allowed from the standard arm to the experimental arm and 27 patients crossed-over. The combination of guadecitabine and carboplatin was found to be effective, however the median progression free survival of 16 weeks when compared to the 9 weeks in the standard treatment arm was not found to be statistically significant [74].

4.2 The administration of epigenetic therapy – better together?

One approach to utilizing epigenetic therapy effectively up front is in alternating treatments of classic chemotherapy and epigenetic therapy. This method was found to be effective and less toxic in clinical translational studies [73, 74]. Sequential administration of classic chemotherapy and epigenetic drugs not only suppresses ovarian cancer growth *in vitro*, but also spares toxicity to normal cells and preserves the healing ability of stem cells [75]. Furthermore, chemotherapy and epigenetic therapy act synergistically allowing smaller doses of both to be administered. In turn, this decreases the toxicity of both chemotherapy and epigenetic therapy [69]. This methodology has yet to be broadly adopted in clinical trials involving epigenetic therapy.

For recurrent disease, epigenetic therapy may have utility. Epigenetic therapy restores platinum sensitivity as both hypermethylation and histone modification contribute to chemoresistance, reversing these epigenetic changes, should reverse the chemoresistance [64]. This has been borne out in the literature as less than 10 percent of platinum resistant patients would be expected to respond to platinum again, yet pretreatment with AZA yields a 22 percent response and decitabine, a 35 percent response [64]. Taxol resistance has not been as heavily explored in the literature as platinum resistance, however, epigenetic therapy, may re-sensitize ovarian cancer to paclitaxel as it does cisplatin. In one preclinical study, the HDACi panobinostat was used to re-sensitize ovarian cancer cell lines that had become resistant to paclitaxel [76]. These researchers were further able to demonstrate that when human ovarian cancer xenografts were implanted in a murine model, panobinostat in combination with cisplatin and paclitaxel was superior in efficacy to cisplatin-paclitaxel or panobinostat alone [76]. Thus, epigenetics may possibly be used upfront to “prime” or increase the efficacy of classic chemotherapy. Additionally, they may be sequenced in between classic chemotherapy and again when patients recur to re-sensitize them to platinum and taxol agents.

5. Future directions in improving patents care outcomes

5.1 Epigenetics and immunotherapy

There is biologic plausibility that epigenetic therapies can prime tumors for a better response to immunotherapy and turn “cold” tumors into “hot” ones [68]. For example, in one murine model, the combination of decitabine and anti-CTLA-4 significantly shrunk tumors and prolonged survival as compared to either agent alone [77]. There is additional preclinical data suggesting that AZA can upregulate T-cells in murine models [78]. Additionally, two clinical trials are currently underway. The results from one study of 75 patients are expected in March 2022 (NCT03206047). Its investigators are looking at AZA and atezolizumab with or without the anti-NY-ESO-1 vaccine (a biologic agent) in women with recurrent platinum resistant ovarian cancer. The other study is looking at guadecitabine with pembrolizumab for recurrent ovarian cancer (NCT02901899). Thirty-five patients have been enrolled in this latter study and results are expected in March 2022.

5.2 Epigenetics and precision medicine

The heterogeneity of ovarian cancer is such that no two tumors are alike, however, tumors expressing similar genetic profiles, have been shown to respond to agents targeting their specific genetics. Recent clinical trials indicate that ovarian cancer patients with homologous recombination deficiency, for example, respond well to PARP inhibition [79, 80]. Newer epigenetic therapies like BET inhibitors, have the ability enhance PARP inhibition [69]. Another clinical challenge in ovarian cancer is the *ARID1A* mutation. Ovarian cancers with this mutation are associated with late-stage disease at diagnosis and early recurrence [81]. Roughly 50 percent of clear cell carcinomas, which are notoriously chemoresistant, harbor this mutation. In one murine model, the HDACi vorinostat was found to be highly effective against ARID1A mutated ovarian cancer [81]. Thus, epigenetics may help further precision medicine and the targeting of actionable mutations.

6. Conclusion

Platinum resistant and recurrent ovarian cancer patients have very little in the way of highly effective treatment. Chemotherapy may be effective for a period of months or a few years for these patients, but it is rarely if ever curable. Epigenetic therapies hold promise, especially in conjunction with other mechanisms, like PARP inhibitors and immunotherapy, but the timing, dosing and patient selection must be fine-tuned before they can enter the mainstream of treatment for ovarian cancer.

Acknowledgements

This work has been funded by The Research Initiative Grant, Camden Health Research Program and Research Grant, The Cooper MD Anderson Cancer Foundation - Pink Roses Teal Magnolias.

Conflict of interest

The authors declare no conflict of interest.

Author details

Courtney Griffiths[1], Michelle Bilbao[1], Lauren Krill[1] and Olga Ostrovsky[2*]

1 Department of Gynecologic Oncology, MD Anderson Cancer Center at Cooper, Camden, NJ, USA

2 Department of Surgical Research, Cooper University Health Care, Camden, NJ, USA

*Address all correspondence to: ostrovsky-olga@cooperhealth.edu

References

[1] Cancer. CGTCAMA 2nd edition. S (MA): SA 2000. TD and C of.

[2] López-Reig R, López-Guerrero JA. The hallmarks of ovarian cancer: proliferation and cell growth. *Eur J Cancer Suppl*. 2020;15:27-37. doi:https://doi.org/10.1016/j.ejcsup.2019.12.001

[3] Momenimovahed Z, Tiznobaik A, Taheri S, Salehiniya H. Ovarian cancer in the world: epidemiology and risk factors. *Int J Womens Health*. 2019;11:287-299. doi:10.2147/IJWH.S197604

[4] Society AC. No Title. Published 2021. https://www.cancer.org/cancer/ovarian-cancer/about/key-statistics.html

[5] Brain KE, Smits S, Simon AE, et al. Ovarian cancer symptom awareness and anticipated delayed presentation in a population sample. *BMC Cancer*. 2014;14:171. doi:10.1186/1471-2407-14-171

[6] Della Pepa C, Tonini G, Pisano C, et al. Ovarian cancer standard of care: are there real alternatives? *Chin J Cancer*. 2015;34(1):17-27. doi:10.5732/cjc.014.10274

[7] Pomel C, Jeyarajah A, Oram D, et al. Cytoreductive surgery in ovarian cancer. *Cancer Imaging*. 2007;7(1):210-215. doi:10.1102/1470-7330.2007.0030

[8] Pokhriyal R, Hariprasad R, Kumar L, Hariprasad G. Chemotherapy Resistance in Advanced Ovarian Cancer Patients. *Biomark Cancer*. 2019;11:1179299X19860815-1179299X19860815. doi:10.1177/1179299X19860815

[9] Matsuo K, Lin YG, Roman LD, Sood AK. Overcoming platinum resistance in ovarian carcinoma. *Expert Opin Investig Drugs*. 2010;19(11):1339-1354. doi:10.1517/13543784.2010.515585

[10] Vasey PA. Resistance to chemotherapy in advanced ovarian cancer: mechanisms and current strategies. *Br J Cancer*. 2003;89 Suppl 3(Suppl 3):S23-8. doi:10.1038/sj.bjc.6601497

[11] Liu MX, Chan D, Ngan H. Gynecology & Obstetrics. *Gynecol Obstet*. Published online 2012:2-5. doi:10.4172/2161-0932.1000e104

[12] Lalwani N, Fasih N. Histologic , Molecular , and Cytogenetic Fea- tures of Ovarian Cancers : Implications for Diagno- sis and Treatment 1. Published online 2011.

[13] Kaku T, Ogawa S, Kawano Y, et al. Histological classification of ovarian cancer. *Med electron Microsc Off J Clin Electron Microsc Soc Japan*. 2003;36(1):9-17. doi:10.1007/s007950300002

[14] Gubbels JA, Claussen N, Kapur AK, Connor JP, Patankar MS. The detection, treatment, and biology of epithelial ovarian cancer. *J Ovarian Res*. 2010;3(1):1-11. doi:10.1186/1757-2215-3-8

[15] Rojas V, Hirshfield KM, Ganesan S, Rodrigucz-Rodriguez L. Molecular characterization of epithelial ovarian cancer: Implications for diagnosis and treatment. *Int J Mol Sci*. 2016;17(12). doi:10.3390/ijms17122113

[16] Manchana T, Phoolcharoen N, Tantbirojn P. BRCA mutation in high grade epithelial ovarian cancers. *Gynecol Oncol Reports*. 2019;29(April):102-105. doi:10.1016/j.gore.2019.07.007

[17] Liu, D., Zhang, XX., Li, MC. *et al.* C/EBPβ enhances platinum resistance of ovarian cancer cells by reprogramming H3K79 methylation. *Nat Commun* **9**, 1739 (2018). https://doi.org/10.1038/s41467-018-03590-5

[18] Glasspool, R., Teodoridis, J. & Brown, R. Epigenetics as a mechanism driving polygenic clinical drug resistance. *Br J Cancer* **94,** 1087-1092 (2006). https://doi.org/10.1038/sj.bjc.6603024

[19] Chang LC, Huang CF, Lai MS, Shen LJ, Wu FL, Cheng WF. Prognostic factors in epithelial ovarian cancer: A population-based study. *PLoS One*. 2018;13(3):e0194993. Published 2018 Mar 26. doi:10.1371/journal.pone.0194993

[20] Ovarian C, Be C, Early F, et al. Ovarian Cancer Early Detection , Diagnosis , and Staging Can Ovarian Cancer Be Found Early ? :1-24.

[21] Bouberhan, S., Pujade-Lauraine, E., & Cannistra, S. A. (2019). Advances in the management of platinum-sensitive relapsed ovarian cancer. *Journal of Clinical Oncology*, *37*(27), 2424-2436. https://doi.org/10.1200/JCO.19.00314

[22] Pujade-Lauraine E, Banerjee S, Pignata S. Management of Platinum-Resistant, Relapsed Epithelial Ovarian Cancer and New Drug Perspectives. *J Clin Oncol*. 2019;37(27):2437-2448. doi:10.1200/JCO.19.00194

[23] Kim S, Han Y, Kim SI, Kim H-S, Kim SJ, Song YS. Tumor evolution and chemoresistance in ovarian cancer. *NPJ Precis Oncol*. 2018;2:20. doi:10.1038/s41698-018-0063-0

[24] Tomao F, D'Incalci M, Biagioli E, Peccatori FA, Colombo N. Restoring platinum sensitivity in recurrent ovarian cancer by extending the platinum-free interval: Myth or reality? *Cancer*. 2017;123(18):3450-3459. doi:10.1002/cncr.30830

[25] Pujade-Lauraine E, Combe P. Recurrent ovarian cancer. *Ann Oncol*. 2016;27(Supplement 1):i63-i65. doi:10.1093/annonc/mdw079

[26] Davis A, Tinker A V, Friedlander M. "Platinum resistant" ovarian cancer: what is it, who to treat and how to measure benefit? *Gynecol Oncol*. 2014;133(3):624-631. doi:10.1016/j.ygyno.2014.02.038

[27] Van Zyl B, Tang D, Bowden NA. Biomarkers of platinum resistance in ovarian cancer: What can we use to improve treatment. *Endocr Relat Cancer*. 2018;25(5):R303-R318. doi:10.1530/ERC-17-0336

[28] Gee ME, Faraahi Z, McCormick A, Edmondson RJ. DNA damage repair in ovarian cancer: Unlocking the heterogeneity. *J Ovarian Res*. 2018;11(1):1-12. doi:10.1186/s13048-018-0424-x

[29] Balch C, Fang F, Matei DE, Huang TH-M, Nephew KP. Minireview: epigenetic changes in ovarian cancer. *Endocrinology*. 2009;150(9):4003-4011. doi:10.1210/en.2009-0404

[30] Li X, Lewis MT, Huang J, et al. Intrinsic resistance of tumorigenic breast cancer cells to chemotherapy. *J Natl Cancer Inst*. 2008;100(9):672-679. doi:10.1093/jnci/djn123

[31] Yu Z, Pestell TG, Lisanti MP, Pestell RG. Cancer stem cells. *Int J Biochem Cell Biol*. 2012;44(12):2144-2151. doi:10.1016/j.biocel.2012.08.022

[32] Steg AD, Bevis KS, Katre AA, et al. Stem cell pathways contribute to clinical chemoresistance in ovarian cancer. *Clin Cancer Res*. 2012;18(3):869-881. doi:10.1158/1078-0432.CCR-11-2188

[33] Kiwerska K. DNA repair in cancer initiation , progression , and therapy — a double-edged sword. Published online 2019:329-334.

[34] Zhang X, Qi Z, Yin H, Yang G. The ranostics Interaction between p53 and Ras signaling controls cisplatin

resistance via HDAC4- and HIF-1 α -mediated regulation of apoptosis and autophagy. 2019;9(4). doi:10.7150/thno.29673

[35] Phi LTH, Sari IN, Yang Y-G, et al. Cancer Stem Cells (CSCs) in Drug Resistance and their Therapeutic Implications in Cancer Treatment. *Stem Cells Int*. 2018;2018:5416923. doi:10.1155/2018/5416923

[36] Handy DE, Castro R, Loscalzo J. Epigenetic modifications: basic mechanisms and role in cardiovascular disease. *Circulation*. 2011;123(19):2145-2156. doi:10.1161/CIRCULATIONAHA.110.956839

[37] Ashraf AHMZ, Afroze SH, Osuji GA, et al. Epigenetic Modifications in Ovarian Cancer : A Review. 2020;4:17-35.

[38] Noble D. Conrad Waddington and the origin of epigenetics. *J Exp Biol*. 2015;218(6):816 LP -818. doi:10.1242/jeb.120071

[39] Yang Q, Yang Y, Zhou N, et al. Epigenetics in ovarian cancer: premise, properties, and perspectives. *Mol Cancer*. 2018;17(1):109. doi:10.1186/s12943-018-0855-4

[40] Sharma S, Kelly TK, Jones PA. Epigenetics in cancer. *Carcinogenesis*. 2010;31(1):27-36. doi:10.1093/carcin/bgp220

[41] Baylin SB, Jones PA. Epigenetic Determinants of Cancer. *Cold Spring Harb Perspect Biol*. 2016;8(9):a019505. doi:10.1101/cshperspect.a019505

[42] Singh A, Gupta S, Sachan M. Epigenetic Biomarkers in the Management of Ovarian Cancer: Current Prospectives. *Front cell Dev Biol*. 2019;7:182. doi:10.3389/fcell.2019.00182

[43] Gooden GC, Legendre C, Spillman M, Goel A, Salhia B. Abstract 3309: Circulating epigenetic biomarkers for the early detection of ovarian cancer. *Cancer Res*. 2018;78(13 Supplement):3309 LP -3309. doi:10.1158/1538-7445.AM2018-3309

[44] Wu T-I, Huang R-L, Su P-H, Mao S-P, Wu C-H, Lai H-C. Ovarian cancer detection by DNA methylation in cervical scrapings. *Clin Epigenetics*. 2019;11(1):166. doi:10.1186/s13148-019-0773-3

[45] Tew BY, Gooden G, Buckley DN, et al. Abstract PR02: Epigenetic biomarkers in cell-free DNA for early detection of high-grade serous ovarian carcinoma. *Clin Cancer Res*. 2020;26(11 Supplement):PR02 LP-PR02. doi:10.1158/1557-3265.LiqBiop20-PR02

[46] Strathdee G, MacKean MJ, Illand M, Brown R. A role for methylation of the hMLH1 promoter in loss of hMLH1 expression and drug resistance in ovarian cancer. *Oncogene*. 1999;18(14):2335-2341. doi:10.1038/sj.onc.1202540

[47] Plumb JA, Strathdee G, Sludden J, Kaye SB, Brown R. Reversal of Drug Resistance in Human Tumor Xenografts by 2′-Deoxy-5-azacytidine-induced Demethylation of the <em>hMLH1</em> Gene Promoter. *Cancer Res*. 2000;60(21):6039 LP -6044. http://cancerres.aacrjournals.org/content/60/21/6039.abstract

[48] Matei D, Fang F, Shen C, et al. Epigenetic Resensitization to Platinum in Ovarian Cancer. *Cancer Res*. 2012;72(9):2197 LP -2205. doi:10.1158/0008-5472.CAN-11-3909

[49] Ramsahoye BH, Biniszkiewicz D, Lyko F, Clark V, Bird AP, Jaenisch R. Non-CpG methylation is prevalent in embryonic stem cells and may be mediated by DNA methyltransferase 3a. *Proc Natl Acad Sci U S A*. 2000;97(10):5237-5242. doi:10.1073/pnas.97.10.5237

[50] Arechederra M, Daian F, Yim A, et al. Hypermethylation of gene body CpG islands predicts high dosage of functional oncogenes in liver cancer. *Nat Commun*. 2018;9(1):3164. doi:10.1038/s41467-018-05550-5

[51] Gujar H, Weisenberger DJ, Liang G. The Roles of Human DNA Methyltransferases and Their Isoforms in Shaping the Epigenome. *Genes (Basel)*. 2019;10(2):172. doi:10.3390/genes10020172

[52] Ibragimova I, Cairns P. Assays for hypermethylation of the BRCA1 gene promoter in tumor cells to predict sensitivity to PARP-inhibitor therapy. *Methods Mol Biol*. 2011;780:277-291. doi:10.1007/978-1-61779-270-0_17

[53] Ehrlich M, Lacey M. DNA hypomethylation and hemimethylation in cancer. *Adv Exp Med Biol*. 2013;754:31-56. doi:10.1007/978-1-4419-9967-2_2

[54] Zhao Z, Shilatifard A. Epigenetic modifications of histones in cancer. *Genome Biol*. 2019;20(1):245. doi:10.1186/s13059-019-1870-5

[55] Strahl BD, Allis CD. The language of covalent histone modifications. *Nature*. 2000;403(6765):41-45. doi:10.1038/47412

[56] Weichert W, Denkert C, Noske A, et al. Expression of class I histone deacetylases indicates poor prognosis in endometrioid subtypes of ovarian and endometrial carcinomas. *Neoplasia*. 2008;10(9):1021-1027. doi:10.1593/neo.08474

[57] Taufiqul Arif KM, Elliot EK, Haupt LM, Griffiths LR. Regulatory mechanisms of epigenetic mirna relationships in human cancer and potential as therapeutic targets. *Cancers (Basel)*. 2020;12(10):1-26. doi:10.3390/cancers12102922

[58] Yao Q, Chen Y, Zhou X. The roles of microRNAs in epigenetic regulation. *Curr Opin Chem Biol*. 2019;51:11-17. doi:10.1016/j.cbpa.2019.01.024

[59] Peng Y, Croce CM. The role of MicroRNAs in human cancer. *Signal Transduct Target Ther*. 2016;1(1):15004. doi:10.1038/sigtrans.2015.4

[60] Chen S-N, Chang R, Lin L-T, et al. MicroRNA in Ovarian Cancer: Biology, Pathogenesis, and Therapeutic Opportunities. *Int J Environ Res Public Health*. 2019;16(9):1510. doi:10.3390/ijerph16091510

[61] Iorio M V, Visone R, Di Leva G, et al. MicroRNA signatures in human ovarian cancer. *Cancer Res*. 2007;67(18):8699-8707. doi:10.1158/0008-5472.CAN-07-1936

[62] Kan CWS, Hahn MA, Gard GB, et al. Elevated levels of circulating microRNA-200 family members correlate with serous epithelial ovarian cancer. *BMC Cancer*. 2012;12:627. doi:10.1186/1471-2407-12-627

[63] F. Lyko and R. Brown, "DNA methyltransferase inhibitors and the development of epigenetic cancer therapies," *Journal of the National Cancer Institute,* vol. 97, no. 20, pp. 1498-1506, 2005.

[64] H. J. Smith, J. M. Straughn, D. J. Buchsbaum, and R. C. Arend, "Epigenetic therapy for the treatment of epithelial ovarian cancer: A clinical review," *Gynecologic oncology reports,* vol. 20, pp. 81-86, 2017.

[65] K. Y. Chan, H. Ozçelik, A. N. Cheung, H. Y. Ngan, and U.-S. Khoo, "Epigenetic factors controlling the BRCA1 and BRCA2 genes in sporadic ovarian cancer," *Cancer research,* vol. 62, no. 14, pp. 4151-4156, 2002.

[66] D. W. Tucker *et al.*, "Epigenetic reprogramming strategies to reverse

global loss of 5-hydroxymethylcytosine, a prognostic factor for poor survival in high-grade serous ovarian cancer," *Clinical Cancer Research,* vol. 24, no. 6, pp. 1389-1401, 2018.

[67] A. Aggarwal, A. Pandurangi, and W. Smith, "Disparities in breast and cervical cancer screening in women with mental illness: a systematic literature review," *American journal of preventive medicine,* vol. 44, no. 4, pp. 392-398, 2013.

[68] D. Matei and K. P. Nephew, "Epigenetic attire in ovarian cancer: the emperor's new clothes," *Cancer research,* vol. 80, no. 18, pp. 3775-3785, 2020.

[69] S. Moufarrij *et al.*, "Epigenetic therapy for ovarian cancer: promise and progress," *Clinical epigenetics,* vol. 11, no. 1, p. 7, 2019.

[70] S. C. Modesitt, M. Sill, J. S. Hoffman, and D. P. Bender, "A phase II study of vorinostat in the treatment of persistent or recurrent epithelial ovarian or primary peritoneal carcinoma: a Gynecologic Oncology Group study," *Gynecologic oncology,* vol. 109, no. 2, pp. 182-186, 2008.

[71] A. A. Mendivil *et al.*, "Increased incidence of severe gastrointestinal events with first-line paclitaxel, carboplatin, and vorinostat chemotherapy for advanced-stage epithelial ovarian, primary peritoneal, and fallopian tube cancer," *International Journal of Gynecologic Cancer,* vol. 23, no. 3, pp. 533-539, 2013.

[72] U. Matulonis *et al.*, "Phase I study of combination of vorinostat, carboplatin, and gemcitabine in women with recurrent, platinum-sensitive epithelial ovarian, fallopian tube, or peritoneal cancer" *Cancer chemotherapy and pharmacology,* vol. 76, no. 2, pp. 417-423, 2015.

[73] S. Fu *et al.*, "Phase Ib-IIa study to reverse platinum resistance by the use of a hypomethylating agent azacitidine in platinum-resistant or refractory epithelial ovarian cancer," *Cancer,* vol. 117, no. 8, p. 1661, 2011.

[74] A. M. Oza *et al.*, "A randomized phase II trial of epigenetic priming with guadecitabine and carboplatin in platinum-resistant, recurrent ovarian cancer," *Clinical Cancer Research,* vol. 26, no. 5, pp. 1009-1016, 2020.

[75] L. Chang, K. Hunter, J. Aikins, S. Brown, and O. Ostrovsky, "Use of Epigenetic Therapy Shortens Duration of Standard Chemotherapy for Ovarian Cancer with Minimal Toxicity to Normal Tissue," *Journal of Cancer Science and Clinical Therapeutics,* vol. 4, no. 2, pp. 100-114, 2020.

[76] L. A. Garrett, W. B. Growdon, B. R. Rueda, and R. Foster, "Influence of a novel histone deacetylase inhibitor panobinostat (LBH589) on the growth of ovarian cancer," *Journal of ovarian research,* vol. 9, no. 1, p. 58, 2016.

[77] L. Wang *et al.*, "Decitabine enhances lymphocyte migration and function and synergizes with CTLA-4 blockade in a murine ovarian cancer model," *Cancer immunology research,* vol. 3, no. 9, pp. 1030-1041, 2015.

[78] M. L. Stone *et al.*, "Epigenetic therapy activates type I interferon signaling in murine ovarian cancer to reduce immunosuppression and tumor burden," *Proceedings of the National Academy of Sciences,* vol. 114, no. 51, pp. E10981-E10990, 2017.

[79] K. Moore *et al.*, "Maintenance olaparib in patients with newly diagnosed advanced ovarian cancer," *New England Journal of Medicine,* vol. 379, no. 26, pp. 2495-2505, 2018.

[80] K. N. Moore *et al.*, "Niraparib monotherapy for late-line treatment of ovarian cancer (QUADRA): a multicentre, open-label, single-arm,

phase 2 trial," *The Lancet Oncology,* vol. 20, no. 5, pp. 636-648, 2019.

[81] T. Fukumoto *et al.*, "Repurposing pan-HDAC inhibitors for ARID1A-mutated ovarian cancer," *Cell reports,* vol. 22, no. 13, pp. 3393-3400, 2018.